SpringerBriefs in Modern Perspectives on Disability Research

This book series on disability research is a comprehensive collection of research on disability and related issues. The series is designed to promote interdisciplinary collaboration and exchange, bringing together scholars and practitioners from different fields to share their perspectives and insights. Disability research is an interdisciplinary field that examines the social, cultural, historical, and political dimensions of disability. It encompasses a wide range of topics, including disability rights, accessibility, assistive technologies, healthcare, education, employment, and social welfare. Disability research scholars employ a range of theoretical and methodological approaches to understand the experiences of people with disabilities, as well as the ways in which disability intersects with other social identities such as race, gender, sexuality, and class.

The series seeks to advance knowledge and understanding of disability by publishing rigorous, innovative, and relevant research. It aims to promote disability rights and social justice by highlighting the ways in which people with disabilities are marginalized and discriminated against in society, and advocating for greater social inclusion and accessibility. The series also seeks to inform policy and practice by disseminating research findings that can help to shape policy decisions and contribute to positive social change.

Getinet Ayano • Christina M. Pollard •
Rosanna Rooney • Rosa Alati

ADHD Across the Lifespan

Disability, Mental Health, and Social Impacts

Springer

Getinet Ayano
Curtin School of Population Health
Curtin University
Bentley, WA, Australia

Rosanna Rooney
Curtin School of Population Health
Curtin University
Bentley, WA, Australia

Christina M. Pollard
Curtin School of Population Health
Curtin University
Bentley, WA, Australia

Rosa Alati
Faculty of Health Sciences, School of Population Health
Curtin University
Perth, WA, Australia

School of Population Health
The University of Queensland
Brisbane, QLD, Australia

Institute for Social Sciences Research
The University of Queensland
Indooroopilly, QLD, Australia

ISSN 3004-9709 ISSN 3004-9717 (electronic)
SpringerBriefs in Modern Perspectives on Disability Research
ISBN 978-981-95-8711-7 ISBN 978-981-95-8712-4 (eBook)
https://doi.org/10.1007/978-981-95-8712-4

This Springer imprint is published by the registered company Springer Nature Singapore Pte Ltd.
The registered company address is: 152 Beach Road, #21-01/04 Gateway East, Singapore 189721, Singapore

Contents

Chapter 1
Introduction to Attention-Deficit Hyperactivity Disorder and Public Health

Abstract This chapter provides a comprehensive introduction to attention-deficit/hyperactivity disorder (ADHD), emphasizing its clinical characteristics, epidemiological patterns, and lifelong impact. ADHD is a prevalent neurodevelopmental condition that affects individuals across different stages of life, influencing academic achievement, occupational success, and overall well-being. Recognizing ADHD as both a medical and public health concern highlights the importance of integrating prevention, intervention, and advocacy to mitigate its negative effects.

By situating ADHD within the broader framework of health systems and policies, this chapter lays a foundation for understanding its multidimensional nature and the critical need for targeted strategies to address its challenges. The discussion underscores the necessity of early identification, equitable access to interventions, and the role of public health initiatives in shaping effective responses.

The chapter is structured into seven key subsections: an overview of ADHD, epidemiology of ADHD, factors influencing ADHD, historical perspectives on ADHD, framing ADHD in the lifespan context, public health implications of ADHD across the lifespan, and the importance of a public health approach. Each section explores specific dimensions of ADHD, providing a detailed examination of its etiology, impact, and management strategies. Through this analysis, the chapter highlights the significance of a comprehensive public health response in addressing ADHD at individual, community, and policy levels.

1.1 Overview of Attention-Deficit Hyperactivity Disorder

Attention-deficit/hyperactivity disorder (ADHD) is a complex neurodevelopmental condition that persists across the lifespan, affecting individuals from childhood to adulthood (APA, 2013; Ayano et al., 2020; Reiersen, 2017; Thapar et al., 2017). The disorder is characterized by considerable heterogeneity in its causes, clinical presentations, and treatment outcomes (APA, 2013; Cortese et al., 2012; Núñez-Jaramillo et al., 2021). It is primarily defined by developmentally inappropriate

G. Ayano et al., *ADHD Across the Lifespan*, SpringerBriefs in Modern Perspectives on Disability Research,
https://doi.org/10.1007/978-981-95-8712-4_1

levels of inattention, hyperactivity, and impulsivity that are pervasive, excessive, and impair functioning across multiple contexts (APA, 2013; Pievsky & McGrath, 2018).

ADHD symptoms are linked to subtle yet widespread alterations in gene expression across multiple brain regions, particularly the caudate and frontal cortex, which play a crucial role in attention control (Berger, 2011; Cortese et al., 2012; Sudre et al., 2023). ADHD is classified into three primary presentations: predominantly inattentive, predominantly hyperactive-impulsive, and combined (APA, 2013; Faraone et al., 2021). Diagnosis relies on standardized criteria outlined in the *Diagnostic and Statistical Manual of Mental Disorders* (DSM-5) and the *International Classification of Diseases* (ICD-11), which emphasize symptom severity, duration, and the extent of functional impairment (APA, 2013; WHO, 2020). Recent advancements in neuroimaging and genetic research have further deepened our understanding of ADHD's biological underpinnings, offering potential avenues for personalized treatment approaches (Zhang et al., 2023).

Although ADHD is commonly perceived as a childhood disorder, it persists into adulthood in a significant proportion of cases, with symptoms often evolving over time (Faraone et al., 2021). While hyperactivity may decline with age, inattention and impulsivity frequently persist, contributing to difficulties in professional, personal, and social domains (Ayano et al., 2023b; Faraone et al., 2021). The global prevalence of ADHD in adults is estimated at approximately 3.1% based on an umbrella review of meta-analytic systematic reviews conducted in 2023 which analyzed data from over 21 million adults across 57 primary studies (Ayano et al., 2023b). Despite this burden, adult ADHD remains underdiagnosed due to reliance on retrospective childhood histories, phenotypic overlap with other psychiatric disorders, limited routine screening in primary care and community settings, and the persistent misconception that ADHD is confined to childhood. Given its persistence and broad cross-cultural impact, improving detection is a public health priority. Untreated adult ADHD is associated with lower occupational attainment, higher risk of workplace accidents, and relationship difficulties, underscoring the need for timely diagnosis and intervention (Able et al., 2007).

The burden of ADHD extends beyond the affected individual, as it can place significant emotional, financial, and physical strain on families and communities (Able et al., 2007; APA, 2013). Prevention and treatment of ADHD remains a critical global mental health priority in, as millions of individuals—many of whom remain undiagnosed and untreated—continue to experience its adverse effects (Ginsberg et al., 2014; Huang et al., 2020). Untreated ADHD in childhood is associated with an increased risk of academic underachievement, juvenile delinquency, and lower socioeconomic attainment in adulthood (Russell et al., 2016), highlighting the importance of early identification, sustained intervention, and comprehensive support systems to mitigate the disorder's long-term consequences. From a public health perspective, comprehensive approaches that incorporate early screening programs, community awareness raising campaigns, and school-based support have demonstrated a reduction in the broader societal burden of ADHD (Schultz & Evans, 2015).

ADHD frequently coexists with other psychiatric conditions, further complicating diagnosis and treatment. Common comorbidities include anxiety disorders (25–50%), depression (10–30%), oppositional defiant disorder (ODD) (40–60%), and substance use disorders (20–30%) (Pliszka, 2020). These co-occurring conditions amplify the challenges faced by individuals with ADHD, reinforcing the need for integrated diagnostic and therapeutic approaches. For example, individuals with both ADHD and anxiety disorders often exhibit heightened emotional dysregulation, necessitating tailored interventions to simultaneously address both conditions (Quenneville et al., 2022). The overlapping symptoms and shared neurobiological mechanisms of ADHD and its comorbidities underscore the importance of adopting a holistic, multidisciplinary approach to ADHD care, particularly as diagnosis is often triggered by functional impairments in academic, occupational, or social settings that prompt individuals or caregivers to seek help for persistent inattention, impulsivity, or emotional dysregulation (French et al., 2021).

1.2 Epidemiology of ADHD: Prevalence and Burden

ADHD is one of the most common neurodevelopmental disorders, estimated to affect approximately 8% of children and adolescents worldwide (Ayano et al., 2023a; Polanczyk et al., 2015). The condition is diagnosed more frequently in males (10%) than in females (5%), with clinical observations showing a male-to-female diagnostic ratio ranging from 2:1 to 9:1 (Ayano et al., 2023a; Polanczyk et al., 2015). However, this difference is partly influenced by variations in symptom presentation. Males are more likely to exhibit overt hyperactivity and impulsivity, which are easily recognizable, whereas females tend to display more inattentive symptoms, often leading to underdiagnosis or misdiagnosis (Ayano et al., 2023a).

Among the three ADHD presentations, the inattentive type (ADHD-I) is the most common, followed by the hyperactive-impulsive (ADHD-HI) and combined (ADHD-C) types (Ayano et al., 2023a). The predominance of inattentive symptoms, particularly in females, may contribute to delays in identification and reduced access to early intervention services.

ADHD prevalence varies significantly across different regions. North America consistently reports higher rates of diagnosis compared to Europe and Asia. These differences are influenced by healthcare infrastructure, diagnostic criteria, access to specialized care, and cultural attitudes toward mental health (Li et al., 2023; Thomas et al., 2015) (Fig. 1.1). In regions where awareness is lower and mental health services are less accessible, ADHD remains underdiagnosed and undertreated (Faraone et al., 2021).

While some individuals experience a reduction in symptoms as they age—often due to brain maturation and improved self-regulation (Faraone et al., 2006; Rubia, 2018)—many continue to struggle with ADHD-related challenges well into adulthood (Asherson et al., 2016). In many cases, hyperactivity diminishes, but inattention and impulsivity persist, affecting educational, occupational, and social

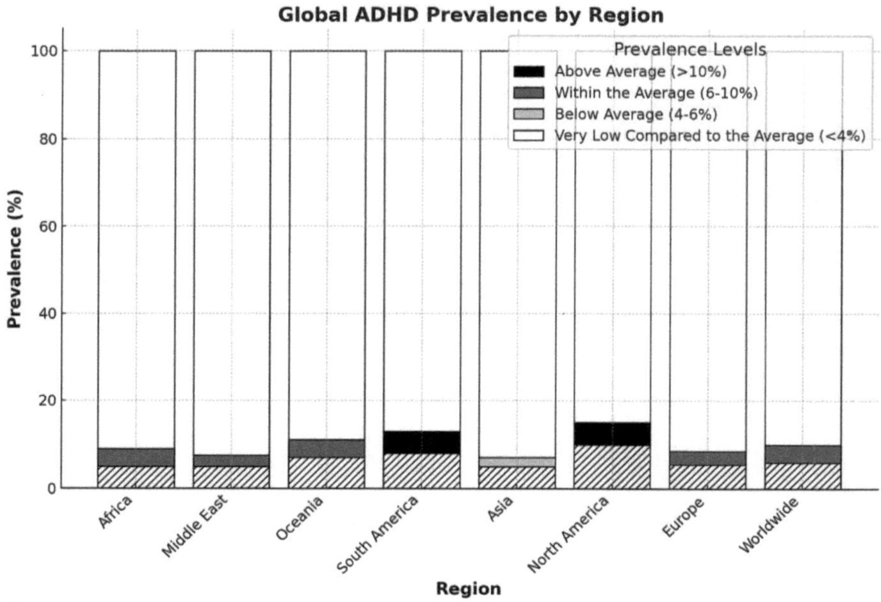

Fig. 1.1 The global prevalence of ADHD by region (Faraone et al., 2021)

functioning. ADHD remains a chronic condition for a significant proportion of individuals, requiring ongoing support and management (Faraone et al., 2021).

1.3 Societal and Economic Burden of ADHD

ADHD impacts not only the individual but also families, communities, and healthcare systems. The disorder is associated with academic difficulties, occupational challenges, and interpersonal conflicts, often leading to long-term disadvantages across various aspects of life. Many individuals with ADHD struggle with time management, organization, impulse control, and maintaining relationships—challenges rooted in executive function deficits—that commonly impair both personal and professional success (Chan & Langberg, 2024).

ADHD frequently occurs alongside other psychiatric conditions, such as anxiety, depression, and oppositional defiant disorder (ODD). These comorbidities increase the complexity of diagnosis and treatment, often requiring multidisciplinary interventions to address overlapping symptoms and challenges (Pliszka, 2020).

The financial burden of ADHD is substantial. Families of children with ADHD face significantly higher expenses for medical care, educational support, and behavioral interventions. A 2019 Australian study involving over 3000 children reported that the average annual societal cost of supporting a child with ADHD was

AUD$15,036, compared to AUD$2848 for a child without ADHD, reflecting significantly higher healthcare, education, and family-related expenses (Zhao et al., 2019). The economic impact extends into adulthood, where individuals with ADHD are at greater risk of lower job attainment and reduced productivity. The overall cost of adult ADHD in the United States alone was estimated at A$124.5 billion (2017 US Dollars) per year in DATE, reflecting lost earnings, healthcare costs, and decreased workplace efficiency (Zhao et al., 2019).

These challenges highlight the urgent need for early intervention, increased public awareness, and improved access to ADHD diagnosis and treatment. Strategies such as early screening programs, school-based interventions, and workplace accommodations can help reduce the long-term burden of ADHD, ensuring better outcomes for individuals and society as a whole.

1.4 Factors Influencing ADHD

ADHD is a multifaceted neurodevelopmental disorder influenced by a combination of genetic, environmental, and psychosocial factors. These influences interact in complex ways, shaping the likelihood of developing ADHD and modulating the severity of symptoms. Understanding these factors is essential for designing effective prevention and intervention strategies.

1.4.1 Genetic Factors

ADHD has a strong genetic basis, with an official that estimated 70–80% of the variation in ADHD traits can be attributed to genetic factors (Faraone et al., 2021). Genome-wide studies identified numerous genetic variants associated with ADHD, each exerting a small effect. Among the most studied are genes involved in dopamine regulation, such as DRD4 and DAT1, which play key roles in the brain's reward and attention pathways (Bonvicini et al., 2016; Sigurdardottir et al., 2016). Rare genetic mutations and chromosomal abnormalities have also been observed in individuals with ADHD, adding to the disorder's genetic complexity (Williams et al., 2010) (Table 1.1).

Large-scale genome-wide association studies (GWAS) have confirmed that ADHD is polygenic, meaning that multiple genetic variations collectively contribute to an individual's risk of developing the disorder (Demontis et al., 2019). Interestingly, genetic risk for ADHD is also associated with subthreshold symptoms in the general population, suggesting that ADHD traits exist on a spectrum rather than as a distinct categorical disorder (Bruxel et al., 2021; Taylor et al., 2019).

Beyond ADHD itself, genetic studies have identified shared genetic links between ADHD and other psychiatric and somatic disorders, including schizophrenia, depression, autism spectrum disorder, migraine, and obesity (Ayano et al.,

Table 1.1 Factors influencing attention-deficit/hyperactivity disorder (ADHD)

Factor type	Risk factors for ADHD	Protective factors for ADHD
Genetic factors	• Family history of ADHD • Specific gene variations (e.g., DRD4, DAT1, COMT)	• Genetic resilience (e.g., certain alleles reducing susceptibility) • Polygenic protective effects
Prenatal factors	• Maternal smoking, alcohol, or drug use during pregnancy • Maternal stress during pregnancy • Hypertensive disorders during pregnancy	• Adequate maternal nutrition (e.g., folate, omega-3) • Supportive social and family environment • Regular prenatal care and monitoring • Absence of pregnancy complications
Perinatal & early life	• Premature birth and low birth weight • Birth complications and hypoxia • Exposure to environmental toxins (e.g., lead, pesticides)	• Maternal cardiovascular health • Skin-to-skin contact and early bonding • Early life environment, breastfeeding
Family & social environment	• Parental mental health problems (e.g., depression, anxiety) • Childhood maltreatment, neglect, or family conflict • Low socioeconomic status, relative disadvantage	• Parental emotional well-being and mental health support • Strong parental involvement, warm parenting • Stable home environment, social support
Psychosocial & behavioral	• High screen time, poor sleep hygiene • Poor diet (e.g., high sugar, ultra-processed foods)	• Positive, consistent parenting practices • Stable and low-stress home environment
School & cognitive environment	• Early academic struggles and school stress • Peer rejection, social isolation and bullying	• Secure parent-child attachment • Early childhood education and cognitive stimulation • Strong caregiver relationships

2025; Faraone et al., 2021). These overlapping genetic influences suggest that ADHD may arise from common biological pathways affecting neurodevelopment and cognitive regulation.

1.4.2 Environmental Factors

1.4.2.1 Prenatal and Perinatal Factors

Early-life exposures, including those occurring in utero, can significantly impact brain development and increase the risk of ADHD. Several prenatal factors have been linked to a higher likelihood of ADHD, including maternal smoking, alcohol, or drug use during pregnancy, which can interfere with fetal brain development and disrupt neurochemical pathways involved in attention and impulse control (Huang et al., 2018; Nilsen & Tulve, 2020) (Table 1.1). Maternal stress, anxiety, and depression have also been associated with elevated ADHD risk in offspring due to altered prenatal stress responses and hormonal changes (Ayano et al., 2021; Tusa et al., 2024). Deficiencies in maternal nutrition, particularly low folate and vitamin D levels, have been associated with an increased likelihood of ADHD (Sucksdorff et al., 2021). Pregnancy complications such as hypertensive disorders, gestational diabetes, and hyperthyroidism may impair fetal neurodevelopment and contribute to later ADHD symptoms (Maher et al., 2018). Perinatal complications—including low birth weight, preterm birth, and birth trauma—have been associated with a heightened risk of ADHD, likely due to their impact on early brain maturation and cognitive development (Momany et al., 2018).

1.4.2.2 Postnatal Environmental Exposures

After birth, children continue to be exposed to environmental risk factors that may shape the trajectory of ADHD symptoms (Table 1.1). Among the most well-documented are exposure to environmental toxins, such as lead, pesticides, and air pollution, which have been associated with increased ADHD symptoms (Braun et al., 2006). Excessive screen time and poor sleep hygiene have also been found to also contribute to attentional difficulties and hyperactive behaviors (Faraone et al., 2021). These findings highlight the importance of minimizing early-life exposures to harmful substances and promoting a healthy developmental environment to reduce ADHD risk.

1.4.2.3 Psychosocial Factors

While ADHD is strongly influenced by biological factors—family dynamics, parenting practices, and social environments also play a role in shaping symptom expression.

Family and Social Environment

Certain psychosocial risk factors have been linked to ADHD severity, including parental mental health issues. Both maternal and paternal depression and anxiety have been associated with greater difficulties in children's emotional regulation and attentional control (Choi et al., 2017; Ouyang et al., 2008; Robinson et al., 2024). Childhood trauma, maltreatment, or neglect can lead to heightened stress responses and behavioral dysregulation (Ouyang et al., 2008). Low socioeconomic status (SES) may limit access to early screening, quality education, and ADHD treatment (Russell et al., 2016). Conversely, protective factors such as strong parental involvement, warm and responsive caregiving, and a structured home environment can help mitigate the effects of ADHD and support positive behavioral outcomes (Shaw et al., 2007) (Table 1.1).

School and Peer Environment

Academic settings can either support or exacerbate ADHD symptoms, depending on the level of structure and accommodation provided. Children with ADHD often face early academic struggles, which can lead to frustration and lower self-esteem (Barry et al., 2002), as well as peer rejection and bullying, which are common due to difficulties in social interactions (Mikami, 2010). Supportive teachers, individualized learning plans, and structured classroom routines can greatly enhance learning outcomes and social adjustment for children with ADHD (DuPaul et al., 2011a, 2011b) (Table 1.1).

1.4.3 Gene-Environment Interactions

The interaction between genetic predispositions and environmental influences plays a critical role in the development of ADHD. Certain environmental stressors may exert a stronger impact on individuals who are genetically predisposed to ADHD. For example, children with specific genetic profiles are more likely to be susceptible to the adverse effects of prenatal toxin exposure, thereby increasing their risk of developing ADHD (Li et al., 2021). Socioeconomic factors may also influence the expression of genetic risk for ADHD. In lower-income environments, genetic influences on ADHD symptoms tend to be more pronounced—possibly due to increased exposure to environmental adversities that exacerbate inherited vulnerabilities (Gould et al., 2018). Additionally, household chaos—characterized by disorganization, high noise levels, and lack of routine—can intensify ADHD symptoms in children with underlying genetic susceptibility (Gould et al., 2018). These findings underscore the importance of examining both biological and environmental contributors in understanding the etiology and manifestation of ADHD. Strategies that address both genetic vulnerability and environmental stressors—such as early intervention, structured home and school environments, and parental education programs—are likely to improve outcomes for individuals with ADHD (Table 1.1).

1.5 Historical Perspectives on ADHD

Symptoms resembling what is now identified as ADHD were described in clinical reports over 200 years ago, reflecting a longstanding recognition of attention and hyperactivity-related difficulties, even prior to the establishment of modern diagnostic criteria (Faraone et al., 2021).

One of the earliest documented descriptions of ADHD-like symptoms dates back to 1775, when German physician Melchior Adam Weikard systematically observed and described inattentive and hyperactive behaviors in children (Lange et al., 2010).

His work laid the foundation for later clinical understandings of attention disorders. In 1798, Scottish physician Alexander Crichton published medical texts discussing attention disturbances, further contributing to early conceptualizations of ADHD (Lange et al., 2010).

The nineteenth and early twentieth centuries saw continued recognition of ADHD-like behaviors. In 1845, Heinrich Hoffmann, who later became head of Germany's first psychiatric hospital in Frankfurt, illustrated hyperactivity and attention deficits in children in his well-known book *Struwwelpeter*, a collection of cautionary tales depicting behaviors associated with ADHD (Hoffmann, 1876). A more formal medical description emerged in 1902, when British physician George Still delivered a series of lectures describing children with persistent difficulties in sustained attention, impulsivity, and self-regulation. His work emphasized the moral and inhibitory aspects of attention disorders, influencing early twentieth-century perspectives (Lange et al., 2010).

By the mid-twentieth century, the term "minimal brain dysfunction" (MBD) was introduced to describe children exhibiting hyperactivity, impulsivity, and inattention. This period marked a shift toward neurological explanations for behavioral disorders. A major breakthrough occurred in 1937, when American physician Charles Bradley discovered that stimulant medications could reduce hyperactivity and inattentive behaviors in children (Bradley, 1937), laying the foundation for modern pharmacological ADHD treatment (Lange et al., 2010).

The latter half of the twentieth century saw ADHD described as a distinct clinical entity. Advances in psychiatric research led to the refinement of diagnostic criteria, culminating in its inclusion in the *Diagnostic and Statistical Manual of Mental Disorders* (DSM) by the American Psychiatric Association—first as "Hyperkinetic Reaction of Childhood" in DSM-II (1968) and later refined as "Attention-Deficit Hyperactivity Disorder" in DSM-III (1980) (American Psychiatric Association, 1968, 1980). The DSM underwent multiple revisions, each refining the understanding of ADHD and its diagnostic framework (APA, 2013; Lange et al., 2010).

Despite historical controversies, ADHD is now widely recognized as a legitimate neurodevelopmental disorder with significant implications for individuals and society. It was first formally introduced in the *Diagnostic and Statistical Manual of Mental Disorders* (DSM-II) in 1968 as "Hyperkinetic Reaction of Childhood," classified under "Disorders Usually First Evident in Infancy, Childhood, or Adolescence." The DSM-III (1980) redefined the condition as "Attention Deficit Disorder (ADD)," with or without hyperactivity, reflecting increased awareness of inattentive symptoms. In DSM-III-R (1987), the term "Attention-Deficit Hyperactivity Disorder (ADHD)" was adopted, and subsequent editions—DSM-IV (1994) and DSM-5 (2013)—further refined the diagnostic criteria, introducing the current subtype classifications: predominantly inattentive, predominantly hyperactive-impulsive, and combined presentation. This historical evolution has shaped contemporary approaches to diagnosis and treatment and underscores the importance of early identification, personalized interventions, and ongoing research to address the disorder's complex and lifelong impact (APA, 2013; Lange et al., 2010).

1.6 How Is ADHD Diagnosed?

Diagnosing ADHD requires a comprehensive evaluation conducted by a qualified healthcare professional, such as a pediatrician, psychologist, or psychiatrist. The process involves detailed clinical interviews with the individual and, when appropriate, parents or caregivers, to gather a thorough history of behaviors and symptoms. The *Diagnostic and Statistical Manual of Mental Disorders*, Fifth Edition (DSM-5) provides standardized criteria for ADHD diagnosis. According to DSM-5, symptoms must be developmentally inappropriate and persist for at least 6 months, be present in multiple settings (e.g., home, school, or workplace), and cause significant impairment in social, academic, or occupational functioning (APA, 2013; Wolraich et al., 2019).

1.6.1 Clinical Approach to ADHD Diagnosis

ADHD cannot be diagnosed solely through rating scales, neuropsychological tests, or neuroimaging techniques. While these tools may offer supportive information, the diagnosis remains clinical, based primarily on observed behaviors and reported histories. Initial concerns regarding the subjectivity of ADHD diagnosis have been addressed through research demonstrating its validity as a neurodevelopmental disorder (Faraone et al., 2021). Studies indicate that trained professionals can reliably diagnose ADHD using standardized criteria, and the diagnosis is predictive of key outcomes such as academic challenges, substance abuse risk, and treatment responsiveness (APA, 2013; Wolraich et al., 2019).

1.6.2 Standardized Diagnostic Guidelines

To enhance diagnostic accuracy, authoritative professional organizations have developed standardized guidelines. For example, the American Academy of Pediatrics (AAP) recommends clinicians evaluate children aged 4–18 years who present with academic or behavioral difficulties for possible ADHD. These guidelines emphasize the necessity of meeting DSM-5 ADHD criteria, the importance of gathering information from multiple sources, including parents and teachers, and the need to consider alternative explanations for the observed behaviors (Wolraich et al., 2019).

1.6.3 Key DSM-5 Criteria for ADHD Diagnosis

The DSM-5 specifies several diagnostic criteria that distinguish ADHD from normal developmental variations. Symptoms must have been present before the age of 12, highlighting ADHD's neurodevelopmental nature. For children up to age 16 years, at least six symptoms of inattention and/or hyperactivity-impulsivity must be present, while for people aged 17 years and over, a minimum of five symptoms are required. Symptoms must persist for at least 6 months and be inconsistent with developmental expectations (APA, 2013; Wolraich et al., 2019). Notably, in 2013, the DSM-5 updated the age-of-onset criterion for ADHD, extending it from before age 7 to before age 12, to more accurately reflect the developmental variability in symptom emergence (APA, 2013; Wolraich et al., 2019).

1.7 Framing ADHD in the Lifespan Context

ADHD is a lifelong neurodevelopmental disorder, with symptom presentation and associated challenges evolving from childhood through adulthood. Understanding ADHD across the lifespan is essential for tailoring interventions and providing appropriate support at different developmental stages.

1.7.1 ADHD in Childhood

In childhood, the hallmark features of ADHD—such as hyperactivity, impulsivity, and inattentiveness—tend to manifest in ways that disrupt learning, strain peer relationships, and challenge parenting strategies. Children with ADHD may struggle to follow instructions, complete tasks, and maintain focus—leading to lower academic achievement and disciplinary action—social difficulties including peer rejection due to impulsivity and challenges in adhering to social norms, and family tensions as parents and siblings cope with behavioral challenges (Ayano et al., 2020, 2023a). Early diagnosis and intervention during this stage are crucial to mitigate these challenges and promote positive developmental outcomes.

1.7.2 ADHD in Adolescence

As individuals transition into adolescence, ADHD symptoms often persist, but hyperactivity tends to diminish, while inattention and impulsivity remain prominent (Turgay et al., 2012). This period introduces new challenges, including increased risk of substance use and engagement in risky behaviors, difficulties with emotional regulation leading to higher rates of anxiety and depression (Groenman et al., 2017). Academic struggles, particularly in time management, organization, and executive functioning, and low self-esteem exacerbated by persistent challenges in education and social interactions emerge. Without appropriate support, adolescents with ADHD may face compromised educational attainment, social difficulties, and heightened vulnerability to mental health comorbidities.

1.7.3 ADHD in Adulthood

In adulthood, ADHD symptoms may become less overt but remain functionally impairing. Adults with ADHD frequently encounter workplace challenges, including job instability and underachievement due to difficulties in sustaining attention and managing responsibilities (Pang et al., 2021). Interpersonal difficulties as inattentiveness and impulsivity contribute to relationship misunderstandings and conflicts (APA, 2013), and mental health comorbidities such as anxiety, depression, and substance use disorders, further exacerbating functional impairments (Barkley et al., 2004). Despite these challenges, many adults remain undiagnosed, often attributing their difficulties to personal failings rather than an underlying neurodevelopmental disorder.

1.7.4 Challenges in Diagnosing ADHD in Adults

Diagnosing ADHD in adults is complex for several reasons: symptom overlap with other psychiatric disorders, making differential diagnosis difficult (APA, 2013; Ginsberg et al., 2014), adaptive coping mechanisms may mask the disorder's manifestations, limited clinician training, and the absence of formal adult diagnostic guidelines. Many adults are misdiagnosed or undiagnosed, leading to delays in accessing appropriate interventions. Although the DSM-5 established standardized diagnostic criteria for adult ADHD, professional organizations continue to work toward improving their implementation and harmonization across clinical settings, thereby enhancing identification and treatment consistency (APA, 2013; Ginsberg et al., 2014).

1.7.5 Persistence of ADHD Across the Lifespan

While ADHD symptoms often diminish with age, research suggests that a large proportion of individuals continue to experience impairments into adulthood. An estimated 40–60% of individuals diagnosed in childhood continue to exhibit ADHD

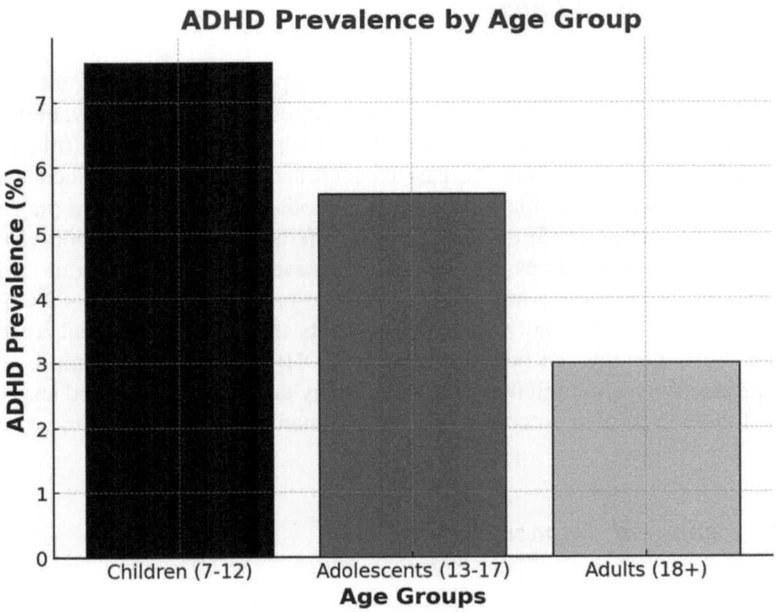

Fig. 1.2 Prevalence of ADHD across the lifespan

symptoms in adulthood (Faraone et al., 2021), with 15% of these still meeting full diagnostic criteria for ADHD (Faraone et al., 2021). ADHD prevalence decreases with age, estimated at 7.6% in children, 5.6% in adolescents, and 3% in adults (Faraone et al., 2021) (Fig. 1.2). This decline may result from symptom attenuation, adaptive coping strategies, or underdiagnosis in older populations.

Figure 1.2 depicts ADHD prevalence across key developmental stages. The highest prevalence is observed among children aged 7–12 years (7.6%), followed by a decline in adolescents aged 13–17 years (5.6%), with further reduction among adults aged 18 years and older (3.0%). This age-related trend is consistent with epidemiological evidence suggesting a progressive decline in the persistence of ADHD symptoms into adulthood (Ayano et al., 2023a; Salari et al., 2023).

1.8 Public Health Implications of ADHD Across the Lifespan

ADHD presents public health challenges that span the lifespan, affecting educational attainment, economic stability, healthcare systems, and social well-being. Addressing these challenges requires multi-strategy, comprehensive and population-wide interventions beyond individual treatment.

1.8.1 Educational Impact

Children and adolescents with ADHD often experience academic difficulties, including higher rates of absenteeism, school dropout, and underachievement (Loe & Feldman, 2007). Difficulties in organization, focus, and impulse control can lead to lower educational attainment, increased disciplinary actions, and strained teacher-student relationships. Early identification and school-based interventions play a crucial role in mitigating these challenges. Multi-tiered systems of support (MTSS) have been effective in addressing the academic and behavioral needs of children with ADHD by providing structured, evidence-based interventions (Stoiber & Gettinger, 2015). Additionally, research suggests that pharmacological treatment and behavioral therapy can help reduce core ADHD symptoms and improve academic productivity, although they may not directly enhance standardized test scores or long-term educational outcomes (Loe & Feldman, 2007).

1.8.2 Economic Impact

ADHD contributes a substantial economic burden related to higher healthcare utilization (e.g., frequent medical visits and treatment), workplace absenteeism and reduced productivity, and higher rates of job instability and lower occupational attainment. In the United States, the annual societal economic burden of ADHD was estimated at US$156 billion in 2018, encompassing direct healthcare, education, caregiving, productivity loss, and unemployment costs (Schein et al., 2022). In Australia, the estimated societal costs of ADHD were AUD$12.76 billion in 2019, with productivity losses accounting for 81% of total financial costs (Sciberras et al., 2022).

Strategies to reduce this economic burden in the workplace setting include flexible schedules, structured task management, vocational training and employment support programs, and policies promoting ADHD-friendly work environments. Untreated ADHD in adults is linked to higher rates of workplace accidents, chronic financial struggles, and reduced lifetime earnings, highlighting the necessity of effective management strategies (Sciberras et al., 2022).

1.8.3 Social Impact

ADHD affects social relationships, family dynamics, and overall well-being, often leading to increased family stress and conflict due to the behavioral challenges associated with ADHD. The social stigma associated with ADHD discourages individuals from seeking diagnosis and treatment, and difficulties in peer interactions increase the risk of social rejection and isolation. Community-based support programs and public awareness campaigns may help reduce stigma and can provide families with resources to effectively manage ADHD-related challenges. Social skills training and peer support networks have been shown to improve interpersonal functioning and quality of life for individuals with ADHD (Markham & Spencer, 2022).

1.8.4 Overall Public Health Burden

In summary, ADHD is not just an individual challenge—it affects families, friends. communities, healthcare systems, and workplaces. A comprehensive public health strategy is essential to effectively manage the disorder across the lifespan (Susan Young et al., 2020).

1.9 Importance of a Public Health Approach

Framing ADHD as a public health issue underscores the need for a comprehensive range of system-wide interventions that extend beyond clinical treatment. A public health approach includes actions to protect, promote, and prevent. For this issue of ADHD this includes a comprehensive portfolio framework of public health interventions from mass communications, to service delivery, programs, policy and resourcing, to advocacy to support change, with an emphasis on addressing inequities and improving health and society-wide outcomes.

1.9.1 Prevention: Primary Prevention Before Disease Onset

Preventative measures focus on reducing modifiable risk factors that contribute to the predisposition and development of ADHD. Prenatal health is a priority, with maternal smoking, drug and alcohol use, and inadequate prenatal care associated with increased risk of ADHD in offspring. Comprehensive public health promotion campaign encouraging cessation of maternal smoking, alcohol and other drug use, and raising awareness of risks related to ADHD offer are a key prevention strategy designed to mitigate these risks. As adverse experiences in early childhood are also associated with higher ADHD prevalence, universal school-based screening programs can be used to identify at-risk children early and facilitate timely intervention (Kim et al., 2022).

1.9.2 Intervention: Secondary Prevention to Reduce Long-Term Impacts

Expanding access to evidence-based treatment is key to reduce ADHD's long-term impact. Multidisciplinary care models that integrate medical, educational, and psychological support have been shown to improve outcomes for individuals with ADHD. Behavioral therapy and cognitive-behavioral interventions can enhance executive function and improve daily functioning (Danciu, 2011). Telehealth platforms have emerged as valuable tools for expanding access to ADHD care, particularly in underserved communities (Lakes et al., 2022).

1.9.3 Advocacy and Policy Change

Public health efforts are required to reduce stigma and promote effective policy options to support individuals with ADHD. Mass communication campaigns can create awareness and correct misconceptions, leading to greater acceptance of ADHD as a legitimate neurodevelopmental disorder. Advocacy can play an important role in influencing policy decisions including funding and resource allocations, commitment to research, ensuring equitable access to treatment and accommodations, and assisting in the identification of, and gaining consensus on the prioritization of effective interventions. The public health approach prioritizes addressing systemic barriers is particularly important for marginalized communities, where ADHD is often underdiagnosed and untreated due to limited access to healthcare and educational resources (Visser et al., 2024).

1.9.4 Implementing a Public Health Framework for ADHD

A public health framework for ADHD should consider policy, systems, and environmental changes to prevent ADHD and increase early identification, access to multidisciplinary and community-based care, educational and workplace accommodations, and equity in diagnosis and treatment access (Rattay & Robinson, 2024).

Summary

This chapter provided an in-depth exploration of ADHD across multiple dimensions, highlighting its clinical characteristics, epidemiology, historical context, diagnostic framework, and public health implications. It began by discussing the clinical presentation and diagnosis of ADHD, emphasizing the core symptoms of inattention, hyperactivity, and impulsivity across the lifespan. The evolution of diagnostic criteria, including updates in the DSM-5, and the challenges associated with adult ADHD diagnosis were also examined. Epidemiological patterns and risk factors were detailed, illustrating global prevalence rates, gender disparities, and the genetic and environmental influences that contribute to the development and persistence of ADHD.

The chapter also traced the historical perspectives on ADHD, documenting how the recognition of attention and hyperactivity disorders has evolved since the eighteenth century to include modern classifications, illustrating shifts in medical and societal understanding. It further outlined the public health burden of ADHD, including its impact on education, economic productivity, and social well-being. The discussion highlighted the importance of early identification, school- and workplace-interventions to mitigate long-term consequences of living with ADHD.

Importantly, the chapter framed ADHD as a public health issue, focusing on the need for prevention, intervention, and advocacy. Policy-driven approaches were emphasized, including universal screening, equitable access to treatment, and stigma reduction strategies, to ensure that individuals with ADHD receive appropriate support across the lifespan. Through a comprehensive analysis, this chapter reinforced the multifaceted nature of ADHD and the importance of adopting a systemic, evidence-based approach to diagnosis, treatment, and public health intervention. In doing so, this chapter lays the groundwork for subsequent chapters by establishing the clinical, epidemiological, and policy foundations upon which more detailed discussions of interventions, lived experiences, and global frameworks are built.

References

Able, S. L., Johnston, J. A., Adler, L. A., & Swindle, R. W. (2007). Functional and psychosocial impairment in adults with undiagnosed ADHD. *Psychological Medicine, 37*(1), 97–107.

American Academy of Pediatrics. Subcommittee on Attention-Deficit/Hyperactivity Disorder and Committee on Quality Improvement. (2001). Clinical practice guideline: Treatment of the school-aged child with attention-deficit/hyperactivity disorder. *Pediatrics, 108*(4), 1033–1044.

American Psychiatric Association. (1968). *Diagnostic and statistical manual of mental disorders* (2nd ed.). Washington, DC: APA.

American Psychiatric Association. (1980). *Diagnostic and statistical manual of mental disorders* (3rd ed.). Washington, DC: APA.

APA. (2013). Diagnostic and statistical manual of mental disorders. *American Psychiatric Association, 21*(21), 591–643.

Asherson, P., Buitelaar, J., Faraone, S. V., & Rohde, L. A. (2016). Adult attention-deficit hyperactivity disorder: Key conceptual issues. *The Lancet Psychiatry, 3*(6), 568–578. https://doi.org/10.1016/s2215-0366(16)30032-3

Ayano, G., Yohannes, K., & Abraha, M. (2020). Epidemiology of attention–deficit/hyperactivity disorder (ADHD) in children and adolescents in Africa: A systematic review and meta–analysis. *Annals of General Psychiatry, 19*(21), 1–10.

Ayano, G., Betts, K., Tait, R., Dachew, B. A., & Alati, R. (2021). Maternal depressive and anxiety symptoms and the risk of attention deficit hyperactivity disorder symptoms in offspring aged 17: Findings from the Raine Study. *Journal of Affective Disorders, 284*, 149–156. https://doi.org/10.1016/j.jad.2021.02.024

Ayano, G., Demelash, S., Gizachew, Y., Tsegay, L., & Alati, R. (2023a). The global prevalence of attention deficit hyperactivity disorder in children and adolescents: An umbrella review of meta-analyses. *Journal of Affective Disorders, 339*, 860–866. https://doi.org/10.1016/j.jad.2023.07.071

Ayano, G., Tsegay, L., Gizachew, Y., Necho, M., Yohannes, K., Abraha, M., Demelash, S., Anbesaw, T., & Alati, R. (2023b). Prevalence of attention deficit hyperactivity disorder in adults: Umbrella review of evidence generated across the globe. *Psychiatry Research, 328*, 115449. https://doi.org/10.1016/j.psychres.2023.115449

Ayano, G., Zena, D., Gizachew, Y., & Tsegay, L. (2025). Neurobiomarkers of psychiatric disorders in children and adolescents and their significance for diagnosis and precision medicine: A narrative review. *NeuroMarkers, 2*(2), 100040. https://doi.org/10.1016/j.neumar.2025.100040

Bradley, C. (1937). The behavior of children receiving Benzedrine. *American Journal of Psychiatry, 94*(3), 577–585.

Barkley, R. A., Fischer, M., Smallish, L., & Fletcher, K. (2004). Young adult follow-up of hyperactive children: Antisocial activities and drug use. *Journal of Child Psychology and Psychiatry, 45*(2), 195–211.

Barry, T. D., Lyman, R. D., & Klinger, L. G. (2002). Academic underachievement and attention-deficit/hyperactivity disorder: The negative impact of symptom severity on school performance. *Journal of School Psychology, 40*(3), 259–283. https://doi.org/10.1016/S0022-4405(02)00100-0

Berger, I. (2011). Diagnosis of attention deficit hyperactivity disorder: Much ado about something. *IMAJ-Israel Medical Association Journal, 13*(9), 571.

Bonvicini, C., Faraone, S., & Scassellati, C. (2016). Attention-deficit hyperactivity disorder in adults: A systematic review and meta-analysis of genetic, pharmacogenetic and biochemical studies. *Molecular Psychiatry, 21*(7), 872–884.

Braun, J. M., Kahn, R. S., Froehlich, T., Auinger, P., & Lanphear, B. P. (2006). Exposures to environmental toxicants and attention deficit hyperactivity disorder in US children. *Environmental Health Perspectives, 114*(12), 1904–1909.

Bruxel, E., Moreira-Maia, C., Akutagava-Martins, G., Quinn, T., Klein, M., Franke, B., Ribasés, M., Rovira, P., Sánchez-Mora, C., & Kappel, D. (2021). Meta-analysis and systematic review of ADGRL3 (LPHN3) polymorphisms in ADHD susceptibility. *Molecular Psychiatry, 26*(6), 2277–2285.

Chan, E. S. M., & Langberg, J. M. (2024). Predicting occupational outcomes for individuals with ADHD: The role of hyperactivity/impulsivity and executive functioning.

Choi, Y., Shin, J., Cho, K. H., & Park, E.-C. (2017). Change in household income and risk for attention deficit hyperactivity disorder during childhood: A nationwide population-based cohort study. *Journal of Epidemiology, 27*(2), 56–62.

Cortese, S., Kelly, C., Chabernaud, C., Proal, E., Di Martino, A., Milham, M. P., & Castellanos, F. X. (2012). Toward systems neuroscience of ADHD: A meta-analysis of 55 fMRI studies. *American Journal of Psychiatry, 169*(10), 1038–1055.

Danciu, E. L. (2011). Multidisciplinary approach of the attention deficit hyperactivity disorder (ADHD) between hope and reality. *Procedia-Social and Behavioral Sciences, 15*, 2967–2971.

Demontis, D., Walters, R. K., Martin, J., Mattheisen, M., Als, T. D., Agerbo, E., Baldursson, G., Belliveau, R., Bybjerg-Grauholm, J., & Bækvad-Hansen, M. (2019). Discovery of the first genome-wide significant risk loci for attention deficit/hyperactivity disorder. *Nature Genetics, 51*(1), 63–75.

Doshi, J. A., Hodgkins, P., Kahle, J., Sikirica, V., Cangelosi, M. J., Setyawan, J., Erder, M. H., & Neumann, P. J. (2012). Economic impact of childhood and adult attention-deficit/hyperactivity disorder in the United States. *Journal of the American Academy of Child & Adolescent Psychiatry, 51*(10), 990–1002.e2. https://doi.org/10.1016/j.jaac.2012.07.008

DuPaul, G. J., Kern, L., Gormley, M. J., & Volpe, R. J. (2011a). Early intervention for young children with ADHD: Academic outcomes for responders to behavioral treatment. *School Mental Health, 3*, 117–126.

DuPaul, G. J., Weyandt, L. L., & Janusis, G. M. (2011b). ADHD in the classroom: Effective intervention strategies. *Theory Into Practice, 50*(1), 35–42. https://doi.org/10.1080/00405841.2011.534935

French, B., Nalbant, G., Wright, H., Sayal, K., Daley, D., Groom, M. J., Cassidy, S., & Hall, C. L. (2021). The impacts associated with having ADHD: *An umbrella review. Neuroscience & Biobehavioral Reviews, 128*, 662–675. https://doi.org/10.1016/j.neubiorev.2021.01.022

Faraone, S. V., Sergeant, J., Gillberg, C., & Biederman, J. (2006). The worldwide prevalence of ADHD: Is it an American condition? *World Psychiatry, 5*(2), 104–113.

Faraone, S. V., Banaschewski, T., Coghill, D., Zheng, Y., Biederman, J., Bellgrove, M. A., Newcorn, J. H., Gignac, M., Al Saud, N. M., Manor, I., Rohde, L. A., Yang, L., Cortese, S., Almagor, D., Stein, M. A., Albatti, T. H., Aljoudi, H. F., Alqahtani, M. M. J., Asherson, P., et al. (2021). The world federation of ADHD international consensus statement: 208 Evidence-based conclusions about the disorder. *Neuroscience & Biobehavioral Reviews, 128*, 789–818. https://doi.org/10.1016/j.neubiorev.2021.01.022

Ginsberg, Y., Quintero, J., Anand, E., Casillas, M., & Upadhyaya, H. P. (2014). Underdiagnosis of attention-deficit/hyperactivity disorder in adult patients: A review of the literature. *The Primary Care Companion for CNS Disorders, 16*(3), 23591.

Gould, K. L., Coventry, W. L., Olson, R. K., & Byrne, B. (2018). Gene-environment interactions in ADHD: The roles of SES and Chaos. *Journal of Abnormal Child Psychology, 46*(2), 251–263. https://doi.org/10.1007/s10802-017-0268-7

Groenman, A. P., Janssen, T. W., & Oosterlaan, J. (2017). Childhood psychiatric disorders as risk factor for subsequent substance abuse: A meta-analysis. *Journal of the American Academy of Child & Adolescent Psychiatry, 56*(7), 556–569.

Hoffmann, H. (1845/1876). *Struwwelpeter*. Frankfurt: Literarische Anstalt.

Huang, L., Wang, Y., Zhang, L., Zheng, Z., Zhu, T., Qu, Y., & Mu, D. (2018). Maternal smoking and attention-deficit/hyperactivity disorder in offspring: A meta-analysis. *Pediatrics, 141*(1), e20172465.

Huang, H., Huang, H., Spottswood, M., & Ghaemi, N. (2020). Approach to evaluating and managing adult attention-deficit/hyperactivity disorder in primary care. *Harvard Review of Psychiatry, 28*(2), 100–106.

Kim, J., Kim, D.-G., & Kamphaus, R. (2022). Early detection of mental health through universal screening at schools. *Georgia Educational Researcher, 19*(1), 62.

Lakes, K. D., Cibrian, F. L., Schuck, S. E., Nelson, M., & Hayes, G. R. (2022). Digital health interventions for youth with ADHD: A mapping review. *Computers in Human Behavior Reports, 6*, 100174.

Lange, K. W., Reichl, S., Lange, K. M., Tucha, L., & Tucha, O. (2010). The history of attention deficit hyperactivity disorder. *ADHD Attention Deficit and Hyperactivity Disorders, 2*(4), 241–255. https://doi.org/10.1007/s12402-010-0045-8

Li, L., Taylor, M. J., Bälter, K., Xie, T., Solberg, B. S., Haavik, J., Arias Vásquez, A., Hartman, C. A., & Larsson, H. (2021). Gene-environment interactions in attention-deficit/hyperactivity disorder symptom dimensions: The role of unhealthy food habits. *Genes (Basel), 13*(1), 47. https://doi.org/10.3390/genes13010047

Li, Y., Yan, X., Li, Q., Li, Q., Xu, G., Lu, J., & Yang, W. (2023). Prevalence and trends in diagnosed ADHD among US children and adolescents, 2017–2022. *JAMA Network Open, 6*(10), e2336872–e2336872. https://doi.org/10.1001/jamanetworkopen.2023.36872

Loe, I. M., & Feldman, H. M. (2007). Academic and educational outcomes of children with ADHD. *Journal of Pediatric Psychology, 32*(6), 643–654.

Maher, G. M., O'Keeffe, G. W., Kearney, P. M., Kenny, L. C., Dinan, T. G., Mattsson, M., & Khashan, A. S. (2018). Association of hypertensive disorders of pregnancy with risk of neurodevelopmental disorders in offspring: A systematic review and meta-analysis. *JAMA Psychiatry, 75*(8), 809–819.

Markham, W. A., & Spencer, N. (2022). Factors that mediate the relationships between household socio-economic status and childhood Attention Deficit Hyperactivity Disorder (ADHD) in children and adolescents: A systematic review. *PLoS One, 17*(3), e0262988. https://doi.org/10.1371/journal.pone.0262988

Mikami, A. Y. (2010). The importance of friendship for youth with attention-deficit/hyperactivity disorder. *Clinical Child and Family Psychology Review, 13*(2), 181–198. https://doi.org/10.1007/s10567-010-0067-y

Momany, A. M., Kamradt, J. M., & Nikolas, M. A. (2018). A Meta-Analysis of the Association Between Birth Weight and Attention Deficit Hyperactivity Disorder. *Journal of Abnormal Child Psychology, 46*(7), 1409–1426. https://doi.org/10.1007/s10802-017-0371-9

Nilsen, F. M., & Tulve, N. S. (2020). A systematic review and meta-analysis examining the interrelationships between chemical and non-chemical stressors and inherent characteristics in children with ADHD. *Environmental Research, 180*, 108884. https://doi.org/10.1016/j.envres.2019.108884

Núñez-Jaramillo, L., Herrera-Solís, A., & Herrera-Morales, W. V. (2021). ADHD: Reviewing the causes and evaluating solutions. *Journal of Personalized Medicine, 11*(3), 166.

Ouyang, L., Fang, X., Mercy, J., Perou, R., & Grosse, S. D. (2008). Attention-deficit/hyperactivity disorder symptoms and child maltreatment: A population-based study. *The Journal of Pediatrics, 153*(6), 851–856.

Pang, X., Wang, H., Dill, S.-E., Boswell, M., Pang, X., Singh, M., & Rozelle, S. (2021). Attention Deficit Hyperactivity Disorder (ADHD) among elementary students in rural China: Prevalence, correlates, and consequences. *Journal of Affective Disorders, 293*, 484–491.

Pievsky, M. A., & McGrath, R. E. (2018). The neurocognitive profile of attention-deficit/hyperactivity disorder: A review of meta-analyses. *Archives of Clinical Neuropsychology, 33*(2), 143–157. https://doi.org/10.1093/arclin/acx055

Pliszka, S. R. (2020). Psychiatric comorbidities in children with attention deficit hyperactivity disorder: Implications for management. *Pediatric Drugs, 5*(11), 741–750. https://doi.org/10.2165/00148581-200305110-00003

Polanczyk, G. V., Salum, G. A., Sugaya, L. S., Caye, A., & Rohde, L. A. (2015). Annual research review: A meta-analysis of the worldwide prevalence of mental disorders in children and adolescents. *Journal of Child Psychology and Psychiatry, 56*(3), 345–365.

Quenneville, A. F., Kalogeropoulou, E., Nicastro, R., Weibel, S., Chanut, F., & Perroud, N. (2022). Anxiety disorders in adult ADHD: A frequent comorbidity and a risk factor for externalizing problems. *Psychiatry Research, 310*, 114423.

Rattay, K., & Robinson, L. R. (2024). Identifying risk factors for attention-deficit/hyperactivity disorder (ADHD): A public health concern and opportunity. *Prevention Science, 25*, 1–8.

Rubia, K. (2018). Cognitive neuroscience of attention deficit hyperactivity disorder (ADHD) and its clinical translation. *Frontiers in Human Neuroscience, 12*, 100.

Reiersen, A. M. (2017). How should we classify complex neurodevelopmental disorders? *Scandinavian Journal of Child and Adolescent Psychiatry and Psychology, 5*(1), 1–2.

Robinson, Z. P., Pelland, J. C., Remmert, J. F., Refalo, M. C., Jukic, I., Steele, J., & Zourdos, M. C. (2024). Exploring the dose–response relationship between estimated resistance training proximity to failure, strength gain, and muscle hypertrophy: A series of meta-regressions. *Sports Medicine, 54*, 2209–2231.

Russell, A. E., Ford, T., Williams, R., & Russell, G. (2016). The association between socioeconomic disadvantage and attention deficit/hyperactivity disorder (ADHD): A systematic review. *Child Psychiatry & Human Development, 47*, 440–458.

Salari, N., Ghasemi, H., Abdoli, N., Rahmani, A., Shiri, M. H., Hashemian, A. H., Akbari, H., & Mohammadi, M. (2023). The global prevalence of ADHD in children and adolescents: A systematic review and meta-analysis. *Italian Journal of Pediatrics, 49*(1), 48. https://doi.org/10.1186/s13052-023-01456-1

Schein, J., Adler, L. A., Childress, A., Cloutier, M., Gagnon-Sanschagrin, P., Davidson, M., Kinkead, F., Guerin, A., & Lefebvre, P. (2022). Economic burden of attentiondeficit/hyperactivity disorder among children and adolescents in the United States: A societal perspective. *Journal of Medical Economics, 25*, 193–205. https://doi.org/10.1080/13696998.2022.2032097

Schultz, B. K., & Evans, S. W. (2015). *A practical guide to implementing school-based interventions for adolescents with ADHD*. Springer.

Sciberras, E., Streatfeild, J., Ceccato, T., Pezzullo, L., Scott, J. G., Middeldorp, C. M., Hutchins, P., Paterson, R., Bellgrove, M. A., & Coghill, D. (2022). Social and economic costs of attention-deficit/hyperactivity disorder across the lifespan. *Journal of Attention Disorders, 26*(1), 72–87.

Shaw, P., Eckstrand, K., Sharp, W., Blumenthal, J., Lerch, J., Greenstein, D., Clasen, L., Evans, A., Giedd, J., & Rapoport, J. (2007). Attention-deficit/hyperactivity disorder is characterized by a delay in cortical maturation. *Proceedings of the National Academy of Sciences, 104*(49), 19649–19654.

Sigurdardottir, H. L., Kranz, G. S., Rami-Mark, C., James, G. M., Vanicek, T., Gryglewski, G., Kautzky, A., Hienert, M., Traub-Weidinger, T., Mitterhauser, M., Wadsak, W., Hacker, M., Rujescu, D., Kasper, S., & Lanzenberger, R. (2016). Effects of norepinephrine transporter gene variants on NET binding in ADHD and healthy controls investigated by PET. *Human Brain Mapping, 37*(3), 884–895. https://doi.org/10.1002/hbm.23071

Stoiber, K. C., & Gettinger, M. (2015). Multi-tiered systems of support and evidence-based practices. In *Handbook of response to intervention: The science and practice of multi-tiered systems of support* (pp. 121–141). Springer.

Sucksdorff, M., Brown, A. S., Chudal, R., Surcel, H.-M., Hinkka-Yli-Salomäki, S., Cheslack-Postava, K., Gyllenberg, D., & Sourander, A. (2021). Maternal vitamin D levels and the risk of offspring attention-deficit/hyperactivity disorder. *Journal of the American Academy of Child & Adolescent Psychiatry, 60*(1), 142–151.e2.

Sudre, G., Gildea, D. E., Shastri, G. G., Sharp, W., Jung, B., Xu, Q., Auluck, P. K., Elnitski, L., Baxevanis, A. D., Marenco, S., & Shaw, P. (2023). Mapping the cortico-striatal transcriptome in attention deficit hyperactivity disorder. *Molecular Psychiatry, 28*(2), 792–800. https://doi.org/10.1038/s41380-022-01844-9

Taylor, M. J., Martin, J., Lu, Y., Brikell, I., Lundström, S., Larsson, H., & Lichtenstein, P. (2019). Association of genetic risk factors for psychiatric disorders and traits of these disorders in a Swedish population twin sample. *JAMA Psychiatry, 76*(3), 280–289.

Thapar, A., Cooper, M., & Rutter, M. (2017). Neurodevelopmental disorders. *The Lancet Psychiatry, 4*(4), 339–346.

Thomas, R., Sanders, S., Doust, J., Beller, E., & Glasziou, P. (2015). Prevalence of attention-deficit/hyperactivity disorder: A systematic review and meta-analysis. *Pediatrics, 135*(4), e994–e1001.

Turgay, A., Goodman, D. W., Asherson, P., Lasser, R. A., Babcock, T. F., Pucci, M. L., Barkley, R., & ADHD Transition Phase Model Working Group. (2012). Lifespan persistence of ADHD: The life transition model and its application. *The Journal of Clinical Psychiatry, 73*(2), 10337.

Tusa, B. S., Alati, R., Ayano, G., Betts, K., Weldesenbet, A. B., & Dachew, B. (2024). The risk of attention deficit hyperactivity disorder symptoms in offspring of mothers with perinatal depression: A systematic review and meta-analysis. *Asian Journal of Psychiatry, 102*, 104261. https://doi.org/10.1016/j.ajp.2024.104261

Visser, M. J., Peters, R. M., & Luman, M. (2024). Understanding ADHD-related stigma: A gender analysis of young adults and key stakeholder perspectives. *Neurodiversity, 2*, 27546330241274664.

WHO. (2020). *World health statistics. 2020.* Retrieved December 30, 2024 from http://www.who.int/gho/publications/world_health_statistics/en

Williams, N. M., Zaharieva, I., Martin, A., Langley, K., Mantripragada, K., Fossdal, R., Stefansson, H., Stefansson, K., Magnusson, P., & Gudmundsson, O. O. (2010). Rare chromosomal deletions and duplications in attention-deficit hyperactivity disorder: A genome-wide analysis. *The Lancet, 376*(9750), 1401–1408.

Wolraich, M. L., Chan, E., Froehlich, T., Lynch, R. L., Bax, A., Redwine, S. T., Ihyembe, D., & Hagan, J. F. (2019). ADHD diagnosis and treatment guidelines: A historical perspective. *Pediatrics, 144*(4), e20191682.

Young, S., Hollingdale, J., Absoud, M., Bolton, P., Branney, P., Colley, W., Craze, E., Dave, M., Deeley, Q., & Farrag, E. (2020). Guidance for identification and treatment of individuals with attention deficit/hyperactivity disorder and autism spectrum disorder based upon expert consensus. *BMC Medicine, 18*, 1–29.

Zhang, W., Sweeney, J. A., Bishop, J. R., Gong, Q., & Lui, S. (2023). Biological subtyping of psychiatric syndromes as a pathway for advances in drug discovery and personalized medicine. *Nature Mental Health, 1*(2), 88–99.

Zhao, X., Page, T. F., Altszuler, A. R., Pelham, W. E., 3rd, Kipp, H., Gnagy, E. M., Coxe, S., Schatz, N. K., Merrill, B. M., Macphee, F. L., & Pelham, W. E., Jr. (2019). Family burden of raising a child with ADHD. *Journal of Abnormal Child Psychology, 47*(8), 1327–1338. https://doi.org/10.1007/s10802-019-00518-5

Chapter 2
The Epidemiology of ADHD Across the Lifespan

Abstract This chapter explores the epidemiology of attention-deficit/hyperactivity disorder (ADHD) across different stages of life, examining how prevalence rates, symptom presentation, and functional impairments evolve from childhood through adulthood. The chapter begins with an analysis of ADHD prevalence in childhood and adolescence, focusing on gender differences, ADHD subtypes, and racial and socioeconomic disparities in diagnosis and treatment access. It then explores the developmental trajectory of ADHD symptoms, detailing how hyperactivity often declines with age, while inattention and impulsivity persist, contributing to lifelong challenges in academic, occupational, and social domains. Discussion also highlights the underdiagnosis and misdiagnosis of ADHD in adults, emphasizing the barriers to healthcare access and disparities in treatment-seeking behavior among different demographic groups.

The impact of comorbid conditions, such as anxiety disorders, depression, and substance use disorders, is explored to underscore the multifaceted burden of ADHD across the lifespan. The chapter further examines treatment patterns and accessibility, discussing regional and socioeconomic differences in medication use, behavioral therapy, and multimodal interventions. Public health initiatives aimed at improving awareness, promoting early diagnosis, and expanding access to ADHD care are also addressed.

By providing a lifespan perspective, this chapter highlights the importance of age-specific interventions, evidence-based treatment strategies, and policy-driven approaches to improving the long-term outcomes of individuals with ADHD.

2.1 Prevalence of ADHD in Childhood and Adolescence

ADHD is a common neurodevelopmental condition affecting children and adolescents worldwide. Estimates suggest that in 2023, around 8% of this age group experience symptoms associated with the disorder, with reported rates ranging from 6 to 10% (Ayano et al., 2023a). This places ADHD among the most frequently identified

G. Ayano et al., *ADHD Across the Lifespan*, SpringerBriefs in Modern Perspectives on Disability Research,
https://doi.org/10.1007/978-981-95-8712-4_2

mental health conditions in young people. Early recognition and swift, well-chosen interventions are pivotal for limiting ADHD's toll—academic underachievement, strained peer relations, and emotional distress. Guided by Pollard's public health planning framework, we follow three disciplined steps: (1) clarify the problem and its determinants; (2) generate a comprehensive menu of options; and (3) rigorously appraise each option for reach, equity, feasibility, and cost-effectiveness (Pollard et al., 2008).

Using this framework, 11 broad intervention types can be deployed: advocacy; legislation and regulation; fiscal or economic levers; organizational or infrastructural support; community capacity-building; education and skills development; social marketing and mass media campaigns; environmental restructuring; service delivery reforms; systematic screening and early detection; and evidence-based clinical treatment. The WHO's *International Classification of Health Interventions* (ICHI) now provides a common taxonomy for coding these approaches, enabling consistent comparison across settings (Fortune et al., 2021).

Because ADHD prevalence and service access vary by gender, age, ethnicity, and geography, selecting the optimal mix from these 11 categories—co-designed with local stakeholders—offers the best chance to achieve culturally responsive, high-impact, and equitable outcomes.

2.1.1 Gender Differences in ADHD

ADHD is identified more often in boys than in girls, with reported diagnosis rates between two and three times higher in males. In the United States, for instance, around 12.9% of boys have been identified with ADHD, compared to 5.6% of girls (Willcutt, 2012). A similar skew is seen in Africa, where prevalence estimates are roughly 10% in boys and 5% in girls (Ayano et al., 2023a). Comparable figures emerge from Asia: a large 2025 national survey of 73,992 Chinese schoolchildren found ADHD rates of 8.1% for boys and 4.6% for girls (Liu et al., 2025).

Several explanations have been proposed for these gender differences in prevalence. One factor is that boys tend to display more noticeable behaviors, such as hyperactivity and impulsivity, which are easily identified in classrooms and other structured environments (Rucklidge, 2010). In contrast, girls more commonly experience inattentive symptoms, which may be less disruptive and go unrecognized for longer periods (Mahone & Wodka, 2008). In some cases, ADHD in girls is mistaken for shyness or anxiety, leading to delays in identification and support (Hinshaw et al., 2022).

Expectations around gender roles may also influence identification rates. Boys who display high-energy levels or difficulty focusing are often referred for assessment sooner, while similar behaviors in girls may be overlooked (Skogli et al., 2013). Biological differences, including brain development and hormonal changes, may also shape how symptoms appear across genders (Martel et al., 2009). Additionally, girls with ADHD are more likely to experience anxiety and mood difficulties, which can lead to misinterpretation of their symptoms (Hinshaw et al., 2022).

Addressing these differences requires greater awareness among educators, healthcare providers, and families to ensure that both boys and girls receive timely and accurate support. Expanding our understanding of how ADHD manifests across the full lifespan—from preschool years (≈2–5 years) and school age (6–12 years), through adolescence (13–17 years), and into adulthood (18 years and beyond)—will allow us to tailor interventions that truly meet the needs of everyone affected.

2.1.2 ADHD Subtypes

ADHD is categorized into three main subtypes: predominantly inattentive (ADHD-I), predominantly hyperactive-impulsive (ADHD-HI), and combined presentation (ADHD-C). Individuals with ADHD-I primarily struggle with focus, organization, and task completion, without being overly active or impulsive. In contrast, those with ADHD-HI are characterized by restlessness, impulsive decision-making, and difficulty staying seated or still. The combined presentation (ADHD-C) involves a mix of inattentive and hyperactive-impulsive symptoms.

Across large population-based samples, the inattentive presentation (ADHD-I) predominates, accounting for roughly 47% of all diagnosed cases, followed by hyperactive-impulsive (ADHD-HI; 34%) and combined (ADHD-C; 21%) (LeRoy et al., 2018). Longitudinal data from the same cohort show that hyperactive-impulsive traits attenuate with age, whereas inattentive symptoms remain comparatively stable. Consequently, children under 10 years are most often classified as ADHD-HI or ADHD-C, but by adolescence—and well into adulthood—the diagnostic center of gravity shifts decisively toward ADHD-I. This developmental pivot has direct clinical implications: screening protocols and intervention priorities must be recalibrated for older age groups to capture persistent inattentive deficits that might otherwise be overlooked (LeRoy et al., 2018).

Understanding these developmental shifts is essential for age-appropriate support. Detecting inattentive features early—because they are the most likely to persist—gives clinicians and educators a window to intervene before those deficits undermine academic achievement, vocational progress, or social relationships later in life.

2.1.3 Geographic and Racial Differences in ADHD

2.1.3.1 ADHD Across Different Regions

ADHD prevalence still shows marked geographic variation, shaped by differences in awareness, service capacity, and screening practices. North America posts some of the highest figures—an estimated 11.4% of U.S. children (3–17 years) have ever

Table 2.1 The prevalence of ADHD in children & adolescents by region

Region	Prevalence (%)	Min (%)	Max (%)	Category
Africa	7.47	5.0	9.0	Within the average
Middle East	6.30	5.0	7.5	Within the average
Oceania	9.00	7.0	11.0	Within the average
South America	10.50	8.0	13.0	Above average
Asia	5.80	5.0	7.0	Below average
North America	12.10	10.0	15.0	Above average
Europe	7.10	5.5	8.5	Within the average
Worldwide	8.00	6.0	10.0	Within the average

received an ADHD diagnosis. A pooled review of Latin-American studies found a similarly elevated rate of ≈11.8% for South America (Willcutt, 2012). At the other extreme, large school-based surveys in East Asia place prevalence nearer 5.8%. Midrange estimates are typical of Europe (≈7.1%), Australia (7.4%), and Africa (≈7.5%) (Ayano et al., 2020; Cénat et al., 2021) (Table 2.1). Regions with few child-mental-health specialists or only sporadic school screening tend to underdiagnose, whereas jurisdictions that embed structured assessments in primary care and education systems register far more cases—underscoring how health-system infrastructure, not biology alone, drives the observed regional spread.

2.1.3.2 Racial and Ethnic Differences

ADHD prevalence varies among different racial and ethnic group. In the United States, ADHD is more common in White (16.6%) and Black (15.9%) children compared to Asian (12.4%) and Hispanic populations (N = 1,613,780) (Cénat et al., 2021). Despite these figures, children from racial and ethnic minority groups are often less likely to be formally diagnosed or to receive treatment.

Several factors are likely to contribute to this gap. Differences in healthcare access, social stigma, and clinician biases may result in some groups receiving less frequent evaluations for ADHD, even when symptoms are present. A large-scale study of 238,000 children aged 3–17 years found that Black, Hispanic, and Asian children were significantly less likely to receive an ADHD diagnosis compared to White children, despite showing similar traits (Shi et al., 2021).

Another factor involves cultural beliefs. In some cultural groups, ADHD symptoms may be viewed as behavioral issues rather than a medical condition, leading to lower rates of diagnosis and treatment-seeking (Ford-Jones, 2015). In addition, families from diverse backgrounds may experience barriers in accessing specialized ADHD services, further delaying identification and support.

2.1.3.3 Understanding Disparities in ADHD Diagnosis

Several large-scale studies, including national health surveys, found that ADHD is identified more frequently in Black and White compared to Hispanic children. However, examining hospital records and healthcare data, the pattern shifts—White children tend to receive more frequent diagnoses and treatment than Black and Hispanic children (Coker et al., 2016).

One possible explanation involves how ADHD is recognized and addressed within different communities. Some families may not seek an ADHD evaluation due to concerns about stigma or potential negative labels. Others may lack access to specialists who can accurately identify ADHD symptoms, leading to underdiagnosis. Additionally, biases in the healthcare system can result in misinterpretation of ADHD behaviors, particularly in children from racial and ethnic minority backgrounds (Faraone et al., 2021).

2.1.3.4 Reducing Gaps in ADHD Diagnosis and Treatment

There are clear disparities in both diagnosis and treatment rates of ADHD across racial and cultural groups. For example, in the United States, ADHD diagnosis rates are highest among White children, followed by Black, Hispanic, and Asian children, highlighting persistent inequities in recognition and access to care (Danielson et al., 2018). These gaps are further compounded by limited mental health services and shortages of ADHD specialists in communities with larger Black, Hispanic, and Native American populations, making timely diagnosis and appropriate treatment more difficult (Coker et al., 2016). Cultural perceptions of ADHD also play a role, as some families may hesitate to pursue diagnosis due to concerns about stigma or discrimination associated with mental health diagnoses (Faraone et al., 2021). Additionally, implicit biases among healthcare providers can affect how symptoms are interpreted, sometimes leading to overdiagnosis in certain populations and underdiagnosis in others (Faraone et al., 2021).

Efforts to increase awareness, improve training for healthcare providers, and expand access to ADHD-related services are critical to ensuring that all children receive appropriate support. Key steps to improve ADHD identification and treatment include expanding ADHD services in underserved areas to ensure early screening and intervention for all children, providing training for educators and healthcare professionals to recognize diverse ADHD presentations—especially in girls and minority groups—and reducing stigma through public health campaigns that encourage families to seek evaluation without fear of negative labeling. By addressing these gaps, it is possible to improve early recognition, diagnosis, and treatment, allowing children and adolescents with ADHD to receive the support they need to thrive in school, at home, and in social settings. However, it is important to note that these diagnosis rates are based on data from 2016 and may not fully reflect more recent trends or interventions aimed at reducing disparities (Danielson et al., 2018).

2.2 Transition of ADHD Symptoms into Adulthood

ADHD has traditionally been regarded as a childhood condition; however, evidence suggests that symptoms frequently persist into adulthood. Studies estimate that around 60% of children diagnosed with ADHD continue to experience symptoms into their mid-20s, with approximately 41% continuing to face functional impairments (Willcutt, 2012). The persistence of ADHD beyond childhood underscores the importance of sustained awareness, support, and treatment strategies tailored to different life stages and cultures.

2.2.1 Changes in Symptom Presentation over Time

ADHD symptoms evolve across the lifespan. In early childhood, hyperactivity and impulsivity are the most noticeable characteristics, often leading to behavioral challenges in school and home environments (Faraone et al., 2021). As individuals transition into adolescence and adulthood, these overt symptoms tend to diminish, while difficulties with inattention, disorganization, and executive function become more prominent (Faraone et al., 2021). Many adults with ADHD struggle with time management, sustained attention, emotional regulation, and task completion (GBD 2019 Mental Disorders Collaborators, 2022). These challenges can impact workplace performance, interpersonal relationships, and overall well-being.

This transition in symptom presentation contributes to diagnostic challenges, as the hyperactivity seen in childhood often shifts to an internal sense of restlessness. Adults with ADHD may experience chronic procrastination, forgetfulness, impulsive decision-making, and difficulties in maintaining routines (Kessler et al., 2006). These issues, if left unrecognized, can contribute to academic struggles, workplace inefficiency, and emotional distress.

2.2.2 Factors Influencing ADHD Persistence

Several factors influence whether or not ADHD symptoms persist into adulthood. The severity of childhood symptoms, presence of coexisting conditions, and access to early interventions all play a role in long-term outcomes. Research indicates that children with pronounced hyperactivity and impulsivity are more likely to experience continued challenges in adulthood (GBD 2019 Mental Disorders Collaborators, 2022). Additionally, children and adolescents with ADHD frequently have co-occurring conditions such as anxiety, depression, and substance use disorders, which can complicate symptom management and increase the risk of social and occupational difficulties (Kessler et al., 2006).

Life transitions, such as entering higher education, joining the workforce, or taking on greater personal responsibilities, may exacerbate ADHD-related challenges. While structured environments—such as schools with clear routines—can help mitigate symptoms, adulthood often demands greater self-regulation and organizational skills. Without appropriate coping mechanisms, adults with ADHD may struggle to meet deadlines, manage finances, and maintain stable relationships. Gender differences also play a role in the persistence of ADHD, with males historically exhibiting more hyperactive symptoms in childhood, while females often present with inattentive symptoms that may go unrecognized and undiagnosed until adulthood.

2.2.3 Neurobiological and Cognitive Considerations

Advances in neuroimaging have demonstrated that ADHD is associated with structural and functional differences in brain regions responsible for executive function, impulse control, and attention regulation (Ayano et al., 2025). Studies show that the prefrontal cortex—critical for planning and decision-making—develops more slowly in individuals with ADHD, contributing to persistent difficulties in focus, organization, and self-discipline (Shaw et al., 2007). Additionally, disruptions in dopamine and norepinephrine pathways play a key role in ADHD, supporting the rationale for pharmacological treatments targeting these neurotransmitter systems (Ayano et al., 2025).

These neurobiological differences help explain why some individuals continue to experience symptoms into adulthood, despite environmental and behavioral adaptations. Understanding the underlying brain mechanisms of ADHD is essential for developing targeted interventions that address not only the behavioral manifestations but also the neurocognitive processes contributing to attention and impulse control deficits (Ayano et al., 2025).

2.2.4 Challenges in Diagnosis and Treatment

A major challenge in ADHD diagnosis among adults is the historical perception that ADHD is a childhood-limited disorder (Faraone et al., 2021). Many adults with ADHD were never formally diagnosed in childhood and may only seek evaluation when they encounter difficulties in academic, professional, or social settings (Ayano et al., 2023b). Furthermore, the symptoms of adult ADHD often overlap with those of anxiety, depression, and other mood disorders, leading to misdiagnosis or delayed diagnosis (Koyuncu et al., 2022).

Effective treatment for adult ADHD requires a multimodal approach. While stimulant medications, such as methylphenidate and amphetamines, remain the primary pharmacological treatment, behavioral interventions also play a crucial role (Hinshaw et al., 2015). Cognitive behavioral therapy (CBT), executive function coaching, and structured organizational strategies have been shown to improve daily functioning and quality of life (Mongia & Hechtman, 2012). Additionally, mindfulness-based therapies and lifestyle modifications—such as exercise, structured routines, and sleep hygiene—can complement medical treatment and enhance self-regulation in people with ADHD (Twiss, 2024)

2.3 Adult ADHD: Prevalence and Health-Seeking Behavior

ADHD in adulthood remains a significant yet underrecognized public health issue. While historically considered a childhood disorder, research now confirms that ADHD frequently persists into adulthood. Global estimates suggest that approximately 3.1% of adults meet the criteria for ADHD, a prevalence that is comparable to, or only slightly lower than, major depressive disorder, which affects around 5% of the adult population (Ayano et al., 2023b). Notably, adult ADHD is more prevalent than several widely recognized psychiatric conditions, including bipolar disorder (1–2%), generalized anxiety disorder (2–3%), and obsessive-compulsive disorder (1–2%) (Steel et al., 2014). Despite its comparable prevalence, ADHD in adulthood has received relatively limited attention from policymakers and healthcare providers, leading to substantial gaps in diagnosis and treatment (Huang et al., 2020).

2.3.1 Prevalence and Underdiagnosis of Adult ADHD

Although ADHD is well-established as a childhood disorder, studies indicate that a significant proportion of individuals continue to experience symptoms beyond adolescence (Di Lorenzo et al., 2021). While childhood ADHD prevalence is estimated to be around 8%, adult ADHD prevalence is lower, likely due to symptom attenuation, coping mechanisms, or diagnostic challenges (Ayano et al., 2023a, 2023b). Longitudinal studies suggest that approximately 60% of those diagnosed in childhood retain symptoms into adulthood, and around 41% continue to experience significant functional impairments (Volkow & Swanson, 2013; Young & Goodman, 2016).

Despite its established prevalence, treatment rates for adult ADHD remain disproportionately low. Studies suggest that between 70 and 90% of adults with ADHD remain undiagnosed or untreated, depending on the region and health system infrastructure (Fayyad et al., 2007; Johnson et al., 2021). This treatment gap is most pronounced in low- and middle-income countries (LMICs), where mental health service availability is severely limited (Alem et al., 2009; Patel et al., 2013). However, even in high-income countries, access challenges persist, including long waiting times for specialist assessment and fragmented service provision (Eke et al., 2020; Matheiken et al., 2024; Smith et al., 2024).

2.3.2 Barriers to Diagnosis and Treatment

Several factors contribute to the persistent underdiagnosis and undertreatment of ADHD in adults:

1. *ADHD as a Childhood-Limited Disorder*:
   Historically, ADHD has been framed as a disorder of childhood, leading to a lack of awareness about its persistence into adulthood (Faraone et al., 2021). Many healthcare providers do not routinely assess adults for ADHD, particularly those presenting with comorbid conditions such as depression or anxiety, further contributing to missed diagnoses.
2. *Diagnostic Challenges in Adults*:
   ADHD in adulthood often manifests differently than in childhood. While hyperactivity and impulsivity tend to decline, inattention, executive dysfunction, and emotional dysregulation become more prominent (Ayano et al., 2023b; Faraone et al., 2021). This change in symptom presentation makes diagnosis complex, especially in the absence of childhood medical records. Moreover, the overlap of ADHD symptoms with other psychiatric disorders increases the risk of misdiagnosis (Montano & Weisler, 2011).
3. *Limited Access to Specialized Care*:
   Access to ADHD-specific care remains limited. Many mental health systems prioritize severe psychiatric disorders, such as schizophrenia and bipolar disorder, leaving ADHD underprioritized (Mellman et al., 2001). In many regions, particularly in LMICs, the availability of ADHD-trained specialists is scarce (Patel et al., 2013). Additionally, long wait times and financial constraints prevent many adults from seeking appropriate evaluation and treatment (Smith et al., 2024).
4. *Stigma and Societal Misconceptions*:
   Public perception of ADHD as a disorder of childhood, combined with stigma around psychiatric conditions, discourages many adults from seeking medical attention (Asherson et al., 2016). Individuals experiencing ADHD-related challenges at work or in relationships may not recognize their symptoms as part of a clinical condition, leading to delays in diagnosis and treatment. A persistent misconception is that ADHD naturally resolves with age, despite substantial evidence demonstrating its continuation into adulthood (Asherson et al., 2016; Faraone et al., 2021; Fayyad et al., 2017).

2.3.3 Addressing the Public Health Burden of Adult ADHD

Given the far-reaching consequences of untreated ADHD in adulthood, a comprehensive public health approach is essential to bridge the diagnosis and treatment gap. Raising awareness among healthcare professionals and the public is a critical first step (Kooij et al., 2019). Education initiatives targeting primary care providers, mental health specialists, and policymakers can help dispel misconceptions and promote routine ADHD screening in adults. Although DSM-5 provides diagnostic criteria for individuals aged 17 and older, the development of supplementary standardized guidelines that emphasize the adult presentation of ADHD could further improve detection and reduce misdiagnosis, while ensuring clinicians are trained to apply these criteria effectively in adulthood remains equally important (Ginsberg et al., 2014a). Expanding access to mental health services is also crucial, as significant disparities in ADHD diagnosis and treatment persist across many regions. Scaling up integrated mental healthcare models and leveraging telemedicine and digital mental health platforms offer promising avenues for increasing access to diagnostic and treatment services (Young et al., 2023). Additionally, reducing stigma and enhancing public health messaging are key components of a successful public health strategy. Campaigns that emphasize ADHD as a legitimate, lifelong neurodevelopmental condition can encourage early recognition and reduce barriers to care. Advocacy efforts should focus on ensuring that adults feel supported in seeking appropriate medical attention and services.

2.4 Age-Dependent Decline of ADHD

ADHD is widely recognized as a neurodevelopmental condition that emerges in early childhood. Its symptom profile and prevalence evolve with age—hyperactivity tends to decline during adolescence, while inattention often persists. Longitudinal research shows a developmental decline in prevalence, with rates estimated at around 8% in childhood, 5–6% in adolescence, and approximately 3% in adulthood (Ayano et al., 2023b; Faraone et al., 2021). This trajectory reflects both true symptom reduction and challenges in adult diagnosis. Although ADHD becomes less prevalent with age, symptoms often transform rather than disappear, highlighting the need for age-specific diagnostic and treatment approaches (Ayano et al., 2023a, 2023b).

2.4.1 Mechanisms Underlying the Age-Related Decline in ADHD Prevalence

The observed reduction in ADHD prevalence over the life course may be attributed to multiple factors, including neurobiological changes, behavioral adaptations, and variations in presentation and diagnostic recognition.

1. *Attenuation of Hyperactive and Impulsive Behaviors*:
   One of the most well-documented changes in ADHD symptomatology over time is the decline of hyperactivity and impulsivity (Biederman et al., 2000). In childhood, these behaviors manifest as excessive movement, difficulty sit-

ting still, and impulsive decision-making. As individuals mature, these outward facing behaviors often decrease, giving way to more subtle forms of restlessness, difficulty with self-regulation, and problems with sustained attention (Faraone et al., 2021). This shift is largely attributed to continued brain development, particularly in the prefrontal cortex, which plays a critical role in executive function (Friedman & Robbins, 2022). While hyperactivity diminishes, difficulties with inattention and executive functioning often persist into adulthood, leading to ongoing challenges in academic, occupational, and personal domains.

2. *Compensatory Coping Mechanisms and Behavioral Adaptation*:
   As individuals with ADHD transition into adulthood, many develop adaptive strategies to manage their symptoms (Sansosti et al., 2017). These may include structured daily routines, selecting work environments that align with their cognitive strengths, and using external organizational aids such as reminders and planners (Heublein, 2023). Over time, these strategies can contribute to the perception of reduced symptoms, even though underlying cognitive and attentional differences persist. While some individuals with ADHD find ways to function effectively, others continue to struggle, particularly in unstructured environments where executive function demands are high.
3. *Diagnostic and Methodological Factors*:
   Variations in diagnostic criteria and clinical recognition of ADHD at different life stages also contribute to the observed decline in prevalence with increasing age (APA, 2013). ADHD often presents differently in adults than in childhood, with less visible hyperactivity and more difficulties related to executive function, emotional regulation, and attentional control (Faraone et al., 2021). Since diagnostic frameworks were originally developed for pediatric ADHD, they may not fully capture the way the condition manifests in adulthood. Furthermore, many adults with ADHD remain undiagnosed due to a reliance on retrospective self-reporting of childhood symptoms, which can be affected by recall bias.
4. *Shifts in Contextual and Psychosocial Demands*:
   During the childhood to adulthood transition, environmental expectations and responsibilities change substantially (Rutter, 1989). Applied structures of the school setting may find, children with ADHD struggling with academic organization, task completion, and peer relationships (APA, 2013), whereas adults often have greater autonomy to select environments that accommodate their needs (Faraone et al., 2021). Some adults with ADHD experience fewer impairments as a result. However, the demands of managing finances, employment, and social relationships in adulthood increase difficulty for some. For other, ADHD-related challenges persist but remain unrecognized, leading to late-life diagnosis or misattribution of symptoms to other mental health conditions.

2.4.2 *Clinical and Public Health Implications*

Understanding the progression of ADHD over the lifespan is essential for optimizing diagnostic and treatment approaches. Despite the reduction in hyperactivity and impulsivity during adulthood many individuals continue to experience executive function difficulties, attentional challenges, and emotional dysregulation into adulthood (Ayano et al., 2023b; Faraone et al., 2021). Effective management requires a lifespan approach that acknowledges the evolving nature of ADHD symptoms, how they respond to environmental conditions, with tailored interventions.

Key considerations for improving ADHD care at different life stages include refining age-appropriate diagnostic criteria to better capture adult ADHD presentations—such as executive dysfunction, emotional dysregulation, and internalized restlessness—to enhance identification and treatment. Enhancing screening and assessment in adults is also vital, as integrating ADHD screening into primary care and psychiatric evaluations can help bridge the diagnostic gap. Tailoring treatment strategies to lifespan needs should incorporate behavioral strategies, workplace accommodations, and executive function training alongside pharmacological interventions when necessary. Finally, ensuring continued access to ADHD care beyond childhood is crucial, as many healthcare systems currently lack adequate services for adults with ADHD. By moving beyond the misconception that ADHD naturally resolves with age, clinicians, researchers, and policymakers can develop more effective public health strategies to support individuals with ADHD throughout their lives.

2.5 Comorbidities and Functional Impairments Across the Lifespan

ADHD is associated with a wide range of co-occurring conditions, spanning both mental and physical health domains (Becker et al., 2012). These comorbidities influence the course of ADHD, affecting diagnosis, treatment outcomes, and overall quality of life (Classi et al., 2012). The nature and impact of these co-occurring conditions vary across developmental stages, underscoring the need for a *lifespan-focused clinical management approach* (Shaw et al., 2012).

2.5.1 *Mental Health Comorbidities*

Individuals with ADHD frequently experience co-occurring mental health conditions that exacerbate core symptoms and contribute to long-term impairment (Shaw et al., 2012). The most prevalent psychiatric comorbidities include anxiety disorders, affecting up to two in five individuals, and depressive disorders, reported in one-quarter of people with ADHD (Bagwell et al., 2006; Zhang et al., 2025). Sleep disturbances, including insomnia and restless legs syndrome, are also common and contribute to cognitive and emotional dysregulation. Additionally, oppositional defiant disorder (ODD) and conduct disorder (CD) are frequently diagnosed in childhood, while bipolar disorder, substance use disorders (SUDs), and autism spectrum disorder (ASD) are frequently observed across the lifespan (Coşkun et al., 2020). These mental health challenges are explored in greater detail in Chap. 3.

2.5.2 Physical Health Comorbidities

Attention-deficit/hyperactivity disorder is also linked to a range of physical health conditions that contribute to healthcare needs and a heightened risk of long-term health complications (Harpin et al., 2013; Jameson et al., 2016). Individuals with ADHD frequently experience metabolic, cardiovascular, respiratory, and neurological conditions, highlighting the complex interaction between neurodevelopmental and systemic health factors (Instanes et al., 2018) (Table 2.2).

Weight concerns, particularly obesity, are commonly reported in individuals with ADHD (Cortese et al., 2016). Difficulties with impulse control, irregular eating patterns, and lower levels of physical activity contribute to an increased likelihood of excessive weight gain (Cortese et al., 2016). Type 2 diabetes is also more common in individuals with ADHD, with behavioral and lifestyle factors playing a role in its development (Cortese et al., 2016).

Cardiovascular conditions, including high blood pressure and an increased likelihood of stroke, are frequently observed in individuals with ADHD (Instanes et al., 2018). Factors such as autonomic nervous system dysfunction and medication effects may contribute to these associations (Zhang et al., 2024). Similarly, respiratory conditions, including asthma, appear to be more common among individuals with ADHD, with possible links to neuroimmune processes (Zhang et al., 2024).

Neurological conditions such as epilepsy and migraines are often reported in individuals with ADHD (Salem et al., 2018) as is the likelihood of experiencing seizures, suggesting a possible overlap in neurodevelopmental mechanisms (Salpekar, 2018). Migraine headaches are also frequently reported, with some evidence pointing to underlying neurochemical factors (Salem et al., 2018).

Gastrointestinal concerns, including irritable bowel syndrome (IBS), are commonly associated with ADHD (Kedem et al., 2020). The role of stress sensitivity and autonomic dysfunction is considered a contributing factor in these digestive issues. Skin conditions, including eczema, are also more frequently noted, possibly influenced by immune system responses and stress-related triggers (Hak et al., 2013).

Beyond chronic conditions, individuals with ADHD are more likely to experience unintentional injuries and accidents (Libutzki et al., 2023). Higher rates of fractures, emergency room visits, and head injuries are reported from childhood onwards. In adulthood, difficulties with attention and impulse control contribute to

Table 2.2 Common physical health comorbidities in ADHD

Condition	Prevalence rate	Clinical implications
Obesity	Adults with ADHD are *70% more likely* to be obese	Impaired impulse control and dysregulated eating patterns contribute to increased obesity risk
Asthma	*14–27%* comorbidity rate	Shared inflammatory and neuroimmune pathways may underlie the ADHD-asthma link
Migraine	Reported in *15–20%* of individuals with ADHD	Evidence suggests dopaminergic dysregulation may contribute to both migraine and ADHD
Epilepsy	Co-occurs in *1–2%* of ADHD cases	ADHD and epilepsy share common neurodevelopmental pathways, requiring careful differential diagnosis
Gastrointestinal disorders	Irritable bowel syndrome (IBS) in *10–15%* of ADHD individuals	Dysregulated autonomic function and stress sensitivity may contribute
Hypertension	Observed in *5–10%* of ADHD cases	Linked to autonomic dysregulation and stimulant medication effects
Type 2 diabetes	*5–10%* comorbidity rate	Impulse control difficulties and metabolic dysfunction may elevate disease risk
Eczema and dermatological conditions	Present in *7–20%* of individuals with ADHD	Immune system dysregulation and stress-related exacerbation of symptoms may be contributing factors
Dental problems	Higher rates of cavities and gum disease (*14–76%* prevalence)	Poor oral hygiene, impulsive dietary habits, and neglect may contribute
Injuries and accidents	Childhood injury rates: *24% in early childhood, 19% in middle childhood, and 31% in adolescence*	Increased impulsivity and inattention raise the risk of unintentional injuries

an increased likelihood of reckless driving, traffic violations, and motor vehicle accidents (Vaa, 2014).

The presence of physical health conditions alongside ADHD highlights the need for a comprehensive approach to healthcare. Addressing both neurodevelopmental and physical health concerns through early identification, tailored lifestyle interventions, and coordinated care can improve long-term outcomes and overall well-being.

2.5.3 *Functional Impairments Across the Lifespan*

Attention-deficit/hyperactivity disorder (ADHD) affects multiple aspects of daily life from childhood through adulthood (Kosheleff et al., 2023). The functional impairments associated with ADHD impact educational attainment, occupational performance, social relationships, financial stability, and overall well-being (Efron et al., 2020; Kosheleff et al., 2023). While the nature and intensity of these difficulties evolve across different life stages, ADHD consistently presents challenges that require targeted interventions to support individuals in achieving their full potential.

2.5.3.1 Academic and Occupational Challenges

Difficulties in school often emerge as one of the earliest signs of ADHD (Ek et al., 2011). Children with ADHD struggle with attention, organization, and impulse control, which can result in lower academic achievement, increased rates of grade repetition, and a higher likelihood of school dropout (Ek et al., 2011). Challenges with task completion, sustained focus, and adherence to classroom rules contribute to academic underperformance. Early intervention strategies, including behavioral therapies, classroom accommodations, and medication, have been shown to improve learning outcomes and reduce the educational gap between children with and without ADHD.

As individuals transition to adolescence and adulthood, ADHD-related challenges shift toward workplace settings (Samosh et al., 2024). Poor time management, disorganization, and difficulties with sustained attention often affect job performance. Individuals with ADHD are more likely to experience frequent job changes, workplace conflicts, and lower overall job stability (CHADD, 2024). Managing professional responsibilities and meeting deadlines can be particularly difficult, reinforcing the need for structured workplace support, coaching, and tailored interventions to improve career success and financial independence.

2.5.3.2 Social and Interpersonal Difficulties

ADHD can significantly impact social interactions from early childhood onward. Many children with ADHD struggle to form and maintain friendships due to impulsive behaviors, difficulty understanding social cues, and challenges in regulating emotions (Dumas, 1998). Peer rejection, social isolation, and difficulties in cooperative play are common, which may contribute to feelings of low self-esteem and frustration.

These difficulties frequently persist into adulthood, affecting romantic relationships, friendships, and family dynamics (Sodano et al., 2019). Adults with ADHD may experience higher rates of marital dissatisfaction, increased relationship conflicts, and difficulties maintaining stable social connections. Emotional dysregulation, impulsivity, and forgetfulness can contribute to misunderstandings and strain interpersonal relationships. Relationship counseling, social skills training, and mindfulness strategies can help mitigate these challenges and improve social functioning (Wehmeier et al., 2010).

2.5.3.3 Financial and Daily Life Challenges

Managing personal finances and daily responsibilities can be particularly difficult for individuals with ADHD (Bangma et al., 2019). Difficulties with planning, organization, and impulse control contribute to financial instability, with individuals experiencing higher rates of impulsive spending, late bill payments, and difficulties maintaining savings (Bangma et al., 2019). Poor budgeting skills and susceptibility to financial mismanagement can lead to long-term economic struggles.

ADHD is also associated with an increased risk of hazardous behaviors, including risky driving and higher rates of traffic violations (Vaa, 2014). Difficulties with attention regulation, impulsivity, and risk assessment contribute to an increased likelihood of motor vehicle accidents. Structured driving programs, behavioral interventions, and medication management may help reduce these risks and promote safer driving habits.

2.5.3.4 Public Health and Clinical Implications

Given the broad-ranging effects of ADHD across the lifespan, comprehensive, multidisciplinary approaches are necessary to mitigate long-term functional impairments. Key strategies to support individuals with ADHD include early screening and intervention in educational settings to prevent long-term academic challenges, cognitive behavioral therapies and executive function training to enhance self-regulation and daily functioning, and workplace accommodations and coaching programs to support career progression and stability. Social skills training and relationship counseling can improve interpersonal connections, while financial literacy programs can assist with budgeting and long-term financial planning. Public safety measures, including structured driving education for individuals with ADHD, are also important. By recognizing ADHD as a condition that persists beyond childhood, healthcare providers, educators, and policymakers can implement strategies that support affected individuals at every stage of life. Addressing these challenges through tailored interventions can improve long-term outcomes, enhance quality of life, and promote greater independence for individuals with ADHD.

2.6 Treatment Patterns and Access to Care

Attention-deficit/hyperactivity disorder (ADHD) remains underdiagnosed and undertreated across various age groups (Ginsberg et al., 2014b). Limited access to healthcare, socioeconomic disparities, cultural perceptions, and systemic biases contribute to significant challenges in diagnosis and treatment (Slobodin & Masalha, 2020). These barriers influence health-seeking behaviors and impact long-term outcomes for individuals with ADHD. Addressing these disparities requires a comprehensive approach that considers differences in treatment accessibility across childhood, adolescence, and adulthood.

2.6.1 Diagnosis and Treatment Gaps

Despite growing awareness, ADHD remains widely underdiagnosed and undertreated, particularly among adolescents and adults (Ginsberg et al., 2014b). A significant proportion of children diagnosed with ADHD do not receive appropriate interventions, while many adults with ADHD remain undiagnosed or receive inadequate care. Disparities in healthcare access, cultural stigma, and systemic biases contribute to these gaps, particularly for individuals from lower-income backgrounds and minority populations.

Key barriers to diagnosis and treatment include limited access to healthcare professionals specializing in ADHD, cultural stigma and misconceptions about ADHD, systemic biases leading to delayed diagnosis and undertreatment, and a lack of affordable and accessible treatment options. Delayed diagnosis and inadequate treatment contribute to persistent academic, occupational, and social impairments. Strengthening early detection programs and improving access to evidence-based interventions are critical in addressing these gaps.

2.6.2 ADHD Treatment Patterns Across Age Groups

Treatment for ADHD typically involves behavioral therapy, medication, or a combination of both, depending on age, symptom severity, and individual needs (Caye et al., 2019; American Academy of Pediatrics. Subcommittee on Attention-Deficit/Hyperactivity Disorder and Committee on Quality Improvement, 2001). However, treatment adherence and accessibility vary significantly across different populations.

2.6.2.1 Pediatric Treatment Patterns

In childhood, a multimodal approach integrating behavioral therapy and pharmacological treatment is the standard recommendation (American Academy of Pediatrics. Subcommittee on Attention-Deficit/Hyperactivity Disorder and Committee on Quality Improvement, 2001). Early intervention has been shown to improve academic performance, social skills, and long-term outcomes (DuPaul et al., 2011). However, treatment rates decline with age, reflecting barriers to sustained ADHD management (Faraone et al., 2021).

Behavioral therapy is recommended as the first-line treatment for young children. School-aged children and adolescents are more likely to receive medication, often in combination with behavioral interventions. Adherence to treatment decreases during adolescence, despite the continued need for symptom management. Many children with ADHD do not receive comprehensive care, further widening academic and social disparities (Faraone et al., 2021). Strengthening support systems within schools and communities is essential to improving long-term outcomes.

2.6.2.2 Adult ADHD Treatment and Discontinuation

Among adults, treatment adherence remains inconsistent, with many discontinuing medication due to side effects, perceived ineffectiveness, or lack of healthcare access (Brikell et al., 2024). Barriers to sustained ADHD treatment in adulthood include limited availability of ADHD specialists for adults, high costs associated with long-term medication use, and concerns regarding stimulant medication misuse and side effects (Brikell et al., 2024).

Adults who continue ADHD treatment report better occupational stability and lower risk of developing comorbid psychiatric conditions (Adamou et al., 2013). Expanding access to specialized care and integrating ADHD management into general healthcare services can improve long-term outcomes for adults with ADHD.

2.6.2.3 Enhancing Lifespan Treatment Strategies

Effective ADHD management requires age-sensitive and sustained interventions that reflect the evolving nature of the disorder across the lifespan. In childhood, a combination of stimulant medication and behavioral interventions—such as behavioral parent training and school-based reinforcement systems—has demonstrated strong efficacy. A meta-analysis by Daley et al. (2014) showed that behavioral interventions significantly improve core ADHD symptoms and academic outcomes when used alongside pharmacotherapy (Daley et al., 2014).

During adolescence, treatment must address emotional regulation difficulties, academic pressures, and evolving peer dynamics. Although fewer clinical trials have targeted this age group, emerging research supports the use of cognitive behavioral therapy (CBT), particularly programs targeting executive function and emotion regulation (Haugan et al., 2022). School accommodations and family involvement remain critical to sustaining engagement and treatment response.

For adults, treatment should be individualized and may include pharmacological support, ADHD coaching, psychoeducation, and workplace accommodations. According to a Cochrane review (Castells et al., 2018), stimulant medications remain effective in reducing core symptoms, but functional improvement often requires non-pharmacologic strategies. Yet many adults face long wait times, diagnostic delays, or stigma-related barriers that hinder access to these services (Asherson et al., 2016; Smith et al., 2024).

Integrated, multidisciplinary treatment models that bring together psychologists, psychiatrists, educators, occupational therapists, and family support workers have shown promise in improving continuity of care and reducing dropout across transitions (Talbott et al., 2021). However, implementation outside of high-resource urban settings remains limited, and further research is needed to establish scalable care pathways for ADHD treatment across the lifespan.

2.6.3 Barriers to ADHD Diagnosis and Treatment

Access to ADHD diagnosis and treatment is highly variable, influenced by regional healthcare disparities and systemic inequities (Zhao et al., 2023). Geographic disparities limit access to ADHD specialists and mental health services in rural and underserved areas. Systemic biases also play a role, with individuals from minority populations often facing delayed diagnosis and reduced likelihood of receiving medication-based treatment. Cultural and socioeconomic factors further complicate access, as stigma surrounding ADHD in certain communities discourages individuals from seeking professional help, leading to underutilization of mental health services. Addressing these disparities requires targeted efforts to ensure equitable screening, diagnosis, and treatment access across all populations.

2.6.4 Public Health and Policy Recommendations

Closing ADHD treatment gaps and addressing healthcare disparities requires a multipronged approach that includes expanding early screening programs to improve ADHD detection rates across all age groups, increasing awareness and reducing stigma through culturally tailored public health campaigns, improving access to ADHD specialists and mental health services, particularly in underserved regions, and enhancing training for primary care providers to facilitate early recognition and diagnosis of ADHD. Additionally, developing policies to ensure equitable treatment access—including insurance coverage for behavioral therapy and medication—is essential. By addressing these barriers, healthcare systems can ensure that individuals with ADHD receive timely, effective, and sustained treatment, thereby improving long-term functional and health outcomes (Brown, 2022; Smith et al., 2024).

Summary

This chapter has provided a comprehensive overview of ADHD across the lifespan, focusing on prevalence, symptom transitions, comorbidities, functional impairments, and access to care. ADHD is a highly prevalent neurodevelopmental disorder that affects individuals from childhood through adulthood. Although symptoms often evolve over time, a substantial proportion of individuals continue to experience challenges, particularly in executive function, emotional regulation, and attention.

ADHD frequently co-occurs with psychiatric and physical health conditions, such as anxiety, depression, substance use disorders, and metabolic issues, which exacerbate difficulties in academic performance, occupational success, interpersonal relationships, and daily functioning. These challenges highlight the importance of comprehensive, lifespan-oriented interventions. However, ADHD remains underdiagnosed and undertreated, especially among adults and marginalized populations, due to limited healthcare access, cultural stigma, and systemic biases.

Management of ADHD typically involves behavioral therapy, medication, and environmental modifications, yet access to effective interventions varies widely across regions and socioeconomic groups. Addressing these gaps requires expanding screening programs, improving diagnostic frameworks, and reducing healthcare disparities to ensure equitable access to ADHD treatment. A public health approach that promotes early intervention, awareness, and sustained support is essential for improving long-term outcomes for individuals with ADHD and their communities.

References

Adamou, M., Arif, M., Asherson, P., Aw, T.-C., Bolea, B., Coghill, D., Guðjónsson, G., Halmøy, A., Hodgkins, P., & Müller, U. (2013). Occupational issues of adults with ADHD. *BMC Psychiatry, 13*, 1–7.

Alem, A., Kebede, D., Fekadu, A., Shibre, T., Fekadu, D., Beyero, T., Medhin, G., Negash, A., & Kullgren, G. (2009). Clinical course and outcome of schizophrenia in a predominantly treatment-naive cohort in rural Ethiopia. *Schizophrenia Bulletin, 35*(3), 646–654.

American Academy of Pediatrics. Subcommittee on Attention-Deficit/Hyperactivity Disorder and Committee on Quality Improvement. (2001). Clinical practice guideline: Treatment of the school-aged child with attention-deficit/hyperactivity disorder. *Pediatrics, 108*(4), 1033–1044.

APA. (2013). Diagnostic and statistical manual of mental disorders. *The American Psychiatric Association, 21*(21), 591–643.

Asherson, P., Buitelaar, J., Faraone, S. V., & Rohde, L. A. (2016). Adult attention-deficit hyperactivity disorder: Key conceptual issues. *The Lancet Psychiatry, 3*(6), 568–578.

Ayano, G., Yohannes, K., & Abraha, M. (2020). Epidemiology of attention-deficit/hyperactivity disorder (ADHD) in children and adolescents in Africa: A systematic review and meta-analysis. *Annals of General Psychiatry, 19*, 21. https://doi.org/10.1186/s12991-020-00271-w

Ayano, G., Demelash, S., Gizachew, Y., Tsegay, L., & Alati, R. (2023a). The global prevalence of attention deficit hyperactivity disorder in children and adolescents: An umbrella review of meta-analyses. *Journal of Affective Disorders, 339*, 860–866. https://doi.org/10.1016/j.jad.2023.07.071

Ayano, G., Tsegay, L., Gizachew, Y., Necho, M., Yohannes, K., Abraha, M., Demelash, S., Anbesaw, T., & Alati, R. (2023b). Prevalence of attention deficit hyperactivity disorder in adults: Umbrella review of evidence generated across the globe. *Psychiatry Research, 328*, 115449. https://doi.org/10.1016/j.psychres.2023.115449

Ayano, G., Zena, D., Gizachew, Y., & Tsegay, L. (2025). Neurobiomarkers of psychiatric disorders in children and adolescents and their significance for diagnosis and precision medicine: A narrative review. *NeuroMarkers, 2*(2), 100040. https://doi.org/10.1016/j.neumar.2025.100040

Bagwell, C. L., Molina, B. S., Kashdan, T. B., Pelham, W. E., Jr., & Hoza, B. (2006). Anxiety and mood disorders in adolescents with childhood attention-deficit/hyperactivity disorder. *Journal of Emotional and Behavioral Disorders, 14*(3), 178–187.

Bangma, D. F., Koerts, J., Fuermaier, A., Mette, C., Zimmermann, M., Toussaint, A. K., Tucha, L., & Tucha, O. (2019). Financial decision-making in adults with ADHD. *Neuropsychology, 33*(8), 1065.

Becker, S. P., Luebbe, A. M., & Langberg, J. M. (2012). Co-occurring mental health problems and peer functioning among youth with attention-deficit/hyperactivity disorder: A review and recommendations for future research. *Clinical Child and Family Psychology Review, 15*, 279–302.

Biederman, J., Mick, E., & Faraone, S. V. (2000). Age-dependent decline of symptoms of attention deficit hyperactivity disorder: Impact of remission definition and symptom type. *American Journal of Psychiatry, 157*(5), 816–818.

Brikell, I., Yao, H., Li, L., Astrup, A., Gao, L., Gillies, M. B., Xie, T., Zhang-James, Y., Dalsgaard, S., & Engeland, A. (2024). ADHD medication discontinuation and persistence across the lifespan: A retrospective observational study using population-based databases. *The Lancet Psychiatry, 11*(1), 16–26.

Brown, Q. (2022). *An investigation that explores the disparities and effects of undiagnosed and undertreatment of ADHD between black and white children*. Alliant International University.

Castells, X., Blanco-Silvente, L., & Cunill, R. (2018). Amphetamines for attention deficit hyperactivity disorder (ADHD) in adults. *Cochrane Database of Systematic Reviews, 8*(8), CD007813. https://doi.org/10.1002/14651858.CD007813.pub3

Caye, A., Swanson, J. M., Coghill, D., & Rohde, L. A. (2019). Treatment strategies for ADHD: An evidence-based guide to select optimal treatment. *Molecular Psychiatry, 24*(3), 390–408.

Cénat, J. M., Blais-Rochette, C., Morse, C., Vandette, M.-P., Noorishad, P.-G., Kogan, C., Ndengeyingoma, A., & Labelle, P. R. (2021). Prevalence and risk factors associated with attention-deficit/hyperactivity disorder among US Black individuals: A systematic review and meta-analysis. *JAMA Psychiatry, 78*(1), 21–28.

CHADD. (2024, October). ADHD Awareness 2024: Awareness is key! *Attention Magazine*. Retrieved from https://chadd.org/attention-article/adhd-awareness-2024-awareness-is-key/

Classi, P., Milton, D., Ward, S., Sarsour, K., & Johnston, J. (2012). Social and emotional difficulties in children with ADHD and the impact on school attendance and healthcare utilization. *Child and Adolescent Psychiatry and Mental Health, 6*, 1–8.

Coker, T. R., Elliott, M. N., Toomey, S. L., Schwebel, D. C., Cuccaro, P., Tortolero Emery, S., Davies, S. L., Visser, S. N., & Schuster, M. A. (2016). Racial and ethnic disparities in ADHD diagnosis and treatment. *Pediatrics, 138*(3), e20160407. https://doi.org/10.1542/peds.2016-0407

Cortese, S., Moreira-Maia, C. R., St Fleur, D., Morcillo-Peñalver, C., Rohde, L. A., & Faraone, S. V. (2016). Association between ADHD and obesity: A systematic review and meta-analysis. *The American Journal of Psychiatry, 173*(1), 34–43. https://doi.org/10.1176/appi.ajp.2015.15020266

Coşkun, M., Güven, G., Alnak, A., & Karayağmurlu, A. (2020). Psychiatric comorbidity and sleep problems in children and adolescents with attention deficit hyperactivity disorder in relation to attention deficit hyperactivity disorder presentation, age and gender. *Journal of Istanbul Faculty of Medicine, 83*(4), 363–372.

Daley, D., van der Oord, S., Ferrin, M., Danckaerts, M., Doepfner, M., Cortese, S., & Sonuga-Barke, E. J. S. (2014). Behavioral interventions in attention-deficit/hyperactivity disorder: A meta-analysis of randomized controlled trials across multiple outcome domains. *Journal of the American Academy of Child & Adolescent Psychiatry, 53*(8), 835–847.e835. https://doi.org/10.1016/j.jaac.2014.05.013

Danielson, M. L., Bitsko, R. H., Ghandour, R. M., Holbrook, J. R., Kogan, M. D., & Blumberg, S. J. (2018). Prevalence of parent-reported ADHD diagnosis and associated treatment among U.S. children and adolescents, 2016. *Journal of Clinical Child & Adolescent Psychology, 47*(2), 199–212. https://doi.org/10.1080/15374416.2017.1417860

Di Lorenzo, R., Balducci, J., Poppi, C., Arcolin, E., Cutino, A., Ferri, P., D'Amico, R., & Filippini, T. (2021). Children and adolescents with ADHD followed up to adulthood: A systematic review of long-term outcomes. *Acta Neuropsychiatrica, 33*(6), 283–298. https://doi.org/10.1017/neu.2021.23

Dumas, M. C. (1998). The risk of social interaction problems among adolescents with ADHD. *Education and Treatment of Children, 21*, 447–460.

DuPaul, G. J., Kern, L., Gormley, M. J., & Volpe, R. J. (2011). Early intervention for young children with ADHD: Academic outcomes for responders to behavioral treatment. *School Mental Health, 3*, 117–126.

Efron, D., Nicholson, J. M., Anderson, V., Silk, T., Ukoumunne, O. C., Gulenc, A., Hazell, P., Jongeling, B., & Sciberras, E. (2020). ADHD at age 7 and functional impairments at age 10. *Pediatrics, 146*(5), e20201061.

Ek, U., Westerlund, J., Holmberg, K., & Fernell, E. (2011). Academic performance of adolescents with ADHD and other behavioural and learning problems—A population-based longitudinal study. *Acta Paediatrica, 100*(3), 402–406. https://doi.org/10.1111/j.1651-2227.2010.02048.x

Eke, H., Ford, T., Newlove-Delgado, T., Price, A., Young, S., Ani, C., Sayal, K., Lynn, R. M., Paul, M., & Janssens, A. (2020). Transition between child and adult services for young people with attention-deficit hyperactivity disorder (ADHD): Findings from a British national surveillance study. *The British Journal of Psychiatry, 217*(5), 616–622. https://doi.org/10.1192/bjp.2019.131

Faraone, S. V., Banaschewski, T., Coghill, D., Zheng, Y., Biederman, J., Bellgrove, M. A., Newcorn, J. H., Gignac, M., Al Saud, N. M., Manor, I., Rohde, L. A., Yang, L., Cortese, S., Almagor, D., Stein, M. A., Albatti, T. H., Aljoudi, H. F., Alqahtani, M. M. J., Asherson, P., … Wang, Y. (2021). The world federation of ADHD international consensus statement: 208 evidence-based conclusions about the disorder. *Neuroscience & Biobehavioral Reviews, 128*, 789–818. https://doi.org/10.1016/j.neubiorev.2021.01.022

Fayyad, J., De Graaf, R., Kessler, R., Alonso, J., Angermeyer, M., Demyttenaere, K., De Girolamo, G., Haro, J. M., Karam, E. G., Lara, C., Lépine, J. P., Ormel, J., Posada-Villa, J., Zaslavsky, A. M., & Jin, R. (2007). Cross-national prevalence and correlates of adult attention-deficit hyperactivity disorder. *The British Journal of Psychiatry, 190*, 402–409. https://doi.org/10.1192/bjp.bp.106.034389

Fayyad, J., Sampson, N. A., Hwang, I., Adamowski, T., Aguilar-Gaxiola, S., Al-Hamzawi, A., Andrade, L. H. S. G., Borges, G., de Girolamo, G., Florescu, S., Gureje, O., Haro, J. M., Hu, C., Karam, E. G., Lee, S., Navarro-Mateu, F., O'Neill, S., Pennell, B.-E., Piazza, M., … WHO World Mental Health Survey Collaborators. (2017). The descriptive epidemiology of DSM-IV adult ADHD in the World Health Organization World Mental Health Surveys. *ADHD Attention Deficit and Hyperactivity Disorders, 9*(1), 47–65. https://doi.org/10.1007/s12402-016-0208-3

Ford-Jones, P. C. (2015). Misdiagnosis of attention deficit hyperactivity disorder: 'Normal behaviour' and relative maturity. *Paediatrics & Child Health, 20*(4), 200–202. https://doi.org/10.1093/pch/20.4.200

Fortune, N., Madden, R., Riley, T., & Short, S. (2021). The International Classification of Health Interventions: An 'epistemic hub'for use in public health. *Health Promotion International, 36*(6), 1753–1764.

Friedman, N. P., & Robbins, T. W. (2022). The role of prefrontal cortex in cognitive control and executive function. *Neuropsychopharmacology, 47*(1), 72–89.

GBD 2019 Mental Disorders Collaborators. (2022). Global regional, and national burden of 12 mental disorders in 204 countries and territories, 1990–2019: A systematic analysis for the Global Burden of Disease Study 2019. *The Lancet Psychiatry, 9*(2), 137–150.

Ginsberg, Y., Quintero, J., Anand, E., Casillas, M., & Upadhyaya, H. P. (2014a). Underdiagnosis of attention-deficit/hyperactivity disorder in adult patients: A review of the literature. *The Primary Care Companion for CNS Disorders, 16*(3), 23591.

Ginsberg, Y., Quintero, J., Anand, E., Casillas, M., & Upadhyaya, H. P. (2014b). Underdiagnosis of attention-deficit/hyperactivity disorder in adult patients: A review of the literature. *The Primary Care Companion for CNS Disorders, 16*(3), 1–8.

Hak, E., de Vries, T. W., Hoekstra, P. J., & Jick, S. S. (2013). Association of childhood attention-deficit/hyperactivity disorder with atopic diseases and skin infections? A matched case-control study using the General Practice Research Database. *Annals of Allergy, Asthma & Immunology, 111*(2), 102–106.e2.

Harpin, V., Mazzone, L., Raynaud, J. P., Kahle, J., & Hodgkins, P. (2013). Long-term outcomes of ADHD: A systematic review of self-esteem and social function. *Journal of Attention Disorders, 20*(4), 295–305. https://doi.org/10.1177/1087054713486516

Haugan, A.-L. J., Sund, A. M., Young, S., Thomsen, P. H., Lydersen, S., & Nøvik, T. S. (2022). Cognitive behavioural group therapy as addition to psychoeducation and pharmacological treatment for adolescents with ADHD symptoms and related impairments: A randomised controlled trial. *BMC Psychiatry, 22*(1), 375. https://doi.org/10.1186/s12888-022-04019-6

Heublein, N. (2023). *Designing a personal knowledge management system for people with ADHD*. Malmö universitet.

Hinshaw, S. P., Arnold, L. E., & For the MTA Cooperative Group. (2015). Attention-deficit hyperactivity disorder, multimodal treatment, and longitudinal outcome: Evidence, paradox, and challenge. *Wiley Interdisciplinary Reviews: Cognitive Science, 6*(1), 39–52.

Hinshaw, S. P., Nguyen, P. T., O'Grady, S. M., & Rosenthal, E. A. (2022). Annual research review: Attention-deficit/hyperactivity disorder in girls and women: Underrepresentation, longitudinal processes, and key directions. *Journal of Child Psychology and Psychiatry, 63*(4), 484–496. https://doi.org/10.1111/jcpp.13480

Huang, H., Huang, H., Spottswood, M., & Ghaemi, N. (2020). Approach to evaluating and managing adult attention-deficit/hyperactivity disorder in primary care. *Harvard Review of Psychiatry, 28*(2), 100–106.

Instanes, J. T., Klungsøyr, K., Halmøy, A., Fasmer, O. B., & Haavik, J. (2018). Adult ADHD and comorbid somatic disease: A systematic literature review. *Journal of Attention Disorders, 22*(3), 203–228.

Jameson, N. D., Sheppard, B. K., Lateef, T. M., Vande Voort, J. L., He, J.-P., & Merikangas, K. R. (2016). Medical comorbidity of attention-deficit/hyperactivity disorder in US adolescents. *Journal of Child Neurology, 31*(11), 1282–1289. https://doi.org/10.1177/0883073816653782

Johnson, J., Morris, S., & George, S. (2021). Misdiagnosis and missed diagnosis of adult attention-deficit hyperactivity disorder. *BJPsych Advances, 27*(1), 60–61. https://doi.org/10.1192/bja.2020.34

Kedem, S., Yust-Katz, S., Carter, D., Levi, Z., Kedem, R., Dickstein, A., Daher, S., & Katz, L. H. (2020). Attention deficit hyperactivity disorder and gastrointestinal morbidity in a large cohort of young adults. *World Journal of Gastroenterology, 26*(42), 6626.

Kessler, R. C., Adler, L., Barkley, R., Biederman, J., Conners, C. K., Demler, O., Faraone, S. V., Greenhill, L. L., Howes, M. J., & Secnik, K. (2006). The prevalence and correlates of adult ADHD in the United States: Results from the National Comorbidity Survey Replication. *American Journal of Psychiatry, 163*(4), 716–723.

Kooij, J. J. S., Bijlenga, D., Salerno, L., Jaeschke, R., Bitter, I., Balázs, J., Thome, J., Dom, G., Kasper, S., Nunes Filipe, C., Stes, S., Mohr, P., Leppämäki, S., Casas, M., Bobes, J., McCarthy, J. M., Richarte, V., Kjems Philipsen, A., Pehlivanidis, A., … Asherson, P. (2019). Updated European Consensus Statement on diagnosis and treatment of adult ADHD. *European Psychiatry, 56*(1), 14–34. https://doi.org/10.1016/j.eurpsy.2018.11.001

Kosheleff, A. R., Mason, O., Jain, R., Koch, J., & Rubin, J. (2023). Functional impairments associated with ADHD in adulthood and the impact of pharmacological treatment. *Journal of Attention Disorders, 27*(7), 669–697. https://doi.org/10.1177/10870547231158572

Koyuncu, A., Ayan, T., Ince Guliyev, E., Erbilgin, S., & Deveci, E. (2022). ADHD and anxiety disorder comorbidity in children and adults: Diagnostic and therapeutic challenges. *Current Psychiatry Reports, 24*(2), 129–140. https://doi.org/10.1007/s11920-022-01324-5

LeRoy, A., Jacova, C., & Young, C. (2018). Neuropsychological performance patterns of adult ADHD subtypes. *Journal of Attention Disorders, 23*(10), 1136–1147. https://doi.org/10.1177/1087054718773927

Libutzki, B., Neukirch, B., Kittel-Schneider, S., Reif, A., & Hartman, C. A. (2023). Risk of accidents and unintentional injuries in men and women with attention deficit hyperactivity disorder across the adult lifespan. *Acta Psychiatrica Scandinavica, 147*(2), 145–154.

Liu, J., Jiang, Z., Li, F., Zheng, Y., Cui, Y., Xu, H., & Li, Y. (2025). Prevalence and comorbidity of attention deficit hyperactivity disorder in Chinese school-attending students aged 6–16: A national survey. *Annals of General Psychiatry, 24*(1), 23. https://doi.org/10.1186/s12991-025-00558-w

Mahone, E. M., & Wodka, E. L. (2008). The neurobiological profile of girls with ADHD. *Developmental Disabilities Research Reviews, 14*(4), 276–284.

Martel, M. M., Klump, K., Nigg, J. T., Breedlove, S. M., & Sisk, C. L. (2009). Potential hormonal mechanisms of attention-deficit/hyperactivity disorder and major depressive disorder: A new perspective. *Hormones and Behavior, 55*(4), 465–479.

Matheiken, S., Erden, M., Krishnadas, R., & Pinto da Costa, M. (2024). Adult attention-deficit hyperactivity disorder: Time for a rethink? *BJPsych Advances, 30*(5), 298–302. https://doi.org/10.1192/bja.2023.54

Mellman, T. A., Miller, A. L., Weissman, E. M., Crismon, M. L., Essock, S. M., & Marder, S. R. (2001). Evidence-based pharmacologic treatment for people with severe mental illness: A focus on guidelines and algorithms. *Psychiatric Services, 52*(5), 619–625. https://doi.org/10.1176/appi.ps.52.5.619

Mongia, M., & Hechtman, L. (2012). Cognitive behavior therapy for adults with attention-deficit/hyperactivity disorder: A review of recent randomized controlled trials. *Current Psychiatry Reports, 14*, 561–567.

Montano, C. B., & Weisler, R. (2011). Distinguishing symptoms of ADHD from other psychiatric disorders in the adult primary care setting. *Postgraduate Medicine, 123*(3), 88–98.

Patel, V., Kieling, C., Maulik, P. K., & Divan, G. (2013). Improving access to care for children with mental disorders: A global perspective. *Archives of Disease in Childhood, 98*(5), 323–327. https://doi.org/10.1136/archdischild-2012-302079

Pollard, C. M., Binns, C. W., & Lewis, J. M. (2008). Selecting interventions to promote fruit and vegetable consumption: From policy to action, a planning framework casestudy in Western Australia. *Australia and New Zealand Health Policy, 5*(1), 27.

Rucklidge, J. J. (2010). Gender differences in attention-deficit/hyperactivity disorder. *Psychiatric Clinics, 33*(2), 357–373.

Rutter, M. (1989). Pathways from childhood to adult life. *Journal of Child Psychology and Psychiatry, 30*(1), 23–51.

Salem, H., Vivas, D., Cao, F., Kazimi, I. F., Teixeira, A. L., & Zeni, C. P. (2018). ADHD is associated with migraine: A systematic review and meta-analysis. *European Child & Adolescent Psychiatry, 27*(3), 267–277. https://doi.org/10.1007/s00787-017-1045-4

Salpekar, J. (2018). Links between epilepsy and ADHD: Time to focus and act. *Epilepsy Currents, 18*(3), 160–161. https://doi.org/10.5698/1535-7597.18.3.160

Samosh, D., Lilius, J., & Atwood, K. (2024). ADHD and career success: Barriers, facilitators, and future research directions. In E. Patton & A. M. Santuzzi (Eds.), *Neurodiversity and work: Employment, identity, and support networks for neurominorities* (pp. 257–281). Springer Nature Switzerland. https://doi.org/10.1007/978-3-031-55072-0_12

Sansosti, F. J., Cimera, R. E., Koch, L. C., & Rumrill, P. (2017). Strategies for ensuring positive transition for individuals with attention-deficit/hyperactivity disorder. *Journal of Vocational Rehabilitation, 47*(2), 149–157. https://doi.org/10.3233/JVR-170891

Shaw, M., Hodgkins, P., Caci, H., Young, S., Kahle, J., Woods, A. G., & Arnold, L. E. (2012). A systematic review and analysis of long-term outcomes in attention deficit hyperactivity disorder: Effects of treatment and non-treatment. *BMC Medicine, 10*(1), 99. https://doi.org/10.1186/1741-7015-10-99

Shaw, P., Eckstrand, K., Sharp, W., Blumenthal, J., Lerch, J. P., Greenstein, D., Clasen, L., Evans, A., Giedd, J., & Rapoport, J. L. (2007, December 4). Attention-deficit/hyperactivity disorder is characterized by a delay in cortical maturation. *Proceedings of the National Academy of Sciences, 104(49)*, 19649–19654. https://doi.org/10.1073/pnas.0707741104. Epub 2007 Nov 16. PMID: 18024590; PMCID: PMC2148343

Shi, Y., Hunter Guevara, L. R., Dykhoff, H. J., Sangaralingham, L. R., Phelan, S., Zaccariello, M. J., & Warner, D. O. (2021). Racial disparities in diagnosis of attention-deficit/hyperactivity disorder in a US National Birth Cohort. *JAMA Network Open, 4*(3), e210321. https://doi.org/10.1001/jamanetworkopen.2021.0321

Skogli, E. W., Teicher, M. H., Andersen, P. N., Hovik, K. T., & Øie, M. (2013). ADHD in girls and boys—Gender differences in co-existing symptoms and executive function measures. *BMC Psychiatry, 13*, 298. https://doi.org/10.1186/1471-244x-13-298

Slobodin, O., & Masalha, R. (2020). Challenges in ADHD care for ethnic minority children: A review of the current literature. *Transcultural Psychiatry, 57*(3), 468–483.

Smith, M. C., Mukherjee, R. A., Müller-Sedgwick, U., Hank, D., Carpenter, P., & Adamou, M. (2024). UK adult ADHD services in crisis. *BJPsych Bulletin, 48*(1), 1–5.

Sodano, S. M., Tamulonis, J. P., Fabiano, G. A., Caserta, A. M., Hulme, K. F., Hulme, K. L., Stephan, G. R., & Tronci, F. (2019). Interpersonal problems of young adults with and without attention-deficit/hyperactivity disorder. *Journal of Attention Disorders, 25*(4), 562–571. https://doi.org/10.1177/1087054718821728

Steel, Z., Marnane, C., Iranpour, C., Chey, T., Jackson, J. W., Patel, V., & Silove, D. (2014). The global prevalence of common mental disorders: A systematic review and meta-analysis 1980–2013. *International Journal of Epidemiology, 43*(2), 476–493.

Talbott, E., De Los Reyes, A., Power, T. J., Michel, J. J., & Racz, S. J. (2021). A team-based collaborative care model for youth with attention-deficit hyperactivity disorder in education and health care settings. *Journal of Emotional and Behavioral Disorders, 29*(1), 24–33.

Twiss, J. R. (2024). *Mindfulness-based cognitive therapy (MBCT) for adults with ADHD: A psychoeducational intervention*. The University of Arizona.

Vaa, T. (2014). ADHD and relative risk of accidents in road traffic: A meta-analysis. *Accident Analysis & Prevention, 62*, 415–425. https://doi.org/10.1016/j.aap.2013.10.003

Volkow, N. D., & Swanson, J. M. (2013). Adult attention deficit–hyperactivity disorder. *New England Journal of Medicine, 369*(20), 1935–1944.

Wehmeier, P. M., Schacht, A., & Barkley, R. A. (2010). Social and emotional impairment in children and adolescents with ADHD and the impact on quality of life. *Journal of Adolescent Health, 46*(3), 209–217. https://doi.org/10.1016/j.jadohealth.2009.09.009

Willcutt, E. G. (2012). The prevalence of DSM-IV attention-deficit/hyperactivity disorder: A meta-analytic review. *Neurotherapeutics, 9*(3), 490–499. https://doi.org/10.1007/s13311-012-0135-8

Young, J. L., & Goodman, D. W. (2016). Adult attention-deficit/hyperactivity disorder diagnosis, management, and treatment in the DSM-5 era. *The Primary Care Companion for CNS Disorders, 18*(6). https://doi.org/10.4088/PCC.16r02000

Young, S., Abbasian, C., Al-Attar, Z., Branney, P., Colley, B., Cortese, S., Cubbin, S., Deeley, Q., Gudjonsson, G. H., Hill, P., Hollingdale, J., Jenden, S., Johnson, J., Judge, D., Lewis,

A., Mason, P., Mukherjee, R., Nutt, D., Roberts, J., … Cocallis, K. (2023). Identification and treatment of individuals with attention-deficit/hyperactivity disorder and substance use disorder: An expert consensus statement. *World Journal of Psychiatry, 13*(3), 84–112. https://doi.org/10.5498/wjp.v13.i3.84

Zhang, L., Li, L., Andell, P., Garcia-Argibay, M., Quinn, P. D., D'Onofrio, B. M., Brikell, I., Kuja-Halkola, R., Lichtenstein, P., Johnell, K., Larsson, H., & Chang, Z. (2024). Attention-deficit/hyperactivity disorder medications and long-term risk of cardiovascular diseases. *JAMA Psychiatry, 81*(2), 178–187. https://doi.org/10.1001/jamapsychiatry.2023.4294

Zhang, Y., Liao, W., Rao, Y., Gao, W., & Yang, R. (2025). Effects of ADHD and ADHD medications on depression and anxiety in children and adolescents: A systematic review and meta-analysis. *Journal of Psychiatric Research, 181*, 623–639. https://doi.org/10.1016/j.jpsychires.2024.12.022

Zhao, X., Hayes, T., Timmons, A. C., Wu, W., & Frazier, S. L. (2023). Unpacking inequities in ADHD diagnosis: Examining individual-level race/ethnicity and state-level online information-seeking patterns. *Administration and Policy in Mental Health and Mental Health Services Research, 50*(4), 576–590. https://doi.org/10.1007/s10488-023-01259-w

Chapter 3
ADHD and Mental Health Comorbidities

Abstract This chapter introduces the intersections between attention-deficit/hyperactivity disorder (ADHD) and mental health comorbidities. It addresses the implications for holistic healthcare needs related to co-occurring psychiatric disorders and the challenges of concurrent mental health conditions. It tells the challenges of individuals who experience ADHD alongside anxiety, depression, and other mental health concerns, illustrating the impact on daily functioning and overall well-being.

The chapter also describes integrated care models applied to ADHD and comorbid conditions, such as multidisciplinary interventions and tailored treatment strategies. Both common and less common comorbidities affect the emotional, cognitive, and social dimensions of individuals with ADHD. Reflective exercises guide you to consider how you will be able to promote mental health and well-being, and minimize the challenges associated with ADHD and its comorbid conditions, to individuals and communities in practice contexts.

3.1 Prevalence and Clinical Overlap of Mental Health Comorbidities in ADHD

The term *comorbidity* refers to the co-occurrence of two or more disorders within the same individual, either simultaneously or within a specific timeframe (Nordgaard et al., 2023). In the context of ADHD, psychiatric comorbidities are common and often complicate diagnosis, treatment, and long-term outcomes (Cuffe et al., 2020). Many individuals with ADHD experience overlapping symptoms with other mental health conditions, increasing the burden of functional impairments across their lifespan (Montano & Weisler, 2011).

Psychiatric comorbidities in ADHD are highly prevalent, with estimates suggesting that over two-thirds of individuals with ADHD meet the diagnostic criteria for at least one additional mental health condition (Choi et al., 2022) (Fig. 3.1). The presence of these comorbid disorders significantly influences symptom expression, treatment response, and overall well-being.

G. Ayano et al., *ADHD Across the Lifespan*, SpringerBriefs in Modern Perspectives on Disability Research,
https://doi.org/10.1007/978-981-95-8712-4_3

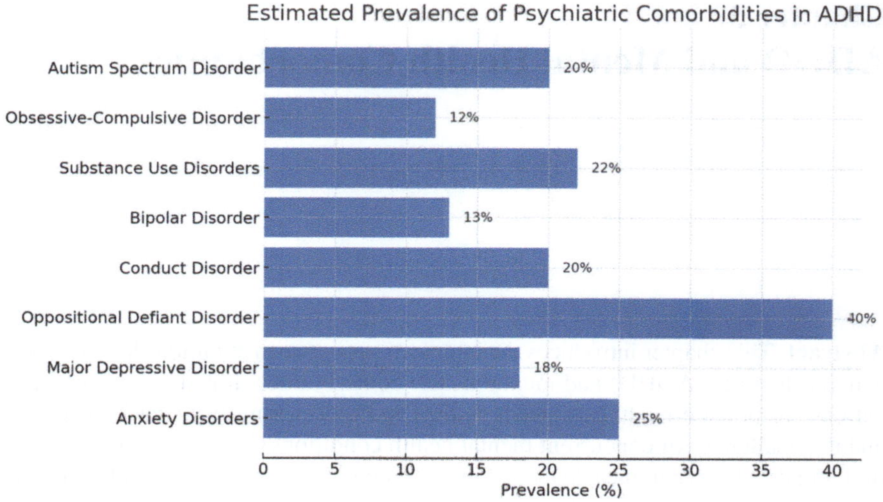

Fig. 3.1 Estimated prevalence of psychiatric comorbidity with ADHD

Anxiety disorders co-occurring with ADHD affect approximately one in four children and adolescents (Choi et al., 2022), while depression is reported in up to one-third of individuals with ADHD (Riglin et al., 2021). Oppositional defiant disorder (ODD) and conduct disorder (CD) are also common, with ODD affecting around 40% of cases and CD present in approximately 20% (Choi et al., 2022). Bipolar disorder shares clinical overlap with ADHD, particularly in mood instability and impulsivity, and is estimated to co-occur in around 10–20% of individuals with ADHD (Asherson et al., 2014). ADHD is also strongly linked to an increased risk of substance misuse, particularly in adolescence and adulthood (Levy et al., 2014). Although less common, obsessive-compulsive disorder (OCD) symptoms can coexist with ADHD, often leading to misinterpretation of compulsive behaviors as impulsivity (Cabarkapa et al., 2019). Furthermore, ADHD and autism spectrum disorder (ASD) frequently co-occur, with approximately 20–40% of children with ASD also meeting the criteria for ADHD (J. C. Visser et al., 2016). The high prevalence of comorbid mental health conditions in individuals with ADHD underscores the need for integrated care approaches that address multiple psychiatric conditions simultaneously. Recognizing these overlapping disorders can improve diagnostic accuracy and treatment outcomes, ensuring that interventions are tailored to the diverse challenges faced by individuals with ADHD across the lifespan. Figure 3.1 shows the estimated prevalence of comorbidities with ADHD.

3.2 Impact of Comorbidities on ADHD Symptomatology

The presence of psychiatric comorbidities in individuals with ADHD can significantly amplify symptom severity, complicates diagnosis, and contributes to greater functional impairments across the lifespan (Abramovitch et al., 2015; Mansour et al., 2017). The interaction between ADHD-related deficits—such as inattention, impulsivity, and executive dysfunction—and co-occurring conditions can exacerbate cognitive, behavioral, and emotional challenges (Taurines et al., 2010). These interplays often lead to heightened academic, occupational, and social difficulties, reinforcing the importance of comprehensive assessment and tailored interventions.

3.2.1 Anxiety Disorders: Amplification of Cognitive and Emotional Dysregulation

Anxiety disorders are among the most frequently co-occurring conditions in individuals with ADHD, profoundly affecting emotional regulation, attentional control, and executive functioning (Kessler et al., 2006). While ADHD is characterized by distractibility and impulsivity, comorbid anxiety introduces excessive worry, cognitive rigidity, and heightened physiological arousal (Bloemsma et al., 2013). These overlapping symptoms can lead to task avoidance, academic underperformance, and social withdrawal (D'Agati et al., 2019). The presence of anxiety can also obscure the recognition of ADHD symptoms, delaying diagnosis and treatment initiation (Faraone et al., 2021). Individuals with both ADHD and anxiety are more likely to experience heightened stress sensitivity and increased healthcare utilization, often requiring a multimodal treatment approach that integrates cognitive behavioral therapy (CBT) and pharmacological interventions (Appolinario et al., 2024).

3.2.2 Mood Disorders: Disruptions in Motivation and Emotional Stability

The co-occurrence of mood disorders, including major depressive disorder (MDD) and bipolar disorder, can substantially worsen ADHD-related impairment (Asherson et al., 2014; Riglin et al., 2021). Depression exacerbates deficits in motivation, working memory and cognitive flexibility, leading to chronic procrastination, low academic achievement, and difficulty maintaining employment (Riglin et al., 2021). The bidirectional relationship between ADHD and depression suggests that untreated ADHD increases vulnerability to recurrent depressive episodes, further impairing social and occupational functioning.

Bipolar disorder presents additional diagnostic and treatment challenges (Brus et al., 2014). Manic episodes can heighten impulsivity, disorganization, and distractibility, whereas depressive episodes further impair executive function and exacerbate emotional dysregulation (Brus et al., 2014). The cyclical nature of mood instability in bipolar disorder complicates ADHD treatment strategies, particularly regarding stimulant use, which may exacerbate mood dysregulation. Individuals with comorbid ADHD and mood disorders face an increased risk of psychiatric hospitalization, social isolation, and long-term disability, underscoring the need for integrated clinical management (Asherson et al., 2014).

3.2.3 *Substance Use Disorders: Increased Risk-Taking and Self-Medication*

ADHD is a well-established risk factor for substance use disorders (SUD), with individuals demonstrating an increased propensity for impulsive decision-making, sensation-seeking behavior, and poor inhibitory control (Levy et al., 2014). Early onset of substance use is common in this population, with an elevated risk of progressing to dependency (Faraone et al., 2015). The presence of SUD further disrupts executive function, exacerbating ADHD-related deficits in attention, memory, and decision-making.

The interplay between ADHD and substance use presents unique treatment challenges (Wilens, 2004). The use of stimulant medication for ADHD in individuals with a history of substance misuse requires careful monitoring to mitigate the risk of diversion and abuse. Furthermore, substance use can mimic or mask ADHD symptoms, leading to misdiagnosis or inappropriate treatment plans. Given the high rates of criminal justice involvement and employment instability among individuals with ADHD and SUD, early intervention programs focusing on behavioral regulation and harm reduction strategies are critical.

3.2.4 *Personality Disorders: Intensification of Emotional Dysregulation and Social Dysfunction*

The co-occurrence of ADHD and personality disorders—particularly borderline personality disorder (BPD) and antisocial personality disorder (ASPD)—significantly worsens emotional regulation, impulsivity, and interpersonal instability (Weiner et al., 2019). BPD, characterized by intense mood swings, fear of abandonment, and self-destructive behaviors, exacerbates the emotional dysregulation inherent in ADHD (Weiner et al., 2019). Individuals with both conditions are at higher risk of self-harm, suicidal behavior, and volatile relationships.

Similarly, ADHD combined with ASPD contributes to heightened aggression, rule-breaking behavior, and an increased likelihood of legal system involvement (Mohr-Jensen et al., 2019). Childhood conduct disorder often precedes this comorbidity, reinforcing the necessity for early behavioral interventions. Individuals with ADHD and co-occurring personality disorders frequently face difficulties in maintaining employment and long-term relationships, highlighting the need for structured, long-term psychosocial support.

3.2.5 *Autism Spectrum Disorder: Increased Social and Cognitive Challenges*

ADHD frequently coexists with autism spectrum disorder (ASD), creating a complex neurodevelopmental profile characterized by deficits in executive functioning, social communication, and sensory processing (Roselló et al., 2017). While ADHD primarily affects impulse control and attentional regulation, ASD introduces additional impairments in social reciprocity, emotional expression, and cognitive flexibility (Roselló et al., 2017). These overlapping difficulties can lead to increased social rejection, higher academic support needs, and challenges in adaptive functioning.

Managing ADHD in the context of ASD requires a nuanced approach, as traditional ADHD interventions—such as stimulant medication and behavioral therapy—may not fully address the social communication deficits and sensory sensitivities associated with ASD. The lifelong functional impact of this comorbidity necessitates early diagnosis and individualized educational, occupational, and social support interventions.

3.2.6 *Obsessive-Compulsive Disorder: Conflicting Treatment Needs*

The co-occurrence of ADHD and obsessive-compulsive disorder (OCD) presents a unique challenge due to their contrasting symptom profiles (Pinto et al., 2016). ADHD is associated with distractibility and impulsivity, whereas OCD is characterized by compulsive behaviors, cognitive inflexibility, and excessive self-regulation. Individuals with both conditions often experience heightened frustration, as ADHD-related impulsivity may interfere with the rigid routines associated with OCD, leading to increased anxiety and distress (APA, 2013).

Treatment strategies must be carefully balanced, as stimulant medications for ADHD may exacerbate compulsions in some individuals, while selective serotonin reuptake inhibitors (SSRIs) used for OCD may contribute to attentional difficulties (Cabarkapa et al., 2019). Behavioral therapy, including exposure and response prevention (ERP) tailored for individuals with ADHD, can help mitigate symptoms and improve daily functioning (Cabarkapa et al., 2019).

3.2.7 *Learning Disabilities: Exacerbation of Academic Impairments*

Learning disabilities commonly co-occur with ADHD, further exacerbating academic difficulties (Semrud-Clikeman & Bledsoe, 2011). Deficits in working memory, processing speed, and reading comprehension contribute to significant educational challenges, often leading to increased frustration, disengagement, and lower self-esteem (APA, 2013). Many individuals with ADHD and learning disabilities struggle with written expression, mathematical reasoning, and sustained attention, resulting in academic underperformance and increased school dropout rates (Sarid & Lipka, 2023).

The long-term implications of this comorbidity extend beyond education, affecting career prospects and financial independence (Pelham et al., 2007). Structured educational interventions, including individualized learning plans (ILPs) and executive function coaching, are essential to improving outcomes for affected individuals. Workplace accommodations (Solberg et al., 2011) and vocational training programs can also facilitate successful transitions into adulthood.

3.3 Diagnostic Challenges and Considerations

The diagnosis of ADHD in adults is frequently complicated by the presence of psychiatric comorbidities, leading to significant rates of underdiagnosis and misdiagnosis (Barkley & Brown, 2008; Nordgaard et al., 2023). About three-quarters of adults with ADHD are estimated to have at least one additional mental health condition, including anxiety disorders, mood disorders, personality disorders, or substance use disorders (Katzman et al., 2017; Nordgaard et al., 2023). These overlapping presentations often obscure the core symptoms of ADHD, delaying recognition and appropriate intervention (Katzman et al., 2017). As a result, many individuals receive treatment targeting secondary psychiatric manifestations rather than the underlying neurodevelopmental disorder, prolonging functional impairments and diminishing overall quality of life.

3.3.1 *Symptom Overlap and Diagnostic Complexity*

ADHD shares several core symptom domains with multiple psychiatric conditions, complicating differentiation (Katzman et al., 2017). Features such as inattention, impulsivity, emotional instability, and restlessness also characterize disorders including generalized anxiety disorder, major depressive disorder, bipolar disorder, and borderline personality disorder (APA, 2013). Consequently, many adults with ADHD are misdiagnosed with primary mood or anxiety disorders, resulting in treatment strategies that fail to address executive dysfunction and attentional deficits (Asherson et al., 2010).

A key distinguishing feature of ADHD is its lifelong trajectory, with symptoms typically emerging in childhood and persisting into adulthood (APA, 2013). In contrast, disorders such as major depression and bipolar disorder tend to have episodic courses (APA, 2013). However, retrospective recall of childhood ADHD symptoms is often unreliable, and adults may attribute lifelong difficulties to external circumstances rather than an underlying disorder. This further complicates diagnostic accuracy, necessitating structured clinical interviews and validated screening tools to distinguish ADHD from overlapping conditions.

In clinical practice, differentiating ADHD from anxiety disorders is particularly challenging. While ADHD-related inattention is driven by distractibility and difficulty sustaining effort, anxiety-related cognitive impairments often stem from excessive worry and hypervigilance (Katzman et al., 2017). Similarly, emotional dysregulation in ADHD may superficially resemble mood swings characteristic of bipolar disorder, yet ADHD lacks the distinct manic and depressive episodes that define bipolar illness (Biederman et al, 2008). Understanding these nuances is crucial for improving diagnostic precision.

3.3.2 Consequences of Misdiagnosis and Underdiagnosis

Diagnostic errors in ADHD have far-reaching consequences, contributing to ineffective treatment approaches, increased psychiatric comorbidities, and heightened socioeconomic burden (Doshi et al., 2012). Misdiagnosis often leads to the prescription of antidepressants, mood stabilizers, or anxiolytics, which may alleviate secondary symptoms but fail to address core executive dysfunction and attentional deficits (Doyle, 2004). This results in persistent difficulties in academic, occupational, and social functioning, reinforcing a cycle of treatment resistance and disability.

Economic analyses underscore the substantial financial burden associated with ADHD misdiagnosis and underdiagnosis. In the United States alone, avoidable healthcare expenditures linked to ADHD misdiagnosis were estimated to exceed US$400 million annually in 2012, primarily due to inappropriate medication use and prolonged psychiatric care (Doshi et al., 2012). Individuals with undiagnosed ADHD often experience higher rates of job instability, lower lifetime earnings, and increased reliance on disability benefits, highlighting the need for more accurate and timely diagnosis (Doshi et al., 2012).

Untreated ADHD is particularly detrimental in populations with co-occurring substance use disorders. The heightened impulsivity associated with ADHD predisposes individuals to early substance experimentation and increased addiction severity (Wilens & Morrison, 2011). Without appropriate ADHD treatment, individuals with comorbid substance use disorders exhibit poorer rehabilitation outcomes, higher relapse rates, and greater engagement with the criminal justice system (Young et al., 2015). Addressing diagnostic gaps in ADHD is therefore critical for mitigating long-term societal costs.

3.3.3 Treatment Challenges in Comorbid ADHD

The presence of psychiatric comorbidities complicates ADHD management, necessitating individualized and multidisciplinary treatment approaches (Caye et al., 2016; Pliszka, 2007). Stimulant medications—considered the first-line pharmacological treatment for ADHD—may exacerbate symptoms of certain comorbid disorders, requiring careful risk-benefit assessment (Wilens et al., 2003). For example, in ADHD co-occurring with bipolar disorder, stimulant use can trigger manic episodes unless stabilized with mood-stabilizing agents. In individuals with generalized anxiety disorder, stimulant medications may heighten physiological arousal and exacerbate worry, requiring dose adjustments or adjunctive anxiolytic therapy. In ADHD with borderline personality disorder, impulsivity and emotional dysregulation are pronounced, necessitating behavioral interventions such as dialectical behavior therapy (DBT) in conjunction with medication. For individuals with co-occurring substance use disorders, stimulant therapy must be carefully monitored due to concerns regarding potential misuse or diversion (Wilens et al., 2003). Non-stimulant alternatives, such as atomoxetine or guanfacine, may be preferable in these cases (Cutler et al., 2022). The interaction between ADHD and its comorbid conditions underscores the necessity of integrated treatment models that address multiple symptom domains while minimizing adverse effects (Pliszka, 2007).

3.3.4 Strategies for Improving Diagnostic Accuracy

Overcoming diagnostic challenges in adult ADHD requires a systematic and multimodal assessment approach (Pliszka, 2007). Comprehensive evaluation should incorporate a detailed clinical history, assessing childhood-onset symptoms and lifelong functional impairments. Structured diagnostic interviews utilizing standardized tools such as the Adult ADHD Self-Report Scale (ASRS) or the Diagnostic Interview for ADHD in Adults (DIVA-5) are required to enhance reliability and differentiate secondary attentional issues to ensure that cognitive deficits are not solely attributable to comorbid conditions such as depression or anxiety. A multidisciplinary team involving psychiatrists, psychologists, and neuropsychologists is essential to facilitate accurate diagnosis and tailored treatment planning. By refining diagnostic protocols and improving clinical awareness of ADHD's neurodevelopmental underpinnings, healthcare providers can reduce misdiagnosis, enhance treatment outcomes, and alleviate the long-term societal burden of ADHD.

3.4 Treatment Approaches for Co-occurring Conditions

The management of ADHD with co-occurring psychiatric conditions necessitates a nuanced, integrated approach that considers the complex interplay of symptom interactions, treatment responsiveness, and potential adverse effects (Caye et al., 2016; Pliszka, 2007). Given the heterogeneity of comorbidities, both pharmacological and psychosocial interventions must be tailored to the specific needs of each patient. A multimodal strategy remains imperative in optimizing clinical outcomes and mitigating long-term functional impairment.

3.4.1 Pharmacological Strategies: Balancing Efficacy and Safety

Treating ADHD in individuals with comorbid anxiety disorders presents a treatment paradox, as stimulant medications—typically first-line for ADHD—may exacerbate anxiety symptoms (Jarrett & Ollendick, 2008). Atomoxetine, a selective norepinephrine reuptake inhibitor (NRI), is often preferred due to its lower propensity to induce anxiety compared to stimulants (Zhang et al., 2025). Extended-release guanfacine or clonidine, both alpha-2 adrenergic agonists, may mitigate hyperactivity and autonomic symptoms of anxiety while providing adjunctive benefits for ADHD (Childress, 2012). Cognitive behavioral therapy (CBT) should be integrated to address cognitive distortions, avoidance behaviors, and attentional biases, thereby augmenting pharmacological efficacy (Safren et al., 2005).

When ADHD co-occurs with major depressive disorder (MDD) or bipolar disorder, precise pharmacologic modulation is necessary to avoid exacerbating mood instability (Clark et al., 2023; Viktorin et al., 2017). In ADHD with MDD, bupropion, a norepinephrine-dopamine reuptake inhibitor (NDRI), may be utilized to target overlapping cognitive and motivational deficits, while selective serotonin reuptake inhibitors (SSRIs) can be co-administered if anxiety symptoms or persistent depressive features are present (Ng, 2017). In ADHD with bipolar disorder, stimulants must be introduced cautiously, only after mood stabilization with first-line treatments such as lithium, valproate, or lamotrigine, and, when appropriate, atypical antipsychotics (e.g., aripiprazole, quetiapine) for more severe symptoms (Girard & Joober, 2017). Adjunctive CBT and dialectical behavior therapy (DBT) should be prioritized to target emotional dysregulation, impulsivity, and maladaptive thought patterns (Saccaro et al., 2024).

Individuals with ADHD exhibit a heightened predisposition toward substance misuse, often engaging in self-medication with stimulants or other psychoactive substances (Palmer et al., 2015). Optimal treatment strategies emphasize non-stimulant medications such as atomoxetine and bupropion, which have lower abuse potential. Lisdexamfetamine, a prodrug stimulant, confers a reduced risk of misuse compared to immediate-release formulations (Levine & Swanson, 2023). Behavioral interventions such as contingency management and motivational interviewing are essential for enhancing medication adherence and promoting abstinence (Parkin et al., 2022). Integrative dual-diagnosis programs that concurrently address ADHD and substance use disorders have demonstrated superior clinical efficacy (Mariani & Levin, 2007).

The intersection of ADHD with borderline personality disorder (BPD) necessitates targeted interventions due to shared impulsivity and emotional dysregulation (Mazyarkin et al., 2019; Storebø et al., 2020). Stimulants should be prescribed judiciously, as they may intensify emotional instability in BPD (Ditrich et al., 2021). Mood stabilizers, such as lamotrigine or lithium, may be indicated to modulate impulsive aggression and affective instability (Pahwa et al., 2020). DBT remains the cornerstone psychosocial intervention, equipping individuals with emotion regulation and interpersonal efficacy skills (Stoffers-Winterling et al., 2022).

Finally, the co-occurrence of ADHD and autism spectrum disorder (ASD) presents distinct neurodevelopmental challenges requiring a multidisciplinary approach (Aishworiya et al., 2022). Stimulants remain the primary pharmacological intervention, although lower doses may be necessary to mitigate irritability or exacerbation of rigidity. Alpha-2 adrenergic agonists, such as guanfacine and clonidine, have shown efficacy in addressing hyperactivity and emotional dysregulation (Harstad et al., 2021). Applied behavior analysis (ABA) and structured behavioral interventions should be prioritized to address deficits in executive function and social communication (Collins et al., 2025). Collaboration among psychiatrists, speech therapists, and occupational therapists is critical to achieving optimal functional outcomes.

3.4.2 Behavioral and Psychosocial Interventions: A Core Component of Treatment

Cognitive behavioral therapy (CBT) is a well-established intervention in the management of ADHD and its comorbidities (Matsumoto et al., 2024). CBT effectively targets executive dysfunction, addressing deficits in time management and organization. It also helps correct maladaptive cognitive distortions that contribute to anxiety and depression, while simultaneously enhancing impulse control and emotional regulation—an especially valuable approach in individuals with ADHD and borderline personality disorder (BPD) comorbidity (Pan et al., 2024). By focusing on these domains, CBT supports the development of adaptive coping mechanisms that are critical for daily functioning.

Mindfulness-based interventions have also emerged as promising therapeutic modalities for ADHD and co-occurring mood disorders. These interventions demonstrate benefits in enhancing attentional control, reducing impulsivity, and lowering affective lability, all while mitigating physiological stress and anxiety (Zylowska et al., 2007). Techniques such as mindfulness-based cognitive therapy (MBCT) and acceptance and commitment therapy (ACT) are increasingly integrated into treatment plans, complementing traditional CBT to foster improved emotional regulation and psychological flexibility (Janssen et al., 2020).

Family and social support interventions play a vital role in managing the interpersonal challenges characteristic of ADHD and its comorbidities. Parent training programs provide caregivers with strategies to manage behavioral difficulties across ADHD, anxiety, and autism spectrum disorder (ASD) presentations (Chronis et al., 2004). Social skills training is especially important for individuals with ADHD-ASD or ADHD-BPD profiles, as these individuals often struggle to navigate peer interactions and maintain relational stability (García-Castellar et al., 2025). Such interventions build essential social competencies, enhancing overall functioning and quality of life.

3.4.3 *Multidisciplinary and Integrated Care Models*

Given the clinical complexity of ADHD when accompanied by psychiatric comorbidities, a comprehensive, multidisciplinary care model is essential (Chaplin, 2018). Interdisciplinary collaboration among primary care physicians, psychiatrists, psychologists, and behavioral therapists ensures cohesive management that addresses the full spectrum of patient needs. Individualized treatment paradigms should be designed based on the severity of symptoms, degree of functional impairment, and patient-specific risk factors. Longitudinal follow-up is crucial to assess treatment response, optimize therapeutic efficacy, and minimize adverse effects. By adopting an integrated care approach, clinicians can provide holistic and sustained support to individuals with ADHD, thereby improving both short-term and long-term outcomes.

3.5 Lifespan Implications of Comorbid ADHD and Mental Health Disorders

The coexistence of ADHD and other psychiatric conditions significantly influences an individual's developmental trajectory, affecting academic, social, occupational, and overall life outcomes (Jangmo et al., 2021; Miranda et al., 2014). These comorbidities often exacerbate ADHD-related impairments, increasing the complexity of diagnosis and treatment. Early detection and intervention are essential to mitigating long-term adverse effects, enhancing functionality, and reducing the burden on healthcare and social support systems (Antai-Otong & Zimmerman, 2016).

3.5.1 *Childhood: Academic and Social Challenges*

Children with ADHD and co-occurring mental health conditions experience profound difficulties in multiple domains, particularly in academic performance, peer relationships, and behavioral regulation (Jangmo et al., 2021).

The combination of inattention, impulsivity, and emotional dysregulation contributes to lower academic achievement, with higher rates of grade retention, special education placement, and disciplinary action. Social difficulties often include peer rejection, bullying victimization, and reduced social reciprocity. Additionally, there is an increased vulnerability to behavioral problems, particularly in cases of comorbid oppositional defiant disorder (ODD) or conduct disorder (CD), which heightens the risk of early delinquency and engagement in health-risk behaviors.

Untreated ADHD and comorbidities in childhood set the stage for long-term functional impairments, necessitating early intervention strategies that include behavioral therapy, family support, and individualized educational planning.

3.5.2 Adolescence: Escalating Risk Factors

As individuals transition into adolescence, the persistence of ADHD symptoms alongside comorbid psychiatric disorders can significantly exacerbate functional impairments (Agnew-Blais et al., 2018). Adolescents with ADHD are at heightened risk for substance use disorders (SUD) due to impulsivity and novelty-seeking behavior, increased academic failure and school dropout rates that further limit future occupational opportunities, and emotional instability that raises the likelihood of self-harm and suicidality, particularly among those with coexisting mood disorders (French et al., 2024). They also experience higher rates of risky behaviors, including delinquency and unsafe sexual practices, contributing to adverse psychosocial outcomes. Without targeted interventions, these adolescents face considerable challenges in establishing autonomy and achieving developmental milestones essential for successful adulthood.

3.5.3 Adulthood: Occupational, Social, and Economic Burden

The long-term consequences of ADHD with comorbid psychiatric disorders persist into adulthood, significantly influencing career stability, relationships, and overall well-being. Adults with ADHD and co-occurring conditions frequently experience occupational difficulties (Miranda et al., 2014), including job instability, chronic underemployment, and financial insecurity due to executive dysfunction and emotional dysregulation. Interpersonal relationships are often strained, with higher rates of divorce, social isolation, and difficulty maintaining stable social networks (Retz et al., 2021; Wiener, 2023). The risk of legal system involvement is also heightened, particularly in individuals with comorbid conduct disorder or antisocial traits, underscoring the necessity of targeted interventions. Additionally, untreated ADHD contributes to an elevated risk of recurrent depressive episodes, substance dependence, and suicidality. Addressing these challenges requires sustained, multidisciplinary interventions that encompass vocational support, social skills training, and ongoing mental healthcare.

3.5.4 A Multidisciplinary Approach for Improved Outcomes

Given the pervasive and enduring impact of ADHD comorbidities, a lifespan-oriented, multidisciplinary treatment model is critical (Jangmo et al., 2021). Effective management requires integrating pharmacological treatment, carefully selecting medications to account for the complexity introduced by co-occurring conditions. Psychotherapy should incorporate evidence-based approaches such as cognitive behavioral therapy (CBT), dialectical behavior therapy (DBT), and mindfulness-based interventions to address emotional dysregulation and maladaptive coping mechanisms. Behavioral and educational interventions are essential for supporting academic, social, and executive functioning challenges from childhood through adulthood. Additionally, strong social support networks and vocational training can facilitate successful transitions into independent living and stable employment, ultimately enhancing long-term outcomes and quality of life for individuals with ADHD.

Summary

This chapter has explored the complex interplay between ADHD and co-occurring mental health disorders, emphasizing their cumulative impact across the lifespan. The high prevalence of psychiatric comorbidities in ADHD, such as anxiety, mood disorders, and substance use disorders, complicates diagnosis and treatment due to overlapping symptoms and the dynamic interaction between ADHD-related inattention, impulsivity, and executive dysfunction with comorbid conditions. These interactions heighten functional impairments across academic, occupational, and social domains.

Diagnostic complexities arise when ADHD symptoms are misinterpreted as mood instability, personality disorders, or secondary attentional difficulties linked to anxiety or depression, highlighting the need for a comprehensive, multimodal diagnostic approach. Treatment must be equally nuanced, balancing pharmacological interventions with evidence-based psychosocial strategies. Pharmacological management should be tailored to address co-occurring conditions, ensuring optimal efficacy while minimizing risks. Therapies such as cognitive behavioral therapy (CBT), dialectical behavior therapy (DBT), and mindfulness-based interventions play critical roles in managing emotional dysregulation and behavioral challenges.

The long-term consequences of untreated ADHD and its comorbidities, including academic difficulties, risk-taking behaviors, and psychiatric deterioration, further underscore the importance of early intervention. A lifespan-oriented, multidisciplinary approach integrating primary care, psychiatry, psychology, and behavioral therapies is essential for optimizing long-term outcomes. Individualized care models that incorporate both medical and social support systems are key to improving functional and psychological well-being. By addressing the complexities of ADHD and its comorbid conditions through precise diagnosis and comprehensive management, this chapter highlights the necessity of a holistic, integrated approach to support affected individuals throughout their lives.

References

Abramovitch, A., Dar, R., Mittelman, A., & Wilhelm, S. (2015). Comorbidity between attention deficit/hyperactivity disorder and obsessive-compulsive disorder across the lifespan: A systematic and critical review. *Harvard Review of Psychiatry, 23*(4), 245–262.

Agnew-Blais, J. C., Polanczyk, G. V., Danese, A., Wertz, J., Moffitt, T. E., & Arseneault, L. (2018). Young adult mental health and functional outcomes among individuals with remitted, persistent and late-onset ADHD. *The British Journal of Psychiatry, 213*(3), 526–534.

Aishworiya, R., Valica, T., Hagerman, R., & Restrepo, B. (2022). An update on psychopharmacological treatment of autism Spectrum disorder. *Neurotherapeutics, 19*(1), 248–262. https://doi.org/10.1007/s13311-022-01183-1

Antai-Otong, D., & Zimmerman, M. L. (2016). Treatment approaches to attention deficit hyperactivity disorder. *Nursing Clinics, 51*(2), 199–211.

APA. (2013). Diagnostic and statistical manual of mental disorders. *American Psychiatric Association, 21*(21), 591–643.

Appolinario, J. C., de Moraes, C. E. F., Sichieri, R., Hay, P., Faraone, S. V., & Mattos, P. (2024). Associations of adult ADHD symptoms with binge eating spectrum conditions, psychiatric and somatic comorbidity, and healthcare utilization. *Brazilian Journal of Psychiatry, 46*, e20243728.

Asherson, P., Adamou, M., Bolea, B., Muller, U., Morua, S. D., Pitts, M., Thome, J., & Young, S. (2010). Is ADHD a valid diagnosis in adults? Yes. *BMJ, 340*, c549. https://doi.org/10.1136/bmj.c549

Asherson, P., Young, A. H., Eich-Höchli, D., Moran, P., Porsdal, V., & Deberdt, W. (2014). Differential diagnosis, comorbidity, and treatment of attention-deficit/hyperactivity disorder in relation to bipolar disorder or borderline personality disorder in adults. *Current Medical Research and Opinion, 30*(8), 1657–1672. https://doi.org/10.1185/03007995.2014.915800

Barkley, R. A., & Brown, T. E. (2008). Unrecognized attention-deficit/hyperactivity disorder in adults presenting with other psychiatric disorders. *CNS Spectrums, 13*(11), 977–984. https://doi.org/10.1017/S1092852900014036

Biederman, J., et al. (2008). Differentiating ADHD from bipolar disorder in children and adolescents. *Journal of Clinical Psychiatry, 69*(9), e25.

Bloemsma, J. M., Boer, F., Arnold, R., Banaschewski, T., Faraone, S. V., Buitelaar, J. K., Sergeant, J. A., Rommelse, N., & Oosterlaan, J. (2013). Comorbid anxiety and neurocognitive dysfunctions in children with ADHD. *European Child & Adolescent Psychiatry, 22*(4), 225–234. https://doi.org/10.1007/s00787-012-0339-9

Brus, M. J., Solanto, M. V., & Goldberg, J. F. (2014). Adult ADHD vs. bipolar disorder in the DSM-5 era: A challenging differentiation for clinicians. *Journal of Psychiatric Practice, 20*(6), 428–437.

Cabarkapa, S., King, J. A., Dowling, N., & Ng, C. H. (2019). Co-morbid obsessive–compulsive disorder and attention deficit hyperactivity disorder: Neurobiological commonalities and treatment implications. *Frontiers in Psychiatry, 10*, 557. https://doi.org/10.3389/fpsyt.2019.00557

Caye, A., Rocha, T. B.-M., Anselmi, L., Murray, J., Menezes, A. M. B., Barros, F. C., Gonçalves, H., Wehrmeister, F., Jensen, C. M., Steinhausen, H.-C., Swanson, J. M., Kieling, C., & Rohde, L. A. (2016). Attention-deficit/hyperactivity disorder trajectories from childhood to Young adulthood: Evidence from a birth cohort supporting a late-onset syndrome. *JAMA Psychiatry, 73*(7), 705–712. https://doi.org/10.1001/jamapsychiatry.2016.0383

Chaplin, S. (2018). Attention deficit hyperactivity disorder: Diagnosis and management. *Progress in Neurology and Psychiatry, 22*(3), 27–29.

Childress, A. C. (2012). Guanfacine extended release as adjunctive therapy to psychostimulants in children and adolescents with attention-deficit/hyperactivity disorder. *Advances in Therapy, 29*(5), 385–400. https://doi.org/10.1007/s12325-012-0020-1

Choi, W.-S., Woo, Y. S., Wang, S.-M., Lim, H. K., & Bahk, W.-M. (2022). The prevalence of psychiatric comorbidities in adult ADHD compared with non-ADHD populations: A systematic literature review. *PLoS One, 17*(11), e0277175. https://doi.org/10.1371/journal.pone.0277175

Chronis, A. M., Chacko, A., Fabiano, G. A., Wymbs, B. T., & Pelham, W. E. (2004). Enhancements to the Behavioral parent training paradigm for families of children with ADHD: Review and future directions. *Clinical Child and Family Psychology Review, 7*(1), 1–27. https://doi.org/10.1023/B:CCFP.0000020190.60808.a4

Clark, A., Tate, B., Urban, B., Schroeder, R., Gennuso, S., Ahmadzadeh, S., McGregor, D., Girma, B., Shekoohi, S., & Kaye, A. D. (2023). Bupropion mediated effects on depression, attention deficit hyperactivity disorder, and smoking cessation. *Health Psychology Research, 11*, 81043. https://doi.org/10.52965/001c.81043

Collins, I. M., Halter, F., Schächinger Tenés, L. T., Lieb, R., & Meyer, A. H. (2025). A meta-analysis of applied behavior analysis-based interventions to improve communication, adaptive, and cognitive skills in children on the autism Spectrum. *Review Journal of Autism and Developmental Disorders.* https://doi.org/10.1007/s40489-025-00506-0

Cuffe, S. P., Visser, S. N., Holbrook, J. R., Danielson, M. L., Geryk, L. L., Wolraich, M. L., & McKeown, R. E. (2020). ADHD and psychiatric comorbidity: Functional outcomes in a school-based sample of children. *Journal of Attention Disorders, 24*(9), 1345–1354.

Cutler, A. J., Mattingly, G. W., Jain, R., & O'Neal, W. (2022). Current and future nonstimulants in the treatment of pediatric ADHD: Monoamine reuptake inhibitors, receptor modulators, and multimodal agents. *CNS Spectrums, 27*(2), 199–207. https://doi.org/10.1017/S1092852920001984

D'Agati, E., Curatolo, P., & Mazzone, L. (2019). Comorbidity between ADHD and anxiety disorders across the lifespan. *International Journal of Psychiatry in Clinical Practice, 23*(4), 238–244.

Ditrich, I., Philipsen, A., & Matthies, S. (2021). Borderline personality disorder (BPD) and attention deficit hyperactivity disorder (ADHD) revisited—A review-update on common grounds and subtle distinctions. *Borderline Personality Disorder and Emotion Dysregulation, 8*(1), 22. https://doi.org/10.1186/s40479-021-00162-w

Doshi, J. A., Hodgkins, P., Kahle, J., Sikirica, V., Cangelosi, M. J., Setyawan, J., Erder, M. H., & Neumann, P. J. (2012). Economic impact of childhood and adult attention-deficit/hyperactivity disorder in the United States. *Journal of the American Academy of Child and Adolescent Psychiatry, 51*(10), 990–1002.e1002. https://doi.org/10.1016/j.jaac.2012.07.008

Doyle, R. (2004). The history of adult attention-deficit/hyperactivity disorder. *Psychiatric Clinics of North America, 27*(2), 203–214. https://doi.org/10.1016/j.psc.2004.01.001

Faraone, S. V., et al. (2015). Attention-deficit/hyperactivity disorder. *Nature Reviews Disease Primers, 1*, 15020.

Faraone, S. V., Banaschewski, T., Coghill, D., Zheng, Y., Biederman, J., Bellgrove, M. A., Newcorn, J. H., Gignac, M., Al Saud, N. M., Manor, I., Rohde, L. A., Yang, L., Cortese, S., Almagor, D., Stein, M. A., Albatti, T. H., Aljoudi, H. F., Alqahtani, M. M. J., Asherson, P., et al. (2021). The world federation of ADHD international consensus statement: 208 evidence-based conclusions about the disorder. *Neuroscience & Biobehavioral Reviews, 128*, 789–818. https://doi.org/10.1016/j.neubiorev.2021.01.022

French, B., Nalbant, G., Wright, H., Sayal, K., Daley, D., Groom, M. J., Cassidy, S., & Hall, C. L. (2024). The impacts associated with having ADHD: An umbrella review. *Frontiers in Psychiatry, 15*, 1343314. https://doi.org/10.3389/fpsyt.2024.1343314

García-Castellar, R., Sánchez-Chiva, D., Roselló-Miranda, B., & Flor-Arasil, P. (2025). Exploring the effectiveness of combining social skills training and two parent programs in improving the social competence of children with attention-deficit/hyperactivity disorder. *Children, 12*(2), 132.

Girard, R., & Joober, R. (2017). Treatment of ADHD in patients with bipolar disorder. *Journal of Psychiatry & Neuroscience, 42*(6), E11–E12. https://doi.org/10.1503/jpn.170097

Harstad, E., Shults, J., Barbaresi, W., Bax, A., Cacia, J., Deavenport-Saman, A., Friedman, S., LaRosa, A., Loe, I. M., Mittal, S., Tulio, S., Vanderbilt, D., & Blum, N. J. (2021). α2-adrenergic agonists or stimulants for preschool-age children with attention-deficit/hyperactivity disorder. *JAMA, 325*(20), 2067–2075. https://doi.org/10.1001/jama.2021.6118

Jangmo, A., Kuja-Halkola, R., Pérez-Vigil, A., Almqvist, C., Bulik, C. M., D'Onofrio, B., Lichtenstein, P., Ahnemark, E., Werner-Kiechle, T., & Larsson, H. (2021). Attention-deficit/hyperactivity disorder and occupational outcomes: The role of educational attainment, comorbid developmental disorders, and intellectual disability. *PLoS One, 16*(3), e0247724.

Janssen, L., de Vries, A. M., Hepark, S., & Speckens, A. E. M. (2020). The feasibility, effectiveness, and process of change of mindfulness-based cognitive therapy for adults with ADHD: A mixed-method pilot study. *Journal of Attention Disorders, 24*(6), 928–942. https://doi.org/10.1177/1087054717727350

Jarrett, M. A., & Ollendick, T. H. (2008). A conceptual review of the comorbidity of attention-deficit/hyperactivity disorder and anxiety: Implications for future research and practice. *Clinical Psychology Review, 28*(7), 1266–1280. https://doi.org/10.1016/j.cpr.2008.05.004

Katzman, M. A., Bilkey, T. S., Chokka, P. R., Fallu, A., & Klassen, L. J. (2017). Adult ADHD and comorbid disorders: Clinical implications of a dimensional approach. *BMC Psychiatry, 17*(1), 302. https://doi.org/10.1186/s12888-017-1463-3

Kessler, R. C., Adler, L., Barkley, R., Biederman, J., Conners, C. K., Demler, O., Faraone, S. V., Greenhill, L. L., Howes, M. J., Secnik, K., Spencer, T., Ustun, T. B., Walters, E. E., & Zaslavsky, A. M. (2006). The prevalence and correlates of adult ADHD in the United States: Results from the National Comorbidity Survey Replication. *The American Journal of Psychiatry, 163*(4), 716–723. https://doi.org/10.1176/ajp.2006.163.4.716

Levine, J., & Swanson, H. (2023). The use of Lisdexamfetamine to treat ADHD in a patient with stimulant (methamphetamine) use disorder. *Case Reports in Psychiatry, 2023*, 5574677. https://doi.org/10.1155/2023/5574677

Levy, S., Katusic, S. K., Colligan, R. C., Weaver, A. L., Killian, J. M., Voigt, R. G., & Barbaresi, W. J. (2014). Childhood ADHD and risk for substance dependence in adulthood: A longitudinal, population-based study. *PLoS One, 9*(8), e105640.

Mansour, R., Dovi, A. T., Lane, D. M., Loveland, K. A., & Pearson, D. A. (2017). ADHD severity as it relates to comorbid psychiatric symptomatology in children with autism Spectrum disorders (ASD). *Research in Developmental Disabilities, 60*, 52–64.

Mariani, J. J., & Levin, F. R. (2007). Treatment strategies for co-occurring ADHD and substance use disorders. *The American Journal on Addictions, 16*(Suppl 1), 45–54; quiz 55-46. https://doi.org/10.1080/10550490601082783

Matsumoto, K., Hamatani, S., Kunisato, Y., & Mizuno, Y. (2024). Components of cognitive-behavioural therapy for mitigating core symptoms in attention-deficit hyperactivity disorder: A systematic review and network meta-analys. *BMJ Mental Health, 27*(1). https://doi.org/10.1136/bmjment-2024-301303

Mazyarkin, Z., Peleg, T., Golani, I., Sharony, L., Kremer, I., & Shamir, A. (2019). Health benefits of a physical exercise program for inpatients with mental health; a pilot study. *Journal of Psychiatric Research, 113*, 10–16. https://doi.org/10.1016/j.jpsychires.2019.03.002

Miranda, A., Berenguer, C., Colomer, C., & Roselló, R. (2014). Influence of the symptoms of attention deficit hyperactivity disorder (ADHD) and comorbid disorders on functioning in adulthood. *Psicothema, 26*(4), 471–476.

Mohr-Jensen, C., Müller Bisgaard, C., Boldsen, S. K., & Steinhausen, H.-C. (2019). Attention-deficit/hyperactivity disorder in childhood and adolescence and the risk of crime in Young adulthood in a Danish Nationwide study. *Journal of the American Academy of Child & Adolescent Psychiatry, 58*(4), 443–452. https://doi.org/10.1016/j.jaac.2018.11.016

Montano, C. B., & Weisler, R. (2011). Distinguishing symptoms of ADHD from other psychiatric disorders in the adult primary care setting. *Postgraduate Medicine, 123*(3), 88–98.

Ng, Q. X. (2017). A systematic review of the use of bupropion for attention-deficit/hyperactivity disorder in children and adolescents. *Journal of Child and Adolescent Psychopharmacology, 27*(2), 112–116. https://doi.org/10.1089/cap.2016.0124

Nordgaard, J., Nielsen, K. M., Rasmussen, A. R., & Henriksen, M. G. (2023). Psychiatric comorbidity: A concept in need of a theory. *Psychological Medicine, 53*(13), 5902–5908. https://doi.org/10.1017/s0033291723001605

Pahwa, M., Nuñez, N. A., Joseph, B., Seshadri, A., Gerberi, D. J., Frye, M. A., & Singh, B. (2020). Efficacy and tolerability of lamotrigine in borderline personality disorder: A systematic review and meta-analysis. *Psychopharmacology Bulletin, 50*(4), 118–136.

Palmer, R. H. C., McGeary, J. E., Heath, A. C., Keller, M. C., Brick, L. A., & Knopik, V. S. (2015). Shared additive genetic influences on DSM-IV criteria for alcohol dependence in subjects of European ancestry. *Addiction, 110*(12), 1922–1931. https://doi.org/10.1111/add.13070

Pan, M.-R., Dong, M., Zhang, S.-Y., Liu, L., Li, H.-M., Wang, Y.-F., & Qian, Q.-J. (2024). One-year follow-up of the effectiveness and mediators of cognitive behavioural therapy among adults with attention-deficit/hyperactivity disorder: Secondary outcomes of a randomised controlled trial. *BMC Psychiatry, 24*(1), 207. https://doi.org/10.1186/s12888-024-05673-8

Parkin, R., Nicholas, F. M., & Hayden, J. C. (2022). A systematic review of interventions to enhance adherence and persistence with ADHD pharmacotherapy. *Journal of Psychiatric Research, 152*, 201–218. https://doi.org/10.1016/j.jpsychires.2022.05.044

Pelham, W. E., Foster, E. M., & Robb, J. A. (2007). The economic impact of attention-deficit/hyperactivity disorder in children and adolescents. *Journal of Pediatric Psychology, 32*(6), 711–727. https://doi.org/10.1093/jpepsy/jsm022

Pinto, R., Monzani, B., Leckman, J. F., Rück, C., Serlachius, E., Lichtenstein, P., & Mataix-Cols, D. (2016). Understanding the covariation of tics, attention-deficit/hyperactivity, and obsessive-compulsive symptoms: A population-based adult twin study. *American Journal of Medical Genetics Part B: Neuropsychiatric Genetics, 171*(7), 938–947. https://doi.org/10.1002/ajmg.b.32436

Pliszka, S. (2007). Practice parameter for the assessment and treatment of children and adolescents with attention-deficit/hyperactivity disorder. *Journal of the American Academy of Child & Adolescent Psychiatry, 46*(7), 894–921. https://doi.org/10.1097/chi.0b013e318054e724

Retz, W., Ginsberg, Y., Turner, D., Barra, S., Retz-Junginger, P., Larsson, H., & Asherson, P. (2021). Attention-deficit/hyperactivity disorder (ADHD), antisociality and delinquent behavior over the lifespan. *Neuroscience & Biobehavioral Reviews, 120*, 236–248. https://doi.org/10.1016/j.neubiorev.2020.11.025

Riglin, L., Leppert, B., Dardani, C., Thapar, A. K., Rice, F., O'Donovan, M. C., Davey Smith, G., Stergiakouli, E., Tilling, K., & Thapar, A. (2021). ADHD and depression: Investigating a causal explanation. *Psychological Medicine, 51*(11), 1890–1897. https://doi.org/10.1017/s0033291720000665

Roselló, B., Berenguer, C., Navío, P., Baixauli, I., & Miranda, A. (2017). Executive functioning, social cognition, pragmatics, and social interaction in attention deficit hyperactivity disorder and autism Spectrum disorder. *Current Developmental Disorders Reports, 4*(3), 72–77. https://doi.org/10.1007/s40474-017-0114-1

Saccaro, L. F., Giff, A., De Rossi, M. M., & Piguet, C. (2024). Interventions targeting emotion regulation: A systematic umbrella review. *Journal of Psychiatric Research, 174*, 263–274. https://doi.org/10.1016/j.jpsychires.2024.04.025

Safren, S. A., Otto, M. W., Sprich, S., Winett, C. L., Wilens, T. E., & Biederman, J. (2005). Cognitive-behavioral therapy for ADHD in medication-treated adults with continued symptoms. *Behaviour Research and Therapy, 43*(7), 831–842. https://doi.org/10.1016/j.brat.2004.07.001

Sarid, M., & Lipka, O. (2023). Students with learning disabilities/attention-deficit/hyperactivity disorder in higher education dealing with remote learning: Lessons learned from COVID-19 era. *Frontiers in Psychology, 14*, 1172771. https://doi.org/10.3389/fpsyg.2023.1172771

Semrud-Clikeman, M., & Bledsoe, J. (2011). Updates on attention-deficit/hyperactivity disorder and learning disorders. *Current Psychiatry Reports, 13*(5), 364–373. https://doi.org/10.1007/s11920-011-0211-5

Solberg, V. S., Phelps, L. A., Haakenson, K. A., Durham, J. F., & Timmons, J. (2011). The nature and use of individualized learning plans as a promising career intervention strategy. *Journal of Career Development, 39*(6), 500–514. https://doi.org/10.1177/0894845311414571

Stoffers-Winterling, J. M., Storebø, O. J., Kongerslev, M. T., Faltinsen, E., Todorovac, A., Sedoc Jørgensen, M., Sales, C. P., Edemann Callesen, H., Pereira Ribeiro, J., Völlm, B. A., Lieb, K., & Simonsen, E. (2022). Psychotherapies for borderline personality disorder: A focused systematic review and meta-analysis. *The British Journal of Psychiatry, 221*(3), 538–552. https://doi.org/10.1192/bjp.2021.204

Storebø, O. J., Stoffers-Winterling, J. M., Völlm, B. A., Kongerslev, M. T., Mattivi, J. T., Jørgensen, M. S., Faltinsen, E., Todorovac, A., Sales, C. P., Callesen, H. E., Lieb, K., & Simonsen, E. (2020). Psychological therapies for people with borderline personality disorder. *Cochrane Database of Systematic Reviews, 5*(5), Cd012955. https://doi.org/10.1002/14651858.CD012955.pub2

Taurines, R., Schmitt, J., Renner, T., Conner, A. C., Warnke, A., & Romanos, M. (2010). Developmental comorbidity in attention-deficit/hyperactivity disorder. *ADHD Attention Deficit and Hyperactivity Disorders, 2*, 267–289.

Viktorin, A., Rydén, E., Thase, M. E., Chang, Z., Lundholm, C., D'Onofrio, B. M., Almqvist, C., Magnusson, P. K., Lichtenstein, P., Larsson, H., & Landén, M. (2017). The risk of treatment-emergent mania with methylphenidate in bipolar disorder. *The American Journal of Psychiatry, 174*(4), 341–348. https://doi.org/10.1176/appi.ajp.2016.16040467

Visser, J. C., Rommelse, N. N. J., Greven, C. U., & Buitelaar, J. K. (2016). Autism spectrum disorder and attention-deficit/hyperactivity disorder in early childhood: A review of unique and shared characteristics and developmental antecedents. *Neuroscience & Biobehavioral Reviews, 65*, 229–263. https://doi.org/10.1016/j.neubiorev.2016.03.019

Weiner, L., Perroud, N., & Weibel, S. (2019). Attention deficit hyperactivity disorder and borderline personality disorder in adults: A review of their links and risks. *Neuropsychiatric Disease and Treatment*, 3115–3129.

Wiener, J. (2023). Social relationships of individuals with ADHD across the lifespan. In J. L. Matson (Ed.), *Clinical handbook of ADHD assessment and treatment across the lifespan* (pp. 517–546). Springer International Publishing. https://doi.org/10.1007/978-3-031-41709-2_20

Wilens, T. E. (2004). Attention-deficit/hyperactivity disorder and the substance use disorders: The nature of the relationship, subtypes at risk, and treatment issues. *Psychiatric Clinics, 27*(2), 283–301.

Wilens, T. E., & Morrison, N. R. (2011). The intersection of attention-deficit/hyperactivity disorder and substance abuse. *Current Opinion in Psychiatry, 24*(4), 280–285. https://doi.org/10.1097/YCO.0b013e328345c956.

Wilens, T. E., Faraone, S. V., Biederman, J., & Gunawardene, S. (2003). Does stimulant therapy of attention-deficit/hyperactivity disorder beget later substance abuse? A meta-analytic review of the literature. *Pediatrics, 111*(1), 179–185. https://doi.org/10.1542/peds.111.1.179

Young, S., Moss, D., Sedgwick, O., Fridman, M., & Hodgkins, P. (2015). A meta-analysis of the prevalence of attention deficit hyperactivity disorder in incarcerated populations. *Psychological Medicine, 45*(2), 247–258. https://doi.org/10.1017/s0033291714000762

Zhang, Y., Liao, W., Rao, Y., Gao, W., & Yang, R. (2025). Effects of ADHD and ADHD medications on depression and anxiety in children and adolescents: A systematic review and meta-analysis. *Journal of Psychiatric Research, 181*, 623–639. https://doi.org/10.1016/j.jpsychires.2024.12.022

Zylowska, L., Ackerman, D. L., Yang, M. H., Futrell, J. L., Horton, N. L., Hale, T. S., Pataki, C., & Smalley, S. L. (2007). Mindfulness meditation training in adults and adolescents with ADHD: A feasibility study. *Journal of Attention Disorders, 11*(6), 737–746. https://doi.org/10.1177/1087054707308502

Chapter 4
ADHD and Suicide Risk Across Life Stages

Abstract Suicide remains a critical public health challenge, with attention-deficit/hyperactivity disorder (ADHD) emerging as a significant risk factor across the lifespan. Individuals with ADHD are disproportionately affected by suicidal ideation, attempts, and completed suicides, with evidence suggesting that impulsivity, emotional dysregulation, and co-occurring psychiatric conditions contribute to heightened vulnerability.

This chapter explores the intersections between ADHD and suicide risk, emphasizing developmental trajectories, underlying neurobiological mechanisms, and the impact of social and environmental stressors. Suicide risk among individuals with ADHD is influenced by a range of factors, including childhood adversity, academic and occupational stressors, interpersonal difficulties, and the presence of mood and anxiety disorders.

Given these complexities, early identification of risk markers and the implementation of targeted interventions are essential. This chapter discusses evidence-based prevention strategies, emphasizing the role of clinical screening, psychological therapies, and pharmacological management in mitigating suicide risk in individuals with ADHD. By adopting a lifespan-oriented approach, clinicians and researchers can enhance understanding and improve outcomes for those most at risk.

4.1 Introduction to ADHD and Suicide Risk

Attention-deficit/hyperactivity disorder (ADHD) is increasingly recognized as a significant risk factor for suicidal behaviors across the lifespan (Ljung et al., 2014; Trivedi et al., 2023). Evidence suggests that individuals with ADHD have a 4.7-fold increased risk of engaging in suicidal behaviors compared to those without ADHD (IRR (incidence rate ratio) = 4.7) (Fitzgerald et al., 2019). This risk is particularly pronounced among females, who exhibit a 9.1-fold higher likelihood of suicidal behavior compared to their non-ADHD counterparts (IRR = 9.1), while males demonstrate a 3.4-fold increased risk (IRR = 3.4) (Fitzgerald et al., 2019).

G. Ayano et al., *ADHD Across the Lifespan*, SpringerBriefs in Modern Perspectives on Disability Research,
https://doi.org/10.1007/978-981-95-8712-4_4

Age is a critical determinant of suicide risk in individuals with ADHD. Young adults aged 20–29 years exhibit the highest vulnerability, with an incidence rate ratio (IRR) of 10.07, reflecting a tenfold increase in suicidal behaviors relative to non-ADHD individuals (Fitzgerald et al., 2019). This underscores the importance of targeted interventions during early adulthood, a life stage characterized by major transitions and increased stress exposure.

The presence of comorbid psychiatric conditions further compounds the risk. Individuals with ADHD and co-occurring mental health disorders have an IRR of 10.43 for suicidal behaviors compared to individuals without ADHD, highlighting the compounded vulnerability within this subgroup (Fitzgerald et al., 2019). The interplay between ADHD, mood instability, and impulsivity, alongside comorbid anxiety, depression, bipolar disorder, or substance use disorders, significantly exacerbates suicide risk (Fitzgerald et al., 2019).

Given these findings, addressing suicide risk in individuals with ADHD requires a comprehensive, lifespan-oriented approach (Balazs & Kereszteny, 2017; Chen et al., 2014; Garas & Balazs, 2022). Early identification of high-risk subgroups—including females, young adults, and those with comorbid psychiatric disorders—is critical. Implementing multimodal interventions that integrate targeted screening, psychiatric management, and tailored prevention programs can play a pivotal role in reducing suicide risk in this vulnerable population.

Effective approaches typically integrate pharmacotherapy (such as stimulants, non-stimulants, mood stabilizers, or antidepressants when indicated) with cognitive behavioral therapy (CBT) aimed at improving emotional regulation, reducing impulsivity, and managing hopelessness (Rice et al., 2024). Family-based interventions help enhance communication and reduce conflict, while crisis management and suicide prevention safety plans address acute risks. Integrated care models that coordinate services between primary care providers, mental health specialists, and social services ensure a cohesive treatment approach (Zhang et al., 2025).

This comprehensive strategy addresses both the core symptoms of ADHD and the broader psychiatric vulnerabilities that contribute to suicidal behaviors, underscoring the necessity of a tailored, interdisciplinary response to this complex public health challenge.

4.2 Suicidal Behavior in Adolescents with ADHD

Adolescence represents a critical developmental window during which individuals with attention-deficit/hyperactivity disorder (ADHD) experience an elevated risk of suicidal behaviors (Austgulen et al., 2023; Fitzgerald et al., 2019). The core symptoms of ADHD—impulsivity, inattention, and hyperactivity—contribute to academic underachievement, social difficulties, and emotional dysregulation, all of which are well-established risk factors for suicidality (Fitzgerald et al., 2019). These vulnerabilities are further compounded by comorbid psychiatric conditions, particularly depression and anxiety disorders, which are disproportionately prevalent among adolescents with ADHD (Fitzgerald et al., 2019).

4.2.1 *Epidemiological Evidence: ADHD and Suicide Attempts in Adolescents*

A nationwide longitudinal study in Sweden found that adolescents with ADHD are at a substantially higher risk of attempting suicide compared to their non-ADHD counterparts (Huang et al., 2018). The relative risk (RR) for suicide attempts in adolescents with ADHD is estimated to be between 3.5 and 5.2, with an even greater risk observed among those with co-occurring mood disorders (Fitzgerald et al., 2019). The presence of comorbid depression increases the likelihood of suicidal behaviors by more than tenfold (adjusted IRR = 10.8), further highlighting the urgent need for early identification and targeted interventions in this population (Fitzgerald et al., 2019).

4.2.2 *The Role of Impulsivity in Suicide Risk*

Impulsivity—a defining feature of ADHD—directly heightens suicide risk by increasing the likelihood of engaging in high-risk behaviors, such as substance use, reckless decision-making, and delinquency (Austgulen et al., 2023; Fitzgerald et al., 2019). Studies indicate that adolescents with ADHD who exhibit higher impulsivity scores are significantly more likely to engage in self-harm or suicide attempts, particularly when experiencing acute distress or interpersonal conflicts (Austgulen et al., 2023; Septier et al., 2019). Emotional dysregulation further amplifies this vulnerability, as difficulties in managing frustration and distress can lead to rapid escalation from suicidal ideation to suicidal action (Septier et al., 2019).

4.2.3 *Protective and Risk-Modifying Factors: The Role of Family and Social Support*

Family dynamics serve as both protective and risk-enhancing factors in adolescent suicide risk (Chou et al., 2016). Supportive family environments—characterized by open communication, emotional validation, and effective problem-solving—are associated with lower suicide risk, including among adolescents with ADHD. For these individuals, consistent parental involvement and monitoring are linked to reduced rates of suicidal ideation and self-harm.

Importantly, clinical guidelines recommend that for adolescents with ADHD and significant functional impairment, pharmacological treatment may be initiated alongside psychosocial interventions once a thorough assessment has been conducted. In these cases, family-based interventions play a dual role—providing emotional stability and enhancing adherence to treatment plans, which in turn can mitigate suicide risk.

These findings underscore the value of integrating family-focused approaches into ADHD care, combining psychoeducation, communication skills training, and, when indicated, timely initiation of medication to address both core ADHD symptoms and associated emotional or behavioral difficulties.

Family context plays a critical role in shaping the mental health outcomes of adolescents with ADHD (Connell et al., 2016). High levels of familial conflict, punitive or authoritarian parenting styles, and limited parental understanding of ADHD symptoms have all been shown to exacerbate psychological distress and elevate risk for suicidal behaviors (Connell et al., 2016). Recent network analyses demonstrate that negative parenting contributes to suicidal ideation indirectly through mechanisms such as affective lability, rumination, anxiety, and depression (Ou et al., 2023). Likewise, a systematic review found that family dysfunction—including inconsistent discipline, poor emotional support, and hostile parent-child interactions—remains a robust predictor of suicidal spectrum behaviors in ADHD, even after accounting for psychiatric comorbidities (Austgulen et al., 2023). These findings underscore the need for family-centered interventions, including psychoeducation about ADHD, parent training to promote supportive parenting practices, and structured family therapy, as integral components of suicide prevention strategies for this high-risk population (Connell et al., 2016). Adolescents with ADHD who perceive parental rejection or experience frequent family conflict are at a threefold higher risk of suicide attempts compared to those raised in more supportive environments. The interplay between ADHD symptoms and family dynamics highlights the need for interventions that not only target the individual but also address family-level risk and protective factors to effectively reduce the risk of suicide in this vulnerable population (Daviss & Diler, 2014).

4.2.4 Clinical Implications: Enhancing Prevention Strategies

Given the heightened risk of suicidality among adolescents with ADHD, multifaceted intervention strategies are required to mitigate suicide risk (Faraone et al., 2021). Behavioral interventions such as cognitive behavioral therapy (CBT) and dialectical behavior therapy (DBT) should be integrated into ADHD treatment to address core issues including impulsivity, emotional dysregulation, and maladaptive coping mechanisms. Emotional regulation training programs that build adaptive coping skills, distress tolerance, and emotional self-regulation have also shown promise in reducing suicide risk in this population (Asarnow et al., 2021).

Family-based psychoeducation and therapy are critical in equipping caregivers with evidence-based parenting strategies that strengthen protective family dynamics and enhance adolescent resilience against suicidal behaviors (Ibrahim et al., 2017). Additionally, schools play a key role in prevention by implementing tailored academic support plans and social skills training to reduce school-related stressors, which are known contributors to suicidality in adolescents with ADHD. Together, these integrated strategies provide a comprehensive framework for reducing suicide risk and promoting well-being among adolescents with ADHD.

4.3 Transition to Adulthood: Persistent Risks

As individuals with attention-deficit/hyperactivity disorder (ADHD) transition into adulthood, the persistence of core symptoms—inattention, hyperactivity, and impulsivity—continues to exacerbate challenges in multiple domains, including employment, interpersonal relationships, and academic or professional achievement (APA, 2013). These ongoing difficulties frequently contribute to psychosocial distress, economic hardship, and increased suicidality.

4.3.1 Epidemiological Evidence: Suicide Risk in Adults with ADHD

A nationwide study in Denmark found that adults with ADHD have a nearly fivefold increased risk (IRR = 4.9) of attempting suicide compared to the general population (Fitzgerald et al., 2019). Notably, this elevated risk persists even after adjusting for psychiatric comorbidities, suggesting that ADHD itself is an independent risk factor for suicidality (Fitzgerald et al., 2019). In cases where ADHD coexists with depression or substance use disorders, the risk escalates further, with adjusted hazard ratios (HR) exceeding 10.0 for suicide attempts and completions (Fitzgerald et al., 2019).

Additionally, a longitudinal cohort study in the United States reported that 48.6% of adults with ADHD experience suicidal ideation at some point in their lives, compared to 14.2% of individuals without ADHD (Jeng et al., 2025). These findings underscore the need for proactive suicide prevention strategies that extend beyond managing co-occurring mental health conditions.

4.3.2 Occupational Challenges and Their Impact on Suicide Risk

Adults with ADHD often encounter significant occupational challenges stemming from difficulties with time management, organization, sustained attention, and impulse control, which frequently impair workplace performance. Studies have shown that adults with ADHD are approximately 60% more likely to experience job instability, including frequent job changes, underemployment, and financial insecurity (Ahlberg et al., 2023). Moreover, these individuals face significantly higher rates of workplace conflicts and terminations, leading to lower self-esteem and chronic stress (Küpper et al., 2012). Occupational instability contributes to an increased risk of hopelessness and suicidal ideation, with an adjusted incidence rate ratio (IRR) of 3.2 among unemployed individuals with ADHD (Ahlberg et al., 2023).

Addressing these challenges requires tailored workplace accommodations, structured coaching programs, and executive function training, which have been identified as critical interventions to reduce occupational stress and enhance job retention among adults with ADHD. By implementing these supports, it is possible to mitigate the risk of suicidal behaviors and improve overall well-being in this vulnerable population.

4.3.3 Interpersonal Dysfunction: A Key Contributor to Suicidality

Impaired emotional regulation, impulsivity, and executive dysfunction frequently result in conflict-laden interpersonal relationships among adults with ADHD, contributing to an elevated risk of suicidality. Studies show that adults with ADHD experience higher rates of marital conflict and divorce, with divorced individuals demonstrating a twofold increase in suicide risk (IRR = 2.1) (Wymbs et al., 2008). Emotion dysregulation further contributes to domestic conflicts, leading to social isolation, loneliness, and relationship dissatisfaction (Fitzgerald et al., 2019). A meta-analysis found that relationship instability is a significant predictor of suicide attempts (OR = 3.5) in adults with ADHD (Fitzgerald et al., 2019). To address these challenges, multimodal interventions—including cognitive behavioral therapy (CBT) for emotional regulation, couple's therapy, and social communication training—are essential to improve interpersonal stability and reduce the risk of suicidal behaviors.

4.3.4 Comprehensive Management Strategies for Suicide Prevention

Given the persistent risks associated with ADHD in adulthood, long-term, integrated care approaches are essential for suicide prevention (Shahidullah et al., 2018). Pharmacological interventions should prioritize long-acting stimulants and non-stimulant medications, such as atomoxetine and extended-release guanfacine, to enhance executive function and manage core symptoms. For individuals with comorbid mood disorders, adjunctive treatment with SSRIs or mood stabilizers can be beneficial.

Psychotherapeutic approaches, including cognitive behavioral therapy (CBT) and dialectical behavior therapy (DBT), effectively target emotional dysregulation and impulsivity, while mindfulness-based interventions may reduce rumination and suicidality in adults with ADHD. Occupational and financial support programs, including executive function coaching, structured workplace accommodations, and financial planning, can mitigate job-related distress and impulsive spending. Interpersonal and social interventions, such as family-based therapy, partner psychoeducation, and peer support groups, are vital for improving relationship stability, reducing social isolation, and enhancing coping mechanisms.

4.4 Gender Differences in Suicide Risk Among ADHD Populations

4.4.1 Epidemiological Evidence of Gender Disparities

Gender plays a pivotal role in the clinical presentation of ADHD and its associated suicide risk. Large-scale national cohort studies from Sweden, Canada, and the United States have consistently demonstrated that females with ADHD face a disproportionately higher risk of suicidality compared to males (Babinski et al., 2020; Leibenluft et al., 2024; Wiglesworth et al., 2023). A Swedish nationwide birth cohort study reported that females with ADHD had a 9.1-fold increased risk of suicidal behavior, whereas males had a 3.4-fold increased risk compared to their non-ADHD counterparts (IRR = 9.1 vs. 3.4, $p < 0.001$) (Fitzgerald et al., 2019).

4.4.2 Internalizing vs. Externalizing Pathways to Suicide Risk

The pathways to suicidal behavior differ significantly between males and females with ADHD, driven by gendered symptom presentations in both ADHD core symptoms and psychiatric comorbidities (Ayano et al., 2023a, 2023b; Balazs & Kereszteny, 2017). Females with ADHD often display an internalizing symptom profile marked by inattention, cognitive fatigue, excessive self-criticism, and emotional dysregulation (Quinn & Madhoo, 2014). These features frequently co-occur with depression, anxiety, and eating disorders—conditions strongly linked to suicidal ideation and self-harm (Miranda et al., 2022).

In contrast, males with ADHD typically present an externalizing symptom profile characterized by hyperactivity, impulsivity, aggression, and oppositional behaviors (Pardini & Fite, 2010). This externalizing pathway increases the risk of conduct disorder (CD), antisocial traits, and substance use disorders (SUDs), all of which are key contributors to impulsive suicide attempts (Miranda et al., 2022; Pardini & Fite, 2010).

4.4.3 Diagnostic Delays and Late Recognition in Females

Females with ADHD often experience delayed diagnosis or misdiagnosis, which increases their exposure to untreated symptoms and heightens suicide risk (Armijo, 2024). Compared to males, females are less likely to exhibit overt hyperactivity and instead present with inattentiveness, emotional sensitivity, and excessive worry, leading to frequent misclassification as generalized anxiety disorder (GAD) or depression (Nussbaum, 2012). A Swedish national birth cohort study found that females diagnosed with ADHD after the age of 18 were 5.7 times more likely to attempt suicide than those diagnosed in childhood (HR = 5.7, 95% CI: 4.2–7.8, $p < 0.001$) (Fitzgerald et al., 2019). Conversely, early ADHD diagnosis was associated with a 40% lower risk of suicide in both males and females, highlighting the protective impact of timely recognition and intervention (Fitzgerald et al., 2019).

4.4.4 Hormonal and Neurobiological Factors Influencing Suicide Risk

Emerging research suggests that hormonal fluctuations across puberty, menstrual cycles, and perimenopause exacerbate ADHD symptoms and emotional instability in females, contributing to higher suicide risk (Rujoiu, 2023). Estrogen and progesterone fluctuations are known to intensify ADHD-related emotional dysregulation, particularly during the premenstrual phase, which can lead to increased impulsivity and depressive episodes in females (Roberts et al., 2018). Adolescent females with ADHD who experience pronounced hormonal variability, especially in the form of estradiol fluctuations, face a greater risk of suicide attempts compared to those with more stable hormonal patterns (Eng, 2024). Hormonal shifts, such as fluctuating estradiol levels, can intensify core ADHD-related challenges like emotional dysregulation and impulsivity, further increasing vulnerability to suicidal behaviors. This connection highlights the importance of considering biological factors, including hormonal variability, when assessing suicide risk in adolescent females with ADHD (Eng, 2024).

4.4.5 Clinical Implications and Gender-Sensitive Suicide Prevention

Given these gender-specific risk factors, suicide prevention strategies must be tailored to address the distinct pathways leading to suicidality in males and females with ADHD.

For Females with ADHD
Prioritize early screening for ADHD in adolescent females presenting with depression and anxiety. Implement integrated treatment approaches that combine ADHD medications—either stimulants or non-stimulants—with evidence-based psychotherapy such as cognitive behavioral therapy (CBT), dialectical behavior therapy (DBT), or acceptance and commitment therapy (ACT). Consider hormonal

modulation strategies, including oral contraceptives or selective serotonin reuptake inhibitors (SSRIs) for premenstrual mood symptoms, to help stabilize emotional fluctuations.

For Males with ADHD

Address impulsivity-driven suicide risk by incorporating emotion regulation and impulse control interventions into ADHD treatment plans. Screen for externalizing comorbidities—including conduct disorder (CD), substance use disorder (SUD), and antisocial personality disorder (ASPD)—which significantly increase the likelihood of impulsive suicide attempts. Strengthen substance use prevention programs targeting ADHD males at risk of self-medicating with alcohol or drugs.

4.5 Impact of Comorbid Psychiatric Disorders on Suicide Risk in ADHD

4.5.1 Epidemiological Evidence: The Amplification of Suicide Risk

The association between ADHD and suicidal behavior is substantially influenced by the presence of psychiatric comorbidities (Austgulen et al., 2023; Balazs & Kereszteny, 2017). Individuals diagnosed solely with ADHD demonstrate an elevated risk of suicidal behavior, with an incident rate ratio (IRR) of 4.09 (95% CI: 3.53–4.73) compared to those without ADHD (Fitzgerald et al., 2019). This risk is notably magnified in the presence of additional psychiatric conditions, where the IRR rises to 10.43 (95% CI: 9.53–11.41) (Fitzgerald et al., 2019). The most elevated risk occurs among individuals with psychiatric disorders other than ADHD, reflected in an IRR of 14.84 (95% CI: 14.52–15.17) (Fitzgerald et al., 2019).

Substance use disorder (SUD) emerges as a particularly potent comorbidity. While those with ADHD alone had an IRR of 2.90 (95% CI: 2.51–3.36), this increased to 21.55 (95% CI: 17.98–25.83) among individuals with both ADHD and SUD (Fitzgerald et al., 2019). Remarkably, this figure aligns closely with individuals with SUD but without ADHD (IRR: 25.12; 95% CI: 24.32–25.95) (Fitzgerald et al., 2019). These findings are consistent with the self-medication hypothesis, suggesting that impulsivity and emotional dysregulation characteristic of ADHD may drive maladaptive substance use, thereby compounding suicide risk.

The interplay between ADHD and neurodevelopmental comorbidities also merits attention. For example, the co-occurrence of ADHD and autism spectrum disorder (ASD) results in a marked increase in suicidality, with an IRR of 4.65 (95% CI: 3.25–6.66), compared to an IRR of 2.63 (95% CI: 2.27–3.05) for ADHD alone (Fitzgerald et al., 2019). Interestingly, those with ASD alone displayed a somewhat lower risk (IRR: 2.31; 95% CI: 1.98–2.71), underscoring a possible synergistic effect when ADHD and ASD co-occur (Fitzgerald et al., 2019).

Furthermore, a cumulative relationship is evident between the number of psychiatric comorbidities and suicide risk. The presence of one comorbid disorder results in an IRR of 4.76 (95% CI: 3.88–5.84); two comorbid disorders, 4.41 (95% CI: 3.47–5.61); and three or more comorbidities elevate the risk further to an IRR of 8.20 (95% CI: 7.36–9.13), relative to individuals without ADHD (Fitzgerald et al., 2019).

These findings collectively highlight the necessity of considering psychiatric comorbidities when assessing suicide risk in individuals with ADHD. From both a clinical and public health perspective, these data emphasize the importance of early identification and comprehensive intervention strategies that address both ADHD and its common comorbidities, particularly SUD and ASD. A multidisciplinary approach, incorporating psychiatric, behavioral, and psychosocial care, is essential to mitigate the heightened risk of suicidality in this vulnerable population.

4.5.2 *The Complex Relationship Between ADHD, Anxiety Disorders, and Suicide Risk*

The interaction between ADHD and anxiety disorders in relation to suicide risk presents a paradoxical pattern in the literature (Austgulen et al., 2023).

Some population-based studies suggest that individuals with ADHD and anxiety disorders have a slightly lower suicide risk compared to those with ADHD alone. For example, a Finnish national psychiatric registry reported that comorbid ADHD and anxiety disorders were associated with a 15% lower risk of suicide attempts (HR = 0.85, 95% CI: 0.78–0.91, $p = 0.004$) compared to ADHD without anxiety (Fitzgerald et al., 2019). This unexpected finding may be attributed to behavioral inhibition mechanisms in anxiety disorders, which could counteract the impulsive, high-risk behaviors commonly observed in ADHD.

However, other studies have found no protective effect of anxiety. For instance, a U.S. cohort reported a 9.95-fold increased suicide risk in individuals with both ADHD and generalized anxiety disorder (GAD) (OR = 9.95, 95% CI: 4.40–22.47, $p < 0.001$) (Yoshimasu et al., 2019).

4.5.3 *Mechanisms Linking Comorbidities to Suicidal Behavior in ADHD*

The cumulative burden of ADHD and psychiatric comorbidities on suicidality is driven by multiple mechanisms, including:

1. **Neurobiological and Executive Dysfunction Pathways:**
   ADHD is associated with prefrontal cortex dysregulation, leading to poor impulse control, emotional instability, and cognitive inflexibility (Arnsten, 2009). When ADHD coexists with major depressive disorder (MDD) or bipolar disorder, dopaminergic and serotonergic dysregulation further amplifies emo-

tional reactivity, increasing the likelihood of suicidal behaviors in response to stressors (van Heeringen & Mann, 2014).

2. **Behavioral and Psychosocial Stressors:**

   Comorbid psychiatric conditions introduce cascading social and occupational impairments, contributing to chronic stress, financial instability, and interpersonal conflicts (Barkley & Fischer, 2010). ADHD with comorbid conduct disorder (CD) or antisocial personality disorder (ASPD) is particularly associated with early-life adversity, substance misuse, and legal problems, all of which elevate suicide risk (Storebø & Simonsen, 2013; Zulauf et al., 2014).

3. **Treatment Gaps and Barriers to Care:**

   Individuals with ADHD and severe comorbidities frequently fall through gaps in mental healthcare systems, with undiagnosed or untreated conditions compounding their suicide risk (Balazs & Kereszteny, 2017). A Canadian healthcare utilization study found that only 36% of adults with ADHD and comorbid MDD received adequate psychiatric treatment, despite their heightened suicide risk (Schein et al., 2024).

4.5.4 Integrated Treatment Approaches for ADHD with Comorbid Disorders

Given the substantial suicide risk associated with comorbid ADHD, a multifaceted, evidence-based treatment strategy is essential (Chaplin, 2018; Wehmeier et al., 2010).

Pharmacological Treatment

ADHD with major depressive disorder (MDD) or bipolar disorder: Stimulant medications should only be introduced after mood stabilization has been achieved using mood stabilizers such as lithium, lamotrigine, or atypical antipsychotics.ADHD with substance use disorders (SUDs): Atomoxetine or bupropion is preferred over stimulant medications due to their lower potential for abuse.

Psychotherapy and Behavioral Interventions

Cognitive behavioral therapy (CBT) and dialectical behavior therapy (DBT) are recommended for emotion regulation and impulse control, particularly in individuals with ADHD and borderline personality traits or a history of recurrent suicidality.

Contingency management and motivational interviewing are critical for addressing ADHD in individuals with substance misuse histories.

Comprehensive Suicide Prevention Strategies

Routine suicide risk screening should be standard practice for individuals with ADHD and psychiatric comorbidities.

Crisis intervention and safety planning must be integrated into ADHD management protocols for high-risk individuals.

4.6 Preventive Strategies and Clinical Implications

4.6.1 Early Identification and Suicide Risk Screening

Comprehensive early identification and systematic suicide risk screening are critical to mitigating suicidality among individuals with ADHD and psychiatric comorbidities (Posner et al., 2011). Given the high prevalence of suicidal ideation and attempts in this population, integrating suicide risk assessment into standard ADHD evaluations is paramount (Crandal et al., 2022; Horowitz et al., 2023). Routine suicidality screening should be mandated for all individuals with ADHD, particularly those with co-occurring depression, anxiety disorders, or substance use disorders (SUDs).

Validated screening instruments, such as the Columbia-Suicide Severity Rating Scale (C-SSRS) and the Suicide Behaviors Questionnaire-Revised (SBQ-R), have demonstrated efficacy in identifying high-risk individuals requiring urgent intervention (Posner et al., 2011). Primary care physicians, psychiatrists, and educators should maintain a high index of suspicion for suicidal behaviors, especially in adolescents, young adults, and females with ADHD, as these subgroups exhibit disproportionately elevated risk (Diamond et al., 2017).

4.6.2 Integrated Multimodal Treatment Approaches

A multifaceted treatment strategy, combining pharmacological and psychosocial interventions, is essential for reducing suicide risk among individuals with ADHD (Chaplin, 2018; Wehmeier et al., 2010).

Pharmacological Interventions

Stimulant and non-stimulant medications help regulate impulsivity and emotional dysregulation, reducing the likelihood of reactive suicidal behaviors.Atomoxetine and bupropion may be preferable for individuals with comorbid substance use disorders due to their lower abuse potential.

Mood stabilizers (e.g., lithium, valproate, or lamotrigine) are indicated when ADHD coexists with bipolar disorder, mitigating mood instability-related suicidality.

Psychotherapeutic and Behavioral Interventions

Cognitive behavioral therapy (CBT) has been extensively validated for individuals with ADHD and co-occurring depression, improving cognitive control, distress tolerance, and suicide prevention skills (Schwenck et al., 2011). Dialectical behavior therapy (DBT), particularly emotion regulation and crisis survival modules, has shown efficacy in individuals with ADHD and borderline personality disorder (BPD), where impulsivity-driven suicidality is pronounced (Schwenck et al., 2011). Behavioral activation strategies are beneficial for individuals with ADHD and anhedonic depression, reducing passive suicidal ideation.

4.6.3 Family and Community-Based Suicide Prevention Interventions

Family environment and social support networks play a pivotal role in mitigating suicide risk among individuals with ADHD (Cai et al., 2023). Parental psychoeducation and training programs equip caregivers with the skills to recognize early warning signs, de-escalate crises, and reinforce adaptive coping strategies.

Family-based interventions, including multisystemic therapy (MST) and functional family therapy (FFT), have demonstrated efficacy in reducing suicidality among adolescents with ADHD and externalizing disorders (Schoenwald & Henggeler, 2005). Community-based support groups and peer mentorship programs provide essential social connectedness, reducing isolation and hopelessness—key risk factors for suicide (Foster et al., 2017; Harrison, 2015). School-based interventions, including mental health literacy programs and structured mentoring for ADHD students, improve self-regulation and resilience, reducing suicide risk (Wasserman et al., 2015).

4.6.4 Suicide Risk Reduction in Schools and Workplaces

Individuals with ADHD face significant academic and occupational challenges, which may exacerbate psychological distress and increase suicide risk.

Educational Accommodations
Schools should implement individualized education plans (IEPs) and behavioral interventions to reduce ADHD-related academic stress.

Executive function coaching and structured learning supports enhance academic engagement, reducing school dropout rates and associated suicide risk.

Anti-bullying initiatives are critical, as individuals with ADHD are disproportionately targeted for peer victimization, a known risk factor for suicidality.

Workplace Adaptations
Adults with ADHD often experience occupational instability, job-related stress, and financial difficulties, all of which are linked to an elevated risk of suicide.

Employers should adopt ADHD-inclusive workplace policies, including flexible schedules, structured task management, and behavioral coaching.

4.6.5 Crisis Intervention and Access to Mental Health Services

For individuals experiencing acute suicidal crises, rapid-access intervention services are essential.

Crisis helplines and mobile psychiatric crisis units should be widely accessible, particularly for young adults with ADHD, who exhibit elevated acute suicide risk.

Digital health solutions, including telepsychiatry, mobile crisis counseling, and AI-driven mental health apps, have emerged as viable tools for supporting high-risk ADHD populations.

Emergency department (ED) suicide prevention protocols should incorporate ADHD-specific risk assessments to ensure that individuals are not prematurely discharged without appropriate follow-up care.

4.6.6 Research and Policy Implications: Addressing ADHD-Related Suicide Disparities

Neurobiological Research Priorities
Further research into dopaminergic and serotonergic dysregulation in ADHD-related suicidality is essential for refining targeted pharmacological interventions.

Addressing ADHD Stigma and Mental Health Disparities
Public health campaigns should increase ADHD awareness and reduce diagnostic stigma, particularly among females, racial minorities, and low-income populations.

Expanding universal ADHD screening programs may improve early detection and access to mental health services, thereby reducing long-term suicide risk.

Summary
This chapter critically examines the association between attention-deficit/hyperactivity disorder (ADHD) and suicide risk, highlighting the developmental trajectory, gender differences, comorbidities, and prevention strategies.

ADHD as a Suicide Risk Factor: Evidence indicates that ADHD significantly increases the risk of suicidal behaviors, with an elevated incidence rate ratio (IRR) for suicide attempts across all age groups. The risk is particularly pronounced in adolescents, young adults, and individuals with psychiatric comorbidities.

Suicide Risk in Adolescents with ADHD: Adolescence represents a critical period where impulsivity, emotional dysregulation, and externalizing behaviors contribute to higher rates of suicidal ideation and attempts. Early intervention and family-based support systems are essential in mitigating this risk.

Transition to Adulthood and Persistent Risks: Adults with ADHD continue to experience occupational instability, interpersonal difficulties, and financial stressors, which exacerbate suicide vulnerability. Integrated workplace interventions and lifelong mental health support are essential for reducing long-term risk.

Gender-Specific Suicide Risk in ADHD: Females with ADHD exhibit disproportionately higher suicide risk, largely due to internalizing symptomatology, underdiagnosis, and co-occurring mood disorders. In contrast, males with ADHD are more likely to present with externalizing behaviors, impulsivity-driven suicidality, and substance use disorders.

Impact of Comorbid Psychiatric Disorders: ADHD frequently coexists with depression, bipolar disorder, anxiety, borderline personality disorder, and substance use disorders, significantly amplifying suicide risk. The presence of multiple comorbidities correlates with exponentially higher suicidal behavior incidence.

Preventive Strategies and Clinical Implications: Early screening, multimodal treatment approaches, and crisis intervention strategies play a pivotal role in suicide prevention. Integrated care models incorporating pharmacological, behavioral, and family-based interventions have demonstrated efficacy in mitigating risk across the lifespan.

This chapter underscores the urgent need for a multidisciplinary, lifespan-oriented approach to address the complex interplay between ADHD and suicidality. Enhancing early detection, targeted interventions, and policy-driven mental health initiatives will be critical in reducing the global burden of ADHD-related suicidality.

References

Ahlberg, R., Du Rietz, E., Ahnemark, E., Andersson, L. M., Werner-Kiechle, T., Lichtenstein, P., Larsson, H., & Garcia-Argibay, M. (2023). Real-life instability in ADHD from young to middle adulthood: A nationwide register-based study of social and occupational problems. *BMC Psychiatry, 23*(1), 336. https://doi.org/10.1186/s12888-023-04713-z

APA. (2013). Diagnostic and statistical manual of mental disorders. *American Psychiatric Association, 21*(21), 591–643.

Armijo, C. (2024). *Leading causes of women going undiagnosed with ADHD and the impacts of going undiagnosed in adulthood California*. State University, Northridge.

Arnsten, A. F. (2009). The emerging neurobiology of attention deficit hyperactivity disorder: The key role of the prefrontal association cortex. *The Journal of Pediatrics, 154*(5), I-S43. https://doi.org/10.1016/j.jpeds.2009.01.018

Asarnow, J. R., Berk, M. S., Bedics, J., Adrian, M., Gallop, R., Cohen, J., Korslund, K., Hughes, J., Avina, C., Linehan, M. M., & McCauley, E. (2021). Dialectical behavior therapy for suicidal self-harming youth: Emotion regulation, mechanisms, and mediators. *Journal of the American Academy of Child & Adolescent Psychiatry, 60*(9), 1105–1115.e1104. https://doi.org/10.1016/j.jaac.2021.01.016

Austgulen, A., Skram, N. K. G., Haavik, J., & Lundervold, A. J. (2023). Risk factors of suicidal spectrum behaviors in adults and adolescents with attention-deficit/hyperactivity disorder—A systematic review. *BMC Psychiatry, 23*(1), 612. https://doi.org/10.1186/s12888-023-05099-8

Ayano, G., Demelash, S., Gizachew, Y., Tsegay, L., & Alati, R. (2023a). The global prevalence of attention deficit hyperactivity disorder in children and adolescents: An umbrella review of meta-analyses. *Journal of Affective Disorders, 339*, 860–866. https://doi.org/10.1016/j.jad.2023.07.071

Ayano, G., Tsegay, L., Gizachew, Y., Necho, M., Yohannes, K., Abraha, M., Demelash, S., Anbesaw, T., & Alati, R. (2023b). Prevalence of attention deficit hyperactivity disorder in adults: Umbrella review of evidence generated across the globe. *Psychiatry Research, 328*, 115449. https://doi.org/10.1016/j.psychres.2023.115449

Babinski, D. E., Neely, K. A., Ba, D. M., & Liu, G. (2020). Depression and suicidal behavior in young adult men and women with ADHD: Evidence from claims data. *The Journal of Clinical Psychiatry, 81*(6), 22578.

Balazs, J., & Kereszteny, A. (2017). Attention-deficit/hyperactivity disorder and suicide: A systematic review. *World Journal of Psychiatry, 7*(1), 44–59. https://doi.org/10.5498/wjp.v7.i1.44

Barkley, R. A., & Fischer, M. (2010). The unique contribution of emotional impulsiveness to impairment in major life activities in hyperactive children as adults. *Journal of the American Academy of Child & Adolescent Psychiatry, 49*(5), 503–513. https://doi.org/10.1016/j.jaac.2010.01.019

Cai, C., Yin, C., Tong, Y., Qu, D., Ding, Y., Ren, D., Chen, P., Yin, Y., An, J., & Chen, R. (2023). Development of the life gatekeeper suicide prevention training programme in China: A Delphi study. *General Psychiatry, 36*(5), e101133. https://doi.org/10.1136/gpsych-2023-101133

Chaplin, S. (2018). Attention deficit hyperactivity disorder: Diagnosis and management. *Progress in Neurology and Psychiatry, 22*(3), 27–29.

Chen, Q., Sjölander, A., Runeson, B., D'Onofrio, B. M., Lichtenstein, P., & Larsson, H. (2014). Drug treatment for attention-deficit/hyperactivity disorder and suicidal behaviour: Register based study. *BMJ, 348*.

Chou, W.-J., Liu, T.-L., Hu, H.-F., & Yen, C.-F. (2016). Suicidality and its relationships with individual, family, peer, and psychopathology factors among adolescents with attention-deficit/hyperactivity disorder. *Research in Developmental Disabilities, 53-54*, 86–94. https://doi.org/10.1016/j.ridd.2016.02.001

Connell, A. M., McKillop, H. N., & Dishion, T. J. (2016). Long-term effects of the family check-up in early adolescence on risk of suicide in early adulthood. *Suicide & Life-Threatening Behavior, 46*(Suppl 1), S15–S22. https://doi.org/10.1111/sltb.12254

Crandal, B. R., Aguinaldo, L. D., Carter, C., Billman, G. F., Sanderson, K., & Kuelbs, C. (2022). Opportunities for early identification: Implementing universal depression screening with a pathway to suicide risk screening in a pediatric health care system. *The Journal of Pediatrics, 241*, 29–35.e21.

Daviss, W. B., & Diler, R. S. (2014). Suicidal behaviors in adolescents with ADHD: Associations with depressive and other comorbidity, parent–child conflict, trauma exposure, and impairment. *Journal of Attention Disorders, 18*(8), 680–690.

Diamond, G. S., Herres, J. L., Ewing, E. S. K., Atte, T. O., Scott, S. W., Wintersteen, M. B., & Gallop, R. J. (2017). Comprehensive screening for suicide risk in primary care. *American Journal of Preventive Medicine, 53*(1), 48–54.

Eng, A. G. (2024). *Hormonal effects on ADHD symptoms in adolescents across the menstrual cycle*. University of Kentucky.

Faraone, S. V., et al. (2021). The World Federation of ADHD International Consensus Statement: 208 evidencebased conclusions about the disorder. *Neuroscience & Biobehavioral Reviews, 128*, 789–818.

Fitzgerald, C., Dalsgaard, S., Nordentoft, M., & Erlangsen, A. (2019). Suicidal behaviour among persons with attention-deficit hyperactivity disorder. *British Journal of Psychiatry, 215*(4), 615–620. https://doi.org/10.1192/bjp.2019.128

Foster, C. E., Horwitz, A., Thomas, A., Opperman, K., Gipson, P., Burnside, A., Stone, D. M., & King, C. A. (2017). Connectedness to family, school, peers, and community in socially vulnerable adolescents. *Children and Youth Services Review, 81*, 321–331.

Garas, P., & Balazs, J. (2022). Long-term suicide risk of children and adolescents with attention deficit and hyperactivity disorder—A systematic review. *European Psychiatry, 65*(S1), S324–S325. https://doi.org/10.1192/j.eurpsy.2022.826

Harrison, K. B. (2015). *The impact of mentoring adolescents with ADHD on life satisfaction in adulthood.* Fielding Graduate University.

Horowitz, L. M., Ryan, P. C., Wei, A. X., Boudreaux, E. D., Ackerman, J. P., & Bridge, J. A. (2023). Screening and assessing suicide risk in medical settings: Feasible strategies for early detection. *Focus, 21*(2), 145–151.

Huang, K.-L., Wei, H.-T., Hsu, J.-W., Bai, Y.-M., Su, T.-P., Li, C.-T., Lin, W.-C., Tsai, S.-J., Chang, W.-H., Chen, T.-J., & Chen, M.-H. (2018). Risk of suicide attempts in adolescents and young adults with attention-deficit hyperactivity disorder: A nationwide longitudinal study. *The British Journal of Psychiatry, 212*(4), 234–238. https://doi.org/10.1192/bjp.2018.8

Ibrahim, M., Russon, J., & Diamond, G. (2017). Attachment-based family therapy for depressed and suicidal adolescents: Development, research and clinical practice. In U. Kumar (Ed.), *Handbook of suicidal behaviour* (pp. 505–521). Springer Singapore. https://doi.org/10.1007/978-981-10-4816-6_27

Jeng, J.-S., Huang, H.-H., Chang, W.-H., Cheng, C.-M., Su, T.-P., Chen, T.-J., Tsai, S.-J., & Chen, M.-H. (2025). Longitudinal study on all-cause and suicide mortality among individuals with attention deficit hyperactivity disorder. *European Child & Adolescent Psychiatry, 34*(3), 1229–1238. https://doi.org/10.1007/s00787-024-02511-w

Küpper, T., Haavik, J., Drexler, H., Ramos-Quiroga, J. A., Wermelskirchen, D., Prutz, C., & Schauble, B. (2012). The negative impact of attention-deficit/hyperactivity disorder on occupational health in adults and adolescents. *International Archives of Occupational and Environmental Health, 85*, 837–847.

Leibenluft, E., Allen, L. E., Althoff, R. R., Brotman, M. A., Burke, J. D., Carlson, G. A., Dickstein, D. P., Dougherty, L. R., Evans, S. C., & Kircanski, K. (2024). Irritability in youths: A critical integrative review. *American Journal of Psychiatry, 181*(4), 275–290.

Ljung, T., Chen, Q., Lichtenstein, P., & Larsson, H. (2014). Common etiological factors of attention-deficit/hyperactivity disorder and suicidal behavior: A population-based study in Sweden. *JAMA Psychiatry, 71*(8), 958–964.

Miranda, J., Barbosa, M., Tarelho, A., & Guedes, R. (2022). Living on the edge: A review on potential risk factors for suicide in adult attention-deficit/hyperactivity disorder. *European Psychiatry, 65*(S1), S184–S184. https://doi.org/10.1192/j.eurpsy.2022.485

Nussbaum, N. L. (2012). ADHD and female specific concerns: A review of the literature and clinical implications. *Journal of Attention Disorders, 16*(2), 87–100.

Ou, W., Yang, Y., Chen, Y., Li, Y., Yang, S., Lu, Y., Li, L., Huang, M., Ma, M., Lv, G., Zhao, X., Qing, Y., Ju, Y., & Zhang, Y. (2023). Bridge symptoms between parenting styles and proximal psychological risk factors associated with adolescent suicidal thoughts: A network analysis. *Child and Adolescent Psychiatry and Mental Health, 17*(1), 129. https://doi.org/10.1186/s13034-023-00674-z

Pardini, D. A., & Fite, P. J. (2010). Symptoms of conduct disorder, oppositional defiant disorder, attention-deficit/hyperactivity disorder, and callous-unemotional traits as unique predictors of psychosocial maladjustment in boys: Advancing an evidence base for DSM-V. *Journal of the American Academy of Child & Adolescent Psychiatry, 49*(11), 1134–1144.

Posner, K., Brown, G. K., Stanley, B., Brent, D. A., Yershova, K. V., Oquendo, M. A., Currier, G. W., Melvin, G. A., Greenhill, L., Shen, S., & Mann, J. J. (2011). The Columbia-suicide severity rating scale: Initial validity and internal consistency findings from three multisite studies with adolescents and adults. *The American Journal of Psychiatry, 168*(12), 1266–1277. https://doi.org/10.1176/appi.ajp.2011.10111704

Quinn, P. O., & Madhoo, M. (2014). A review of attention-deficit/hyperactivity disorder in women and girls: Uncovering this hidden diagnosis. *The Primary Care Companion for CNS Disorders, 16*(3), 27250. https://doi.org/10.4088/PCC.13r01596

Rice, K. M., Peltzman, T., Gottlieb, D., Shiner, B., & Watts, B. V. (2024). Stimulant medication and suicide mortality in attention-deficit hyperactivity disorder. *BJPsych Open, 10*(1), e33. https://doi.org/10.1192/bjo.2023.643

Roberts, B., Eisenlohr-Moul, T., & Martel, M. M. (2018). Reproductive steroids and ADHD symptoms across the menstrual cycle. *Psychoneuroendocrinology, 88*, 105–114.

Rujoiu, P. B. (2023). *The effect of sex hormones on attention-deficit/hyperactivity disorder symptoms in women: A systematic review.*

Schein, J., Cloutier, M., Gauthier-Loiselle, M., Bungay, R., Chen, K., Chan, D., & Childress, A. (2024). Health care resource utilization and costs associated with psychiatric comorbidities in adult patients with attention-deficit/hyperactivity disorder. *Journal of Managed Care & Specialty Pharmacy, 30*(6), 588–598.

Schoenwald, S. K., & Henggeler, S. W. (2005). Multisystemic therapy for adolescents with serious externalizing problems. In *Handbook of clinical family therapy* (pp. 103–127). John Wiley & Sons, Inc.

Schwenck, C., Schmitt, D., Sievers, S., Romanos, M., Warnke, A., & Schneider, W. (2011). Cognitive and emotional empathy in children with ADHD and conduct disorder. *Zeitschrift fur Kinder-und Jugendpsychiatrie und Psychotherapie, 39*(4), 265–276.

Septier, M., Stordeur, C., Zhang, J., Delorme, R., & Cortese, S. (2019). Association between suicidal spectrum behaviors and attention-deficit/hyperactivity disorder: A systematic review and meta-analysis. *Neuroscience & Biobehavioral Reviews, 103*, 109–118.

Shahidullah, J. D., Carlson, J. S., Haggerty, D., & Lancaster, B. M. (2018). Integrated care models for ADHD in children and adolescents: A systematic review. *Families, Systems & Health, 36*(2), 233.

Storebø, O. J., & Simonsen, E. (2013). The association between ADHD and antisocial personality disorder (ASPD): A review. *Journal of Attention Disorders, 20*(10), 815–824. https://doi.org/10.1177/1087054713512150

Trivedi, C., Nandakumar, A. L., Yousefzadehfard, Y., Goriparthi, T. S., Chaudhari, G., Vora, D., Mansuri, Z., & Jain, S. (2023). Suicide risk among adolescents with ADHD: An overview from the national inpatient sample data set. *The Journal of Nervous and Mental Disease, 211*(3), 216–220.

van Heeringen, K., & Mann, J. J. (2014). The neurobiology of suicide. *The Lancet Psychiatry, 1*(1), 63–72. https://doi.org/10.1016/S2215-0366(14)70220-2

Wasserman, D., Hoven, C. W., Wasserman, C., Wall, M., Eisenberg, R., Hadlaczky, G., Kelleher, I., Sarchiapone, M., Apter, A., Balazs, J., Bobes, J., Brunner, R., Corcoran, P., Cosman, D., Guillemin, F., Haring, C., Iosue, M., Kaess, M., Kahn, J.-P., et al. (2015). School-based suicide prevention programmes: The SEYLE cluster-randomised, controlled trial. *The Lancet, 385*(9977), 1536–1544. https://doi.org/10.1016/S0140-6736(14)61213-7

Wehmeier, P. M., Schacht, A., & Barkley, R. A. (2010). Social and emotional impairment in children and adolescents with ADHD and the impact on quality of life. *Journal of Adolescent Health, 46*(3), 209–217. https://doi.org/10.1016/j.jadohealth.2009.09.009

Wiglesworth, A., Falke, C. A., Fiecas, M., Luciana, M., Cullen, K. R., & Klimes-Dougan, B. (2023). Brain signatures in children who contemplate suicide: Learning from the large-scale ABCD study. *Psychological Medicine, 53*(5), 2164–2173.

Wymbs, B. T., Pelham, W. E., Jr., Molina, B. S., Gnagy, E. M., Wilson, T. K., & Greenhouse, J. B. (2008). Rate and predictors of divorce among parents of youths with ADHD. *Journal of Consulting and Clinical Psychology, 76*(5), 735–744. https://doi.org/10.1037/a0012719

Yoshimasu, K., Barbaresi, W. J., Colligan, R. C., Voigt, R. G., Killian, J. M., Weaver, A. L., & Katusic, S. K. (2019). Psychiatric comorbidities modify the association between childhood ADHD and risk for suicidality: A population-based longitudinal study. *Journal of Attention Disorders, 23*(8), 777–786. https://doi.org/10.1177/1087054717718264

Zhang, L., Zhu, N., Sjölander, A., Nourredine, M., Li, L., Garcia-Argibay, M., Kuja-Halkola, R., Brikell, I., Lichtenstein, P., D'Onofrio, B. M., Larsson, H., Cortese, S., & Chang, Z. (2025). ADHD drug treatment and risk of suicidal behaviours, substance misuse, accidental injuries, transport accidents, and criminality: Emulation of target trials. *BMJ, 390*, e083658. https://doi.org/10.1136/bmj-2024-083658

Zulauf, C. A., Sprich, S. E., Safren, S. A., & Wilens, T. E. (2014). The complicated relationship between attention deficit/hyperactivity disorder and substance use disorders. *Current Psychiatry Reports, 16*(3), 436. https://doi.org/10.1007/s11920-013-0436-6

Chapter 5
ADHD as a Disability: Legal, Social, and Educational Implications

Abstract This chapter explores the classification of attention-deficit/hyperactivity disorder (ADHD) as a disability and examines its legal, social, and educational implications. While ADHD is widely recognized as a neurodevelopmental condition that affects cognitive, emotional, and behavioral functioning, its status as a disability remains subject to debate across different jurisdictions. The extent to which individuals with ADHD receive legal protections, educational accommodations, and workplace adjustments is largely influenced by policy frameworks, cultural perceptions, and institutional practices.

The chapter analyzes how ADHD is defined within international disability laws, including frameworks such as the United Nations Convention on the Rights of Persons with Disabilities (UNCRPD) and national legislative systems. Particular attention is given to inconsistencies in disability recognition, highlighting how variations in diagnostic criteria and policy implementation affect individuals' access to education, employment, and social support systems.

Emphasis is placed on the educational impact of ADHD, including the barriers faced by students and the role of inclusive education policies in mitigating academic disadvantages. Additionally, the chapter examines workplace challenges, exploring the extent to which employees with ADHD benefit from anti-discrimination laws, reasonable accommodations, and employer support programs.

By integrating legal analysis, policy evaluation, and real-world case studies, this chapter provides a comprehensive perspective on ADHD as a disability. The discussion underscores the need for greater legislative clarity, enhanced institutional support, and advocacy efforts to ensure that individuals with ADHD receive equitable access to education, employment, and social resources.

G. Ayano et al., *ADHD Across the Lifespan*, SpringerBriefs in Modern Perspectives on Disability Research,
https://doi.org/10.1007/978-981-95-8712-4_5

5.1 Legal Recognition of ADHD as a Disability

The legal classification of attention-deficit/hyperactivity disorder (ADHD) as a disability varies widely across jurisdictions, impacting individuals' access to legal protections, accommodations, and essential services (U.S. Department of Justice, 2022; McCoy et al., 2023; Østerud, 2023; Weyandt & Dupaul, 2008).

While some countries explicitly recognize ADHD within disability legislation, others only provide classification when ADHD results in severe and persistent functional impairment support (McCoy et al., 2023; Østerud, 2023; Weyandt & Dupaul, 2008).

This inconsistency affects individuals' ability to secure educational support, workplace adjustments, and anti-discrimination protections.

5.1.1 ADHD in Disability Laws and Policies

In the United States, ADHD qualifies as a disability under the Americans with Disabilities Act (ADA, 1990) if it "substantially limits one or more major life activities," including learning, working, or social functioning. This classification provides individuals with legal protection against discrimination and ensures access to reasonable accommodations in both employment and educational settings (U.S. Department of Justice, 2022).

Additionally, ADHD is recognized under the "Other Health Impairment" (OHI) category in the Individuals with Disabilities Education Act (IDEA, 1975; amended 2004), enabling students to qualify for Individualized Education Programs (IEPs) or 504 Plans that provide structured educational support (Social Security Administration, 2023).

In the United Kingdom, ADHD is considered a disability under the Equality Act 2010 if it has a "substantial and long-term adverse effect" on an individual's ability to carry out daily activities. This Act mandates reasonable adjustments in employment, education, and public services to prevent discrimination and promote inclusivity (UK Government, 2010).

Australia's approach is more variable. Under the Disability Discrimination Act (DDA, 1992), ADHD is not automatically classified as a disability; individuals must demonstrate severe and permanent functional impairment to qualify for accommodations under this legislation (Australian Human Rights Commission, 2023). The National Disability Insurance Scheme (NDIS, 2013) does not typically provide funding for ADHD alone, but individuals with significant impairments may be eligible for support under Psychosocial Disability or Neurodevelopmental Disorders. Access to services under the NDIS is highly inconsistent and requires extensive documentation (National Disability Insurance Scheme (NDIS, 2022).

Furthermore, support for students with ADHD varies by state and territory, with some jurisdictions offering Individualized Education Plans (IEPs) or school-based adjustments. ADHD is not universally classified as a disability in Australian schools, and eligibility often depends on the severity of functional impairment (Department of Education Western Australia, 2022).

In the European Union, ADHD recognition and support differ significantly across member states. While countries such as Sweden and Denmark provide robust legal protections and educational accommodations, other nations offer limited recognition and inconsistent access to services (European Commission, 2021). Although the European Disability Strategy 2021–2030 aims to harmonize disability rights across the EU, ADHD-specific policies remain underdeveloped, resulting in disparities in workplace inclusion and educational opportunities (European Parliament, 2021).

5.1.2 Variability in Legal Definitions and Access to Support

The classification of ADHD as a disability is inconsistent across global legal frameworks, affecting individuals' ability to secure accommodations and financial support. In many jurisdictions, ADHD is only recognized as a disability when it is accompanied by severe, persistent functional impairment that significantly impacts education, employment, or daily living (Australian Human Rights Commission, 2012; European Parliament, 2021). This variability leads to inequities in disability benefits, insurance coverage, and legal protections.

Differences in Eligibility Criteria

In the United States, ADHD is considered a disability under the ADA if it "substantially limits major life activities," such as learning, working, or social functioning. However, access to Social Security Disability Insurance (SSDI) is rare and requires extensive evidence of functional impairment (Department of Education (USA), 2020; Social Security Administration, 2023).

In the United Kingdom, the Equality Act 2010 provides legal protections for individuals with ADHD, but securing accommodations often depends on the discretion of employers and educational institutions (U.S. Department of Justice, 2022).

Australia's approach is more restrictive; ADHD is not automatically classified as a disability under the Disability Discrimination Act (DDA, 1992) or the National Disability Insurance Scheme (NDIS, 2013). Only individuals who can demonstrate severe and permanent functional impairment qualify for disability support, resulting in inconsistent access to services (Australian Human Rights Commission, 2012; National Disability Insurance Scheme (NDIS, 2022).

Within the European Union, ADHD recognition varies significantly between member states. Sweden and Denmark offer robust accommodations, while countries like France and Italy provide limited legal recognition and inconsistent support (European Parliament, 2021).

Bureaucratic Barriers to Disability Status
Bureaucratic barriers further complicate the process of obtaining disability status for ADHD. Stringent and subjective eligibility assessments often require extensive clinician evaluations and administrative approvals, resulting in inconsistent determinations. Applicants must submit comprehensive medical and psychological assessments, often involving multiple specialist reports, making the process both costly and time-intensive. Additionally, limited public awareness and institutional knowledge about ADHD as a disability contribute to underdiagnosis and inadequate accommodations in workplaces and educational settings.

5.1.3 Legal Protections Against Discrimination

Despite legal frameworks designed to prevent discrimination, individuals with ADHD frequently experience challenges in education, employment, and healthcare (Australian Human Rights Commission, 2012; European Parliament, 2021). Enforcement of these protections is often inconsistent, leaving many individuals struggling to secure reasonable accommodations, job opportunities, and adequate support (McCoy et al., 2023; Østerud, 2023; Weyandt & Dupaul, 2008).

In the educational sector, students with ADHD theoretically qualify for individualized learning plans and classroom accommodations in many countries. However, inconsistent ADHD recognition frequently results in limited access to special education services and insufficient teacher training (Department of Education (USA), 2020; Department of Education Western Australia, 2022). In the United States, the IDEA (2004) and Section 504 of the Rehabilitation Act (1973) mandate accommodations such as extra test time and specialized instruction, but implementation varies widely by district (U.S. Department of Justice, 2022). In Australia, ADHD is not automatically covered under the National Disability Insurance Scheme (NDIS, 2013), restricting access to individualized school support (NDIS, 2022).

In the workplace, the ADA (1990) in the U.S.A. and the Equality Act 2010 in the UK provide legal protections against discrimination. Nonetheless, employees with ADHD often encounter stigma and may hesitate to disclose their diagnosis due to fears of job repercussions (Hotte-Meunier et al., 2024). Employers in many countries lack sufficient training on ADHD-related accommodations, contributing to inconsistent enforcement of workplace adjustment (Hotte-Meunier et al., 2024; Østerud, 2023).

Healthcare access presents another challenge. Individuals with ADHD frequently encounter difficulties in obtaining consistent medical care, particularly for medication, therapy, and disability benefits (McKenna et al., 2024). In some European nations, ADHD-related treatments are not fully covered by national health systems, creating financial barriers that limit access to essential care (Baweja et al., 2021).

Advocacy efforts continue to prioritize the standardization of ADHD classification as a disability on a global scale, aiming to strengthen workplace accommodations, reduce employment discrimination, and promote comprehensive public awareness campaigns to combat ADHD stigma.

5.2 Social Implications of ADHD as a Disability

The classification of attention-deficit/hyperactivity disorder (ADHD) as a disability has profound social implications, shaping public perceptions, stigma, and the lived experiences of individuals affected by the condition. Despite increasing awareness, misconceptions and societal biases continue to influence how individuals with ADHD navigate education, employment, healthcare, and social relationships (European Parliament, 2021; National Disability Insurance Scheme (NDIS, 2022).

5.2.1 Stigma and Misconceptions

ADHD remains widely misunderstood, with persistent myths regarding its origins, severity, and impact. Common misconceptions include the belief that ADHD is a result of laziness, poor discipline, or bad parenting, rather than a neurodevelopmental condition with a biological basis (Hinshaw & Scheffler, 2014). Additionally, ADHD is often perceived as an excuse for inattention or hyperactivity rather than recognized as a disorder characterized by executive function deficits affecting focus, impulse control, and emotional regulation (National Disability Insurance Scheme (NDIS, 2022). Another widespread misconception is that ADHD is overdiagnosed, particularly in children, despite evidence that ADHD remains underdiagnosed and undertreated in adults, women, and minority populations (Asherson et al., 2016; Sayal et al., 2018).

Impact of Stigma on Diagnosis and Treatment

Societal stigma frequently discourages individuals from seeking professional diagnosis or treatment due to fears of judgment, discrimination, or negative labeling (Corrigan et al., 2014). Parents of children with ADHD may delay seeking help, fearing their child will be perceived as disruptive in school settings (Sciutto & Eisenberg, 2007). Adults with ADHD may also avoid disclosure in workplace or healthcare settings to prevent being perceived as incompetent or unreliable (Faraone et al., 2021).

In workplace and educational settings, employers and educators often misinterpret ADHD symptoms as carelessness, lack of motivation, or irresponsibility (Faraone et al., 2021). Adults with ADHD frequently report negative workplace experiences, including dismissal, denied promotions, or reduced responsibilities (Erskine et al., 2016). Similarly, university students with ADHD often struggle to access accommodations due to skepticism about ADHD as a legitimate disability (Erskine et al., 2016).

The psychosocial consequences of these negative perceptions can be profound. Persistent societal judgment can lead to low self-esteem, anxiety, and depression among individuals with ADHD (Erskine et al., 2016; Klein et al., 2012). Social isolation is also common, as individuals with ADHD often feel misunderstood or judged by peers, family, and colleagues (Corrigan et al., 2014).

5.2.2 *Impact on Mental Health and Self-Identity*

The psychological and emotional consequences of ADHD-related stigma extend beyond discrimination, profoundly affecting an individual's mental health, self-esteem, and self-identity (Klein et al., 2012; Shaw et al., 2007). Many individuals with ADHD experience chronic self-doubt, internalized stigma, and difficulties in self-acceptance, particularly if diagnosed later in life (Erskine et al., 2016; Faraone et al., 2021).

Repeated negative feedback from teachers, peers, and employers can reinforce feelings of incompetence, increasing self-doubt and low self-worth (Corrigan et al., 2014). Individuals diagnosed in adulthood often grapple with regret and self-criticism over past difficulties that were previously unexplained (Asherson et al., 2016). Additionally, ADHD is frequently associated with higher rates of comorbid anxiety and depressive disorders, exacerbated by negative social interactions and perceived inadequacy (Barkley & Brown, 2008; Shaw et al., 2007). Fear of judgment or failure can contribute to avoidant behaviors in work and social settings, limiting opportunities for success and validation (Faraone et al., 2021).

Imposter syndrome is a common experience among individuals with ADHD, particularly those with high academic or professional achievements, who often feel their success is undeserved (Young & Goodman, 2016). This phenomenon is linked to masking behaviors, where individuals overcompensate through perfectionism or excessive work efforts to hide their struggles (F. Mowlem et al., 2019).

The classification of ADHD as a disability carries both positive and negative implications for self-identity and mental well-being. On the positive side, recognizing ADHD as a disability can validate lived experiences, providing relief and affirmation that reframes struggles as legitimate neurodevelopmental challenges rather than personal failures (Hinshaw & Scheffler, 2014). Legal recognition can also lead to improved access to workplace adjustments, educational accommodations, and disability benefits (Asherson et al., 2016). Moreover, a formal diagnosis can reduce self-blame by helping individuals understand their challenges as neurobiological rather than character flaws, fostering greater self-compassion (Corrigan et al., 2014).

However, there are potential negative effects associated with the disability label. Some individuals internalize negative stereotypes, perceiving themselves as "less capable" because of the disability classification (F. Mowlem et al., 2019). Fear of workplace discrimination or bias may also lead individuals to conceal their diagnosis, limiting access to necessary accommodations (Faraone et al., 2021). Additionally, some individuals may overidentify with ADHD, attributing all their difficulties to the disorder rather than recognizing areas for skill development and adaptation (Faraone et al., 2021).

5.3 ADHD in Education: Challenges and Accommodations

Attention-deficit/hyperactivity disorder (ADHD) significantly influences educational experiences, often posing challenges for students navigating traditional learning environments. The core symptoms of ADHD—inattention, impulsivity, and hyperactivity—can hinder academic achievement, affect classroom behavior, and contribute to higher dropout rates (Faraone et al., 2021; Sayal et al., 2018). However, with appropriate accommodations and targeted interventions, students with ADHD can achieve academic success and develop skills to enhance their educational outcomes (Hosseinnia et al., 2024; Raggi & Chronis, 2006).

5.3.1 Impact of ADHD on Learning and Academic Performance

ADHD disrupts conventional classroom engagement, as inattention, impulsivity, and hyperactivity interfere with students' ability to absorb and retain information (APA, 2013). Inattention challenges students' ability to maintain focus, follow multistep instructions, and complete tasks, leading to missed information, inconsistent performance, and incomplete assignments (Faraone et al., 2021). Impulsivity manifests as difficulty filtering thoughts before speaking or acting, often resulting in disruptive behavior, interruptions, and challenges adhering to classroom norms (George J DuPaul et al., 2011). Hyperactivity, characterized by an inability to remain still for prolonged periods, can cause restlessness, fidgeting, and reduced engagement in sedentary learning activities (Sayal et al., 2018). These issues not only impact academic performance but also influence peer relationships, teacher perceptions, and self-confidence (F. Mowlem et al., 2019).

Research demonstrates that students with ADHD experience lower academic achievement, increased grade retention, and a higher likelihood of school dropout (Karlsberg Bennett et al., 2020). Even when controlling for cognitive ability, students with ADHD tend to underperform in standardized tests and coursework across subjects like reading, writing, and mathematics (Galéra et al., 2009). Adolescents with ADHD are also two to three times more likely to repeat a grade or leave school early (George J. DuPaul et al., 2011). College students with ADHD report greater struggles with time management, independent learning, and sustained attention, leading to lower graduation rates compared to their neurotypical peers (Sedgwick-Müller et al., 2022).

Many academic struggles in ADHD stem from executive function (EF) deficits, which affect organization, time management, and working memory (Kofler et al., 2019). Students with ADHD often have difficulties managing assignments, planning long-term projects, and maintaining consistent study routines. Poor estimation of time required for tasks leads to chronic procrastination and inconsistent study habits (Chacko et al., 2024). Working memory limitations can make it challenging to retain information, follow multistep instructions, and solve complex problems, further impairing academic performance (Alderson et al., 2013). Without targeted support, these challenges can accumulate over time, increasing educational disengagement and mental health risks such as anxiety and depression (F. Mowlem et al., 2019).

5.3.2 Educational Accommodations and Legal Protections

Students with ADHD benefit from individualized support strategies to mitigate the impact of executive dysfunction and promote academic success. Many countries have enacted policies to protect students' educational rights, but implementation remains inconsistent (George J DuPaul et al., 2011; Sayal et al., 2018).

Legal frameworks supporting ADHD accommodations vary across countries. In the United States, the Individuals with Disabilities Education Act (IDEA, 2004) enables students with ADHD to qualify for Individualized Education Programs (IEPs) under the category of Other Health Impairment (OHI), providing specialized instruction and behavioral interventions (Department of Education (USA), 2020; U.S. Department of Justice, 2022). Additionally, Section 504 of the Rehabilitation Act (1973) ensures reasonable accommodations, such as extended test time and classroom modifications, even if students do not qualify for IDEA services (U.S. Department of Justice, 2022).

In the United Kingdom, the Special Educational Needs and Disability (SEND) Code of Practice (2015) outlines provisions for SEN support, including modified classroom instruction, behavioral interventions, and exam accommodations (UK Government, 2010). Education, Health, and Care Plans (EHCPs) provide legally binding educational support for students with significant impairments (Department for Education, 2022).

In Australia, the Disability Discrimination Act (DDA, 1992) protects students with ADHD from discrimination but does not automatically classify ADHD as a disability, requiring severe impairment for eligibility (Australian Human Rights Commission, 2012). State-based Special Educational Needs (SEN) programs offer varying levels of support, with inconsistent access to accommodations depending on the (Department of Education Western Australia, 2022).

The European Union's European Disability Strategy 2021–2030 aims to harmonize disability rights but lacks consistent ADHD-specific policies, leading to variations in educational support across member states (European Commission, 2021).

Common ADHD accommodations in schools include extra time on exams and assignments, which helps students compensate for working memory deficits and time management difficulties (Cole et al., 2024). Preferential seating, placing students close to the teacher, minimizes distractions and improves focus (George J. DuPaul et al., 2011). Modified workloads, which break tasks into smaller components, support task initiation and completion (Kofler et al., 2019). Assistive technology, such as digital tools, can aid organization, time management, and note-taking (Advokat et al., 2010). Additionally, behavioral support plans that incorporate structured self-regulation strategies have been shown to improve classroom engagement and academic performance (George J. DuPaul et al., 2011).

5.3.3 Challenges in Implementation

Despite legal protections, many students fail to receive adequate support due to systemic barriers, underdiagnosis, and limited school resources (George J DuPaul et al., 2011; Erskine et al., 2016). Underdiagnosis and late identification remain significant challenges, especially among females, high-achieving students, and ethnic minorities, delaying appropriate interventions and accommodations (!!! INVALID CITATION!!!). Without timely diagnosis, these students often navigate educational challenges without necessary support.

Limited school resources further complicate the provision of effective accommodations. Public schools frequently struggle with insufficient funding and a lack of trained personnel to implement individualized interventions, undermining efforts to support students with ADHD (Faraone et al., 2021). Educator training deficits also contribute to inconsistent support, as many teachers lack formal ADHD training and may misinterpret symptoms as behavioral problems rather than recognizing them as neurodevelopmental challenges (F. Mowlem et al., 2019).

Transitioning to higher education introduces additional barriers. Universities often rely on self-advocacy models, requiring students to navigate support services independently—an approach that places considerable demands on individuals already struggling with executive function deficits (Advokat et al., 2010). Increased academic demands in college settings, which emphasize greater independence and self-regulation, can exacerbate ADHD-related difficulties (Gee et al., 2020). These challenges collectively contribute to lower college completion rates among students with ADHD; fewer than 15% of students with ADHD complete a degree, compared to nearly 50% of their neurotypical peers (Kuriyan et al., 2013; Sedgwick-Müller et al., 2022).

5.4 ADHD and Employment: Workplace Challenges and Legal Protections

Attention-deficit/hyperactivity disorder (ADHD) significantly impacts occupational functioning, contributing to higher job turnover, lower job satisfaction, and workplace difficulties associated with executive dysfunction, time management challenges, and interpersonal conflicts (Barkley & Brown, 2008; Faraone et al., 2021). While legal protections exist in various jurisdictions, inconsistent recognition of ADHD as a workplace disability and stigma associated with disclosure create additional barriers to career stability and professional advancement (Young et al., 2020; Doyle, 2020).

5.4.1 ADHD and Occupational Functioning

Adults with ADHD often struggle with key workplace competencies due to core symptoms of inattention, impulsivity, and hyperactivity (Advokat et al., 2010). Time management and meeting deadlines can be particularly challenging, as individuals with ADHD frequently underestimate task duration, procrastinate, and struggle with prioritization. These issues often lead to missed deadlines and increased workplace stress (Barkley, 2018; Kofler et al., 2019). Organizational difficulties and challenges with multitasking are also common; executive function deficits can affect task planning, goal-setting, and project management, making it difficult to juggle multiple responsibilities effectively (Asherson et al., 2021).

Impulsivity may manifest as difficulty regulating emotions in high-pressure situations, which can negatively impact professional relationships. Moreover, sustaining attention on repetitive or low-stimulation tasks is often a significant barrier, as individuals with ADHD may find routine, detail-oriented work particularly challenging. This can result in inattentiveness and increased error rates, further exacerbating workplace difficulties (Faraone et al., 2021).

ADHD's impact on career outcomes is substantial. Higher job turnover is frequently observed, as individuals with ADHD may experience workplace conflicts, underperformance, or difficulty adapting to rigid work structures (Barkley & Brown, 2008). Lower job satisfaction and performance ratings are also common, with ADHD-related challenges often highlighted in performance reviews, overshadowing strengths such as creativity and problem-solving skills (Young et al., 2020). Additionally, difficulties in task completion, emotional regulation, and interpersonal communication contribute to increased workplace stress and comorbid mental health challenges, including anxiety and depression (Faraone et al., 2021).

5.4.2 Workplace Accommodations and Support

Legal frameworks mandate reasonable accommodations for employees with disabilities, including ADHD, in several countries (Doyle, 2020; Faraone et al., 2021). Despite these protections, many employees with ADHD do not request accommodations due to concerns about stigma, discrimination, or job security (Young et al., 2020).

In the United States, the Americans with Disabilities Act (ADA, 1990) requires employers to provide reasonable accommodations for individuals whose ADHD substantially limits major life activities (U.S. Department of Justice, 2022). Additionally, the Rehabilitation Act of 1973 prohibits discrimination against employees with ADHD in federally funded organizations. In the United Kingdom, the Equality Act (2010) mandates that employers implement reasonable workplace adjustments for employees with ADHD to ensure equal participation (UK Government, 2010). In Australia, the Disability Discrimination Act (DDA, 1992) protects employees with ADHD, though eligibility for accommodations typically depends on demonstrating severe functional impairment (Australian Human Rights Commission, 2023). Within the European Union, the European Disability Strategy 2021–2030 promotes workplace inclusion for neurodivergent individuals, but ADHD accommodations vary significantly across member states (European Commission, 2021).

Effective workplace accommodations for ADHD focus on reducing distractions, improving time management, and enhancing task organization. Flexible work schedules and remote work options can help mitigate executive function challenges and allow employees to work during periods of peak focus (Barkley, 2018; Weyandt & DuPaul, 2006). Structured task management systems and time supports, such as checklists and reminders, assist with prioritization and completion of work tasks (Doyle, 2020; Young et al., 2020). Providing noise reduction strategies and designated quiet workspaces can reduce environmental distractions and promote sustained attention (Asherson et al., 2021). Clear, written instructions and job expectations help ensure that employees understand their responsibilities and can organize their work effectively (DuPaul et al., 2011; Kofler et al., 2019).

5.4.3 Disclosure and Workplace Discrimination

The decision to disclose ADHD in the workplace is complex, carrying both potential benefits and risks. While disclosure can facilitate access to accommodations and legal protections, concerns about stigma and career limitations remain significant (Doyle, 2020; Young et al., 2020). Disclosure can be a pathway to workplace accommodations under disability legislation, providing necessary supports for improved job performance through structured workflows and management adjustments (Doyle, 2020; Weyandt & DuPaul, 2006). It also grants legal protection against discrimination, allowing employees to challenge unfair treatment (Faraone et al., 2021).

However, there are notable risks associated with disclosure. Individuals with ADHD may be overlooked for promotions or leadership roles due to stigma and misconceptions about their capabilities (Mowlem et al., 2019). Some employees face direct or indirect workplace discrimination, including micromanagement or exclusion from career opportunities (Asherson et al., 2021; Young et al., 2020). Additionally, concerns about job security and workplace culture, particularly in high-pressure environments, can deter disclosure.

Despite existing legal protections, cases of workplace discrimination persist, highlighting gaps in employer compliance and enforcement (Faraone et al., 2021). Legal frameworks provide protections against ADHD-related discrimination. In the United States, the Americans with Disabilities Act (1990) and the Rehabilitation Act (1973) mandate reasonable accommodations and prohibit workplace discrimination (U.S. Department of Justice, 2022). The United Kingdom's Equality Act (2010) requires employers to make reasonable adjustments for employees with ADHD (UK Government, 2010). In Australia, the Disability Discrimination Act (1992) protects against workplace discrimination, though accommodations often require demonstration of severe functional impairment (Australian Human Rights Commission, 2023). Within the European Union, the European Disability Strategy (2021–2030) promotes inclusion for neurodivergent individuals, but ADHD-specific implementation remains inconsistent (European Commission, 2021).

Landmark legal cases demonstrate the challenges employees face. In the United States, a 2019 lawsuit resulted in a $400,000 settlement after an employee with ADHD was denied accommodations and subsequently terminated. In the United Kingdom, a 2021 employment tribunal ruled in favor of a software engineer whose employer failed to provide reasonable adjustments. In Australia, a 2022 case involved an employee filing a complaint after being denied remote work accommodations (Australian Human Rights Commission, 2023). Despite these legal victories, many cases go unreported due to fear of employer retaliation and the complexity of legal proceedings (Doyle, 2020).

5.5 Policy and Future Directions

As awareness of attention-deficit/hyperactivity disorder (ADHD) grows, urgent policy reforms are needed to establish consistent legal recognition, improve workplace accommodations, and ensure equitable access to support services worldwide (Doyle, 2020; Faraone et al., 2021). Disparities in ADHD classification and disability status directly affect individuals' access to educational adjustments, workplace protections, and financial support (Asherson et al., 2021; Young et al., 2020). Advocacy groups continue to push for standardized policies that guarantee individuals with ADHD the necessary accommodations and legal protections to enhance their quality of life and productivity.

5.5.1 *Establishing Global Recognition of ADHD as a Disability*

The legal classification of ADHD as a disability varies across jurisdictions, shaping individuals' access to special education services, workplace accommodations, and government assistance programs (Australian Human Rights Commission, 2023; European Commission, 2021). These disparities have far-reaching consequences, leading to inconsistent support systems and unmet needs.

In the United States, ADHD is recognized as a disability under the Americans with Disabilities Act (ADA, 1990) and the Individuals with Disabilities Education Act (IDEA, 2004), allowing eligible students to access Individualized Education Programs (IEPs) and employees to receive reasonable accommodations (U.S. Department of Justice, 2022). In the United Kingdom, the Equality Act (2010) recognizes ADHD as a disability if it has a substantial and long-term impact on daily functioning. Individuals with severe ADHD may qualify for Special Educational Needs (SEN) programs and workplace adjustments (UK Government, 2010).

In Australia, ADHD is not automatically classified as a disability under the Disability Discrimination Act (DDA, 1992) or the National Disability Insurance Scheme (NDIS, 2013), limiting access to consistent accommodations. Recognition often depends on state-specific policies, which can result in unequal access to services (Australian Human Rights Commission, 2023; Department of Education Western Australia, 2022). Within the European Union, ADHD recognition and support policies vary across member states. While Sweden and Denmark provide extensive accommodations, many other countries lack ADHD-specific legal protections. The European Disability Strategy (2021–2030) aims to improve uniformity in disability rights but has yet to establish ADHD-focused policies (European Parliament, 2021).

The impact of inconsistent ADHD recognition is substantial. In countries where ADHD lacks formal recognition, individuals face barriers in obtaining disability benefits, financial aid, insurance coverage, and mental health care, limiting their ability to thrive (Faraone et al., 2021; Young et al., 2020). Students in countries with weaker ADHD policies often experience lower academic achievement and higher dropout rates due to inadequate educational support (DuPaul et al., 2011; Sayal et al., 2018). In the workplace, employees in regions with limited ADHD protections struggle with job security, career advancement, and stigma, which may discourage them from disclosing their diagnosis or seeking necessary accommodations (Doyle, 2020; Asherson et al., 2021).

5.5.2 Expanding Access to Educational and Workplace Accommodations

Systematic reforms in education and employment settings are critical to ensuring equitable access to accommodations for individuals with ADHD (Faraone et al., 2021; Young et al., 2020). Expanding ADHD-specific policies in schools and workplaces can improve long-term academic and professional outcomes, fostering greater inclusion and success.

In educational settings, mandatory ADHD training for educators should be prioritized to enhance the identification of ADHD, reduce stigma, and improve classroom accommodations (DuPaul et al., 2011; Zentall, 2012). Teacher training programs that incorporate ADHD-inclusive teaching strategies can empower educators to better support students with ADHD. Standardized academic support frameworks should also be implemented, incorporating Universal Design for Learning (UDL) approaches, alternative assessment methods, and assistive technologies to provide equitable opportunities for all students (Barkley, 2018; Kofler et al., 2019). Expanding school-based mental health services is equally important, as strengthened mental health support can facilitate early ADHD diagnosis and intervention, leading to improved academic outcomes and reduced dropout rates (Sayal et al., 2018).

In workplace settings, traditional disability frameworks often fail to address the specific challenges faced by employees with ADHD. Tailored accommodations, including flexible work schedules, structured task management systems, and quiet workspaces, are essential for supporting employees effectively (Asherson et al., 2021; Doyle, 2020). Corporate neurodiversity initiatives implemented by companies such as Microsoft and JPMorgan Chase have demonstrated the benefits of ADHD-inclusive hiring practices, highlighting the value of fostering neurodivergent-friendly workplaces. Additionally, implementing manager training programs on ADHD can reduce stigma and enhance support for employees with ADHD, ultimately improving productivity and job retention (Young et al., 2020).

5.5.3 Increasing Public Awareness and Reducing Stigma

Despite growing recognition of ADHD as a neurodevelopmental condition, stigma remains a significant barrier to diagnosis, treatment, and social inclusion (Faraone et al., 2021; Young et al., 2020). Public health campaigns, targeted awareness initiatives, and policy-driven mental health funding are crucial for combating misinformation and improving ADHD literacy.

Effective public health strategies can help dispel myths and misconceptions about ADHD, emphasizing that it is a legitimate neurodevelopmental disorder rather than a product of poor parenting or lack of discipline (Doyle, 2020; Sayal et al., 2018). Campaigns that highlight scientific findings and lived experiences can challenge stereotypes and reduce blame toward affected individuals and their families. Encouraging early diagnosis and intervention, particularly among adults, women, and minority groups, is essential to ensure timely access to support services (Mowlem et al., 2019). Many individuals in these groups remain underdiagnosed, leading to unnecessary challenges in educational and occupational settings.

Integrating ADHD-inclusive messaging into national mental health initiatives can further normalize the condition and promote acceptance of neurodiversity (Asherson et al., 2021). National health agencies should prioritize ADHD education alongside other mental health conditions, ensuring that ADHD is not marginalized within broader mental health frameworks. By combining these approaches, policymakers and advocates can foster a more supportive and inclusive environment for individuals with ADHD.

5.5.4 Future Research on ADHD and Disability Rights

Further research is needed to evaluate the effectiveness of ADHD policies, accommodations, and legal protections across different regions. A priority area of inquiry should be the long-term impact of ADHD accommodations on employment and educational outcomes. Examining how workplace and educational supports influence career progression, academic success, and overall well-being will help policymakers refine interventions and ensure that accommodations truly promote equity (Faraone et al., 2021; Weyandt & DuPaul, 2006).

Comparative analysis of ADHD-related disability laws is also essential for identifying best practices and gaps in protection. Evaluating legal frameworks such as the Americans with Disabilities Act (U.S.A.), the Equality Act (UK), and EU disability policies will enable researchers and advocates to recommend harmonized standards that promote consistent support for individuals with ADHD across different contexts (European Commission, 2021; Young et al., 2020).

Finally, research exploring neurodiversity advocacy and policy evolution is critical for understanding the role of ADHD within the broader neurodiversity movement and its implications for disability rights and public policy. This research can inform future initiatives aimed at fostering inclusion and reducing stigma in educational, occupational, and social settings (Doyle, 2020).

Summary

This chapter has explored the impact of ADHD across different aspects of society, focusing on education, employment, and legal protections. It highlights the challenges individuals with ADHD face in these domains and the policy reforms needed to ensure equitable access to support services.

In education, students with ADHD experience significant learning challenges due to inattention, impulsivity, and executive function deficits. Educational accommodations, such as extended test times, structured learning environments, and teacher training, are crucial for improving academic outcomes and promoting student success (Barkley, 2018; DuPaul et al., 2011).

Within the workplace, adults with ADHD often encounter difficulties in maintaining employment, navigating workplace relationships, and managing time effectively. Legal frameworks, including the Americans with Disabilities Act (ADA) in the United States and the Equality Act in the United Kingdom, provide workplace protections. However, inconsistent enforcement and stigma continue to be barriers to career advancement for individuals with ADHD (Doyle, 2020; Young et al., 2020).

Global disparities in the recognition of ADHD as a disability affect individuals' access to accommodations and support services. Advocacy efforts aim to promote policy consistency, workplace inclusivity, and public awareness to reduce stigma and improve outcomes (Asherson et al., 2021; European Commission, 2021).

Future directions and research should focus on expanding ADHD-specific policies in schools and workplaces, increasing public education, and enhancing neurodiversity initiatives to improve outcomes for individuals with ADHD. Ongoing research is essential to guide evidence-based interventions and policy reforms that can foster a more supportive environment (Faraone et al., 2021).

By addressing these issues through legal recognition, improved accommodations, and public awareness campaigns, societies can create a more inclusive environment that supports individuals with ADHD in achieving their full potential.

References

Advokat, C., Lane, S. M., & Luo, C. (2010). College students with and without ADHD: Comparison of self-report of medication usage, study habits, and academic achievement. *Journal of Attention Disorders, 15*(8), 656–666. https://doi.org/10.1177/1087054710371168

Alderson, R. M., Kasper, L. J., Hudec, K. L., & Patros, C. H. (2013). Attention-deficit/hyperactivity disorder (ADHD) and working memory in adults: A meta-analytic review. *Neuropsychology, 27*(3), 287.

APA. (2013). Diagnostic and statistical manual of mental disorders. *American Psychiatric Association, 21*(21), 591–643.

Asherson, P., Buitelaar, J., Faraone, S. V., & Rohde, L. A. (2016). Adult attention-deficit hyperactivity disorder: Key conceptual issues. *The Lancet Psychiatry, 3*(6), 568–578. https://doi.org/10.1016/s2215-0366(16)30032-3

Asherson, P., Buitelaar, J., Faraone, S. V., & Rohde, L. A. (2021). Adult attention-deficit hyperactivity disorder: Key conceptual issues. *The Lancet Psychiatry, 8*(7), 568–578.

Australian Human Rights Commission. (2012). Disability rights: Students with ADHD. https://humanrights.gov.au/our-work/disability-rights.

Australian Human Rights Commission. (2023). Disability discrimination act 1992. https://humanrights.gov.au/our-work/disability-rights/disability-discrimination-act-1992.

Barkley, R. A., & Brown, T. E. (2008). Unrecognized attention-deficit/hyperactivity disorder in adults presenting with other psychiatric disorders. *CNS Spectrums, 13*(11), 977–984. https://doi.org/10.1017/S1092852900014036

Barkley, R. A. (2018). *Attention-deficit hyperactivity disorder: A handbook for diagnosis and treatment* (4th ed.). Guilford Press.

Baweja, R., Soutullo, C. A., & Waxmonsky, J. G. (2021). Review of barriers and interventions to promote treatment engagement for pediatric attention deficit hyperactivity disorder care. *World Journal of Psychiatry, 11*(12), 1206–1227. https://doi.org/10.5498/wjp.v11.i12.1206

Cole, A. M., Chan, E. S. M., Gaye, F., Harmon, S. L., Kofler, M. J. (2024). The role of working memory and organizational skills in academic functioning for children with attention-deficit/hyperactivity disorder. *Neuropsychology, 38*(6), 487–500. https://doi.org/10.1037/neu0000960. Epub 2024 Jul 11. PMID: 38990684; PMCID: PMC11469574.

Chacko, A., Merrill, B. M., Kofler, M. J., & Fabiano, G. A. (2024). Improving the efficacy and effectiveness of evidence-based psychosocial interventions for attention-deficit/hyperactivity disorder (ADHD) in children and adolescents. *Translational Psychiatry, 14*(1), 244. https://doi.org/10.1038/s41398-024-02890-3

Corrigan, P. W., Druss, B. G., & Perlick, D. A. (2014). The impact of mental illness stigma on seeking and participating in mental health care. *Psychological Science in the Public Interest, 15*(2), 37–70.

Department for Education. (2022). Education, health, and care plans: Overview. https://www.gov.uk/government/publications/send-code-of-practice-0-to-25

Department of Education (USA). (2020). Students with ADHD and section 504: A resource guide. https://www2.ed.gov/about/offices/list/ocr/docs/504-resource-guide-201612.pdf

Department of Education Western Australia. (2022). Inclusive education policy. https://www.education.wa.edu.au/inclusive-education-policy

Doyle, N. (2020). Neurodiversity at work: A biopsychosocial model and the impact on working adults. *British Medical Bulletin, 135*(1), 108–125. https://doi.org/10.1093/bmb/ldaa021

DuPaul, G. J., Kern, L., Gormley, M. J., & Volpe, R. J. (2011). Early intervention for young children with ADHD: Academic outcomes for responders to behavioral treatment. *School Mental Health, 3*, 117–126.

DuPaul, G. J., Weyandt, L. L., & Janusis, G. M. (2011). ADHD in the classroom: Effective intervention strategies. *Theory Into Practice, 50*(1), 35–42. https://doi.org/10.1080/00405841.2011.534935

Erskine, H. E., Norman, R. E., Ferrari, A. J., Chan, G. C., Copeland, W. E., Whiteford, H. A., & Scott, J. G. (2016). Long-term outcomes of attention-deficit/hyperactivity disorder and conduct disorder: A systematic review and meta-analysis. *Journal of the American Academy of Child and Adolescent Psychiatry, 55*(10), 841–850. https://doi.org/10.1016/j.jaac.2016.06.016

European Commission. (2021). Union of equality: European disability strategy 2021–2030. https://ec.europa.eu/social/main.jsp?catId=1202&langId=en2021

European Parliament. (2021). The European disability strategy 2021–2030: Towards a barrier-free Europe for persons with disabilities. https://www.europarl.europa.eu/doceo/document/TA-9-2021-0314_EN.html

Faraone, S. V., Banaschewski, T., Coghill, D., Zheng, Y., Biederman, J., Bellgrove, M. A., Newcorn, J. H., Gignac, M., Al Saud, N. M., Manor, I., Rohde, L. A., Yang, L., Cortese, S., Almagor, D., Stein, M. A., Albatti, T. H., Aljoudi, H. F., Alqahtani, M. M. J., Asherson, P., et al. (2021). The world federation of ADHD international consensus statement: 208 evidence-based conclusions about the disorder. *Neuroscience & Biobehavioral Reviews, 128*, 789–818. https://doi.org/10.1016/j.neubiorev.2021.01.022

Galéra, C., Melchior, M., Chastang, J. F., Bouvard, M. P., & Fombonne, E. (2009). Childhood and adolescent hyperactivity-inattention symptoms and academic achievement 8 years later: The GAZEL youth study. *Psychological Medicine, 39*(11), 1895–1906. https://doi.org/10.1017/s0033291709005510

Gee, B., Reynolds, S., Carroll, B., Orchard, F., Clarke, T., Martin, D., Wilson, J., & Pass, L. (2020). Practitioner review: Effectiveness of indicated school-based interventions for adolescent

depression and anxiety–a meta-analytic review. *Journal of Child Psychology and Psychiatry, 61*(7), 739–756.
Hinshaw, S. P., & Scheffler, R. M. (2014). *The ADHD explosion: Myths, medication, money, and today's push for performance*. Oxford University Press.
Hosseinnia, M., Mazaheri, M. A., & Heydari, Z. (2024). Educational intervention of parents and teachers for children with attention deficit hyperactivity disorder. *Journal of Education Health Promotion, 13*, 53. https://doi.org/10.4103/jehp.jehp_1816_22
Hotte-Meunier, A., Sarraf, L., Bougeard, A., Bernier, F., Voyer, C., Deng, J., El Asmar, S., Stamate, A. N., Corbière, M., Villotti, P., & Sauvé, G. (2024). Strengths and challenges to embrace attention-deficit/hyperactivity disorder in employment—A systematic review. *Neurodiversity, 2*, 27546330241287655. https://doi.org/10.1177/27546330241287655
Karlsberg Bennett, J., O'Neill, S., Rajendran, K., & Halperin, J. M. (2020). Do preschoolers' neuropsychological functioning and hyperactivity/inattention predict social functioning trajectories through childhood? *Journal of Pediatric Psychology, 45*(7), 793–802. https://doi.org/10.1093/jpepsy/jsaa053
Klein, R. G., Mannuzza, S., Olazagasti, M. A. R., Roizen, E., Hutchison, J. A., Lashua, E. C., & Castellanos, F. X. (2012). Clinical and functional outcome of childhood attention-deficit/hyperactivity disorder 33 years later. *Archives of General Psychiatry, 69*(12), 1295–1303.
Kofler, M. J., Irwin, L. N., Soto, E. F., Groves, N. B., Harmon, S. L., & Sarver, D. E. (2019). Executive functioning heterogeneity in pediatric ADHD. *Journal of Abnormal Child Psychology, 47*, 273–286.
Kuriyan, A. B., Pelham, W. E., Molina, B. S. G., Waschbusch, D. A., Gnagy, E. M., Sibley, M. H., Babinski, D. E., Walther, C., Cheong, J., Yu, J., & Kent, K. M. (2013). Young adult educational and vocational outcomes of children diagnosed with ADHD. *Journal of Abnormal Child Psychology, 41*(1), 27–41. https://doi.org/10.1007/s10802-012-9658-z
McCoy, R. T., Joseph, R., & Bongar, B. (2023). Americans with disabilities act. In *Encyclopedia of domestic violence* (pp. 1–15). Springer.
McKenna, K., Wanni Arachchige Dona, S., Gold, L., Dew, A., & Le, H. N. D. (2024). Barriers and enablers of service access and utilization for children and adolescents with attention deficit hyperactivity disorder: A systematic review. *Journal of Attention Disorders, 28*(3), 259–278. https://doi.org/10.1177/10870547231214002
Mowlem, F., Agnew-Blais, J., Taylor, E., & Asherson, P. (2019). Do different factors influence whether girls versus boys meet ADHD diagnostic criteria? Sex differences among children with high ADHD symptoms. *Psychiatry Research, 272*, 765–773. https://doi.org/10.1016/j.psychres.2018.12.128
National Disability Insurance Scheme. (NDIS). (2022). *National disability insurance scheme act 2013*. https://www.ndis.gov.au/about-us/governance/legislation
National Disability Insurance Scheme. (NDIS). (2022). NDIS Annual Report 2021–2022. Australian Government.
Østerud, K. L. (2023). Mental illness stigma and employer evaluation in hiring: Stereotypes, discrimination and the role of experience. *Sociology of Health & Illness, 45*(1), 90–108. https://doi.org/10.1111/1467-9566.13544
Raggi, V. L., & Chronis, A. M. (2006). Interventions to address the academic impairment of children and adolescents with ADHD. *Clinical Child and Family Psychology Review, 9*, 85–111.
Sayal, K., Prasad, V., Daley, D., Ford, T., & Coghill, D. (2018). ADHD in children and young people: Prevalence, care pathways, and service provision. *The Lancet Psychiatry, 5*(2), 175–186.
Sedgwick-Müller, J. A., Müller-Sedgwick, U., Adamou, M., Catani, M., Champ, R., Gudjónsson, G., Hank, D., Pitts, M., Young, S., & Asherson, P. (2022). University students with attention deficit hyperactivity disorder (ADHD): A consensus statement from the UK adult ADHD network (UKAAN). *BMC Psychiatry, 22*(1), 292. https://doi.org/10.1186/s12888-022-03898-z
Shaw, P., Eckstrand, K., Sharp, W., Blumenthal, J., Lerch, J., Greenstein, D., Clasen, L., Evans, A., Giedd, J., & Rapoport, J. (2007). Attention-deficit/hyperactivity disorder is characterized by a delay in cortical maturation. *Proceedings of the National Academy of Sciences, 104*(49), 19649–19654.

Sciutto, M. J., & Eisenberg, M. (2007). Evaluating the evidence for and against the overdiagnosis of ADHD. *Journal of Attention Disorders, 11*(2), 106–113.

Social Security Administration. (2023). ADHD and disability benefits. https://www.ssa.gov/

U.S. Department of Justice. (2022). Americans with Disabilities Act (ADA). https://www.ada.gov/

UK Government. (2010). Equality Act 2010. https://www.legislation.gov.uk/ukpga/2010/15/contents

Weyandt, L. L., & DuPaul, G. J. (2006). ADHD in college students: Developmental findings. *Journal of Attention Disorders, 10*(1), 9–19.

Weyandt, L. L., & Dupaul, G. J. (2008). ADHD in college students: Developmental findings. *Developmental Disabilities Research Reviews, 14*(4), 311–319. https://doi.org/10.1002/ddrr.38

Young, J. L., & Goodman, D. W. (2016). Adult attention-deficit/hyperactivity disorder diagnosis, management, and treatment in the DSM-5 era. *Prim Care Companion CNS Disord, 18*(6). https://doi.org/10.4088/PCC.16r02000

Young, S., Adamo, N., Ásgeirsdóttir, B. B., Branney, P., Beckett, M., Colley, W., Cubbin, S., Deeley, Q., Farrag, E., Gudjonsson, G., Hill, P., Hollingdale, J., Kilic, O., Lloyd, T., Mason, P., Paliokosta, E., Perecherla, S., Sedgwick, J., Skirrow, C., … Asherson, P. (2020). Females with ADHD: An expert consensus statement taking a lifespan approach providing guidance for the identification and treatment of attention-deficit/hyperactivity disorder in girls and women. *BMC Psychiatry, 20*, 404.

Zentall, S. S. (2012). *ADHD and education: Foundations, characteristics, methods, and collaboration*. Pearson.

Chapter 6
Social and Economic Impact of ADHD Across the Lifespan

Abstract This chapter provides an overview of the social and economic consequences of ADHD across the lifespan, highlighting the far-reaching effects on individuals, families, and society. It explores how ADHD, particularly when left untreated, can contribute to academic struggles, social challenges, and employment instability, ultimately shaping long-term financial and health-related outcomes.

The discussion extends to the broader societal implications of ADHD, including its impact on healthcare systems, education, and the workforce. Special attention is given to the cumulative burden on families, the social stigma associated with the disorder, and the economic costs incurred through lost productivity, increased healthcare utilization, and interactions with the criminal justice system.

Importantly, this chapter also examines potential protective factors and strategies that can mitigate the negative consequences of ADHD, emphasizing the role of early intervention, workplace accommodations, and policy-driven initiatives. By critically analyzing the social and economic dimensions of ADHD, this chapter encourages readers to consider the broader implications of the disorder and the opportunities for improving outcomes across different life stages.

6.1 Childhood and Adolescence: Academic and Emotional Challenges

Attention-deficit/hyperactivity disorder (ADHD) emerges early in life, profoundly shaping a child's experiences in academic, social, and familial settings. Characterized by persistent inattention, hyperactivity, and impulsivity, ADHD presents significant challenges in learning, peer relationships, and emotional regulation. These difficulties, if unaddressed, often compound over time, affecting long-term outcomes in education, mental health, and overall well-being (Faraone et al., 2021; Barkley, 2018).

The burden of ADHD extends beyond the individual and can place considerable strain on families. Parents often struggle with increased stress, disrupted family dynamics, and the complex task of navigating educational and healthcare systems to

G. Ayano et al., *ADHD Across the Lifespan*, SpringerBriefs in Modern Perspectives on Disability Research,
https://doi.org/10.1007/978-981-95-8712-4_6

secure appropriate support (Johnston & Chronis-Tuscano, 2021). Without early identification and targeted intervention, ADHD can lead to poor academic performance, social isolation, emotional dysregulation, and an elevated risk of comorbid mental health conditions (Asherson et al., 2016). This section critically examines these challenges and their long-term implications.

6.1.1 Academic Underachievement and Learning Difficulties

Children with ADHD frequently struggle with sustained attention, organization, and task completion, leading to academic underachievement and diminished self-confidence compared to their peers (DuPaul et al., 2017). Difficulties with concentration and cognitive processing are common, as inattention impairs reading comprehension, problem-solving, and working memory, making it challenging for children to follow lessons and retain new information (Sayal et al., 2018). Executive function deficits also contribute to disorganized study habits, misplaced assignments, and difficulties meeting deadlines (Biederman et al., 2006).

Children with ADHD experience higher rates of grade repetition due to academic struggles are more likely to be placed in special education programs (Weyandt & DuPaul, 2006). In the United States, Individualized Education Programs (IEPs) and Section 504 Plans provide accommodations such as extended test time and modified instruction, but access varies widely based on school policies and available resources (U.S. Department of Education, 2021).

Adolescents with ADHD exhibit higher dropout rates, often driven by academic frustration, disciplinary actions, and inadequate support systems (Faraone et al., 2021). Structured learning environments, comprehensive teacher training, and the integration of assistive technologies can help mitigate these challenges, promoting academic engagement and improving long-term educational attainment (DuPaul & Stoner, 2014).

6.1.2 Behavioral and Social Challenges

ADHD profoundly impacts behavioral regulation and peer interactions, increasing the likelihood of disciplinary actions, social rejection, and difficulty forming meaningful relationships (Barkley, 2018). Children with ADHD are at heightened risk of disciplinary actions, as they are three times more likely than their peers to receive detentions, suspensions, or expulsions due to impulsivity and difficulties adhering to school rules (Sayal et al., 2018). Unfortunately, schools with rigid disciplinary policies often penalize ADHD-related behaviors rather than implementing strategies to support self-regulation and positive behavior (DuPaul et al., 2017).

Peer rejection and social isolation are also common experiences for children with ADHD. Difficulties abiding with social norms, emotional regulation, and impulse control often lead to peer conflict and exclusion from social groups, undermining social development and self-esteem (Mowlem et al., 2019). Many children with ADHD also experience higher rates of bullying, which can contribute to heightened anxiety, withdrawal, and further reduced self-esteem (Young et al., 2020). Importantly, evidence shows that targeted social skills training and behavioral interventions can significantly improve peer relationships and reduce social difficulties in children with ADHD (Evans et al., 2018; Mowlem et al., 2019).

Additionally, ADHD is associated with an increased risk of oppositional defiant disorder (ODD) and conduct disorder (CD). Up to half of the children with ADHD develop comorbid disruptive behavior disorders, which increase the risk of chronic school difficulties and negative interactions with authority figures (Faraone et al., 2021).

Early intervention strategies, including social skills training and behavioral therapy, have been shown to effectively manage social difficulties by fostering peer relationships and reducing disruptive behaviors, even though ADHD symptoms may persist (Evans et al., 2018; Jensen-Doss & Hawley, 2010). These interventions can help children develop appropriate social behaviors, improve emotional regulation, and promote successful integration into school and community settings.

6.1.3 Emotional Dysregulation and Mental Health Risks

Children with ADHD often struggle to manage their emotions, leading to increased frustration, mood instability, and difficulty coping with stress (Barkley, 2018). Emotional dysregulation can manifest as sudden outbursts of anger, irritability, or sadness, contributing to challenges in academic and social settings.

Low self-esteem and negative self-perception are common among children with ADHD. Persistent negative feedback from teachers, parents, and peers can reinforce feelings of incompetence and self-doubt, compounding academic and social struggles (Mowlem et al., 2019). Children with ADHD may avoid academic and social challenges in an effort to prevent failure or embarrassment, further limiting their opportunities for growth and success (Asherson et al., 2016).

Children and adolescents with ADHD are also at higher risk of developing anxiety and depression. Research suggests they are twice as likely to develop anxiety disorders and three times more likely to experience depression compared to their neurotypical peers (Faraone et al., 2021). Of particular concern is that emotional hypersensitivity and difficulty processing criticism can increase vulnerability to self-harm and suicidal ideation, particularly among those who lack adequate treatment or support (Sayal et al., 2018).

Behavioral therapy (Evans et al., 2018), social-emotional learning programs (Lawson et al., 2019), and school-based mental health services (Power et al., 2009) can help children with ADHD develop resilience and adaptive coping strategies. These interventions are crucial for improving mental health outcomes by fostering supportive environments that promote emotional well-being.

6.1.4 Family Strain and Parent–Child Conflict

The challenges associated with ADHD extend beyond the affected individual, placing significant emotional and logistical strain on families (Johnston & Chronis-Tuscano, 2021). Frequent parent–child conflicts are common, as parents often struggle to manage impulsivity, emotional outbursts, and school-related challenges. These daily frustrations can lead to power struggles that strain the parent–child relationship (DuPaul & Stoner, 2014). Additionally, differences in parenting approaches—such as varying levels of tolerance or inconsistent discipline—can exacerbate family conflict and contribute to inconsistent support for the child with ADHD (Johnston & Chronis-Tuscano, 2021).

Parental stress and caregiver burnout are important concerns. Parents of children with ADHD report higher levels of stress, exhaustion, and depressive symptoms compared to parents of neurotypical children, often feeling overwhelmed by the demands of managing ADHD-related behaviors and navigating support systems (Biederman et al., 2006). Families with limited financial resources including single-parent households face heightened difficulties accessing specialized care and educational support, further compounding stress and feelings of isolation (Johnston & Chronis-Tuscano, 2021).

Strained sibling relationships frequently develop within families affected by ADHD. Siblings of children with ADHD may feel overshadowed or neglected as parental attention is often directed toward managing ADHD-related challenges (DuPaul & Stoner, 2014). Over time, this dynamic can foster resentment, emotional distancing, and tension within the family unit, undermining sibling bonds and family cohesion (Mowlem et al., 2019).

Structured behavioral strategies (Fabiano et al., 2009), parent training programs (Daley et al., 2014), and family therapy (Chronis-Tuscano et al., 2013) can alleviate familial stress and create a more supportive home environment. These interventions empower parents with effective management strategies, foster understanding among siblings, and enhance the overall well-being of the entire family.

6.1.5 Looking Ahead: ADHD's Impact Beyond Childhood

While childhood is the foundational period for ADHD-related challenges, the consequences extend well beyond adolescence. Difficulties in academic performance, social integration, and emotional regulation influence future career opportunities, financial stability, and overall adult mental health (Barkley, 2018; Faraone et al., 2021). As individuals with ADHD transition into adulthood, they often encounter employment instability, strained relationships, and economic disadvantage, all of which contribute to broader societal costs and long-term disparities (Asherson et al., 2016). Recognizing the life course implications of ADHD underscores the need for early interventions and sustained support to enhance outcomes across multiple domains.

The next section will explore how ADHD continues to shape life trajectories in adulthood, examining its impact on workplace productivity, financial independence, and broader social inclusion.

6.2 Adulthood: Long-Term Individual and Family Challenges

While often perceived as a childhood disorder, a significant proportion of individuals with ADHD continue to experience substantial challenges into adulthood, affecting multiple domains of their life, including employment, relationships, financial stability, and mental health (Faraone et al., 2021; Asherson et al., 2016). The transition to adulthood introduces new complexities, as the structured academic support available during childhood is no longer present, necessitating self-management of symptoms in professional, financial, and personal spheres (Barkley, 2018).

This section examines the persistent impact of ADHD in adulthood, with a focus on employment challenges, relationship difficulties, risk-taking behaviors, and co-occurring psychiatric disorders. Emphasizing the need for tailored interventions, we explore strategies that support long-term well-being and functional outcomes for adults with ADHD.

6.2.1 Employment Challenges and Workplace Instability

Adults with ADHD face significantly higher rates of job instability, underemployment, and workplace conflict due to difficulties with executive functioning, task organization, and interpersonal communication (Kessler et al., 2005; Young et al., 2020). Frequent job changes and employment instability are common, as individuals with ADHD are more likely to change jobs frequently and face higher rates of unemployment and job loss compared to their neurotypical peers (Faraone et al., 2021). Symptoms such as inattention, impulsivity, and difficulty with time management contribute to decreased workplace productivity and increased financial insecurity (Asherson et al., 2016).

Underemployment and career stagnation are also prevalent challenges. Many adults with ADHD are employed in roles below their skill level due to difficulties navigating structured work environments, completing administrative tasks, and maintaining prolonged focus (Biederman et al., 2006). Research indicates that ADHD is associated with lower lifetime earnings and reduced career progression, further impacting financial stability and quality of life (Klein et al., 2012).

Workplace conflicts and interpersonal difficulties are common among adults with ADHD. Impulsivity and emotional dysregulation often lead to miscommunication, difficulty responding to constructive criticism, and frustration with colleagues and supervisors (Barkley, 2018). These challenges are compounded in rigid corporate environments, leading to an increased likelihood of workplace disputes and disciplinary actions (Young et al., 2020).

Conversely individuals with ADHD can thrive in creative, fast-paced, and entrepreneurial settings where adaptability and innovation are valued. Workplace accommodations, such as structured task management, flexible schedules, and ADHD coaching, can improve career stability and long-term outcomes, empowering adults with ADHD to leverage their strengths and achieve professional success (Asherson et al., 2016).

6.2.2 Relationship Difficulties and Family Dynamics

Interpersonal relationships, particularly romantic partnerships and family interactions, are significantly affected by ADHD due to emotional sensitivity, impulsivity, and inconsistent communication patterns (Biederman et al., 2006; Barkley, 2018). Higher divorce rates and marital distress are common, with adults with ADHD being twice as likely to experience divorce compared to those without ADHD. This increased risk is largely attributed to difficulties in managing household responsibilities, emotional reactivity, and communication breakdowns (Young et al., 2020). Impulsivity and poor emotional regulation often lead to misunderstandings and conflicts, further straining long-term relationships (Asherson et al., 2016).

Social isolation and difficulty maintaining friendships are also prevalent among adults with ADHD. Difficulties in reading social cues, remembering commitments, and regulating emotions can place strain on friendships, sometimes resulting in social withdrawal and feelings of isolation (Kessler et al., 2005). Adults with ADHD frequently report heightened loneliness and a history of interpersonal rejection, which can contribute to emotional distress and exacerbate symptoms of ADHD (Barkley, 2018).

Parenting challenges and intergenerational ADHD risk add further complexity to family dynamics. Parents with ADHD often struggle to maintain consistent discipline, organization, and emotional regulation, particularly when raising children who also have ADHD (Johnston & Chronis-Tuscano, 2021). Given the strong genetic basis of ADHD, children of adults with ADHD have an increased likelihood of developing the disorder, which can amplify family stress and caregiving demands (Faraone et al., 2021).

ADHD-informed relationship counselling and structured parenting interventions can help address these challenges by enhancing communication, reducing stress, and improving overall family functioning (Young et al., 2020). These supports can foster healthier relationships and a more stable home environment for families affected by ADHD.

6.2.3 Risk-Taking Behaviors and Impulsivity in Adulthood

Adults with ADHD exhibit a heightened tendency for impulsive decision-making, increasing their vulnerability to financial mismanagement, substance use disorders, and legal complications (Barkley, 2018). Financial instability and impulsive spending are common, as difficulties with delayed gratification and long-term planning contribute to excessive credit card debt, financial mismanagement, and overall economic instability (Doyle, 2020). Employment instability further exacerbates financial stress, compounding mental health challenges and reducing overall quality of life (Young et al., 2020).

The prevalence of substance use disorders is consistently higher among adults with ADHD compared to the general population, with studies reporting a two- to threefold increase (Katzman et al., 2017; Miranda et al., 2016). Individuals with ADHD are particularly vulnerable to substance use disorders (SUDs) involving alcohol, nicotine, and stimulants, often as a means of self-medicating symptoms or coping with stress (Asherson et al., 2016). Impulsivity and sensation-seeking tendencies further elevate the risk of substance dependence and related health complications (Kessler et al., 2005).

Reckless driving and legal issues are additional concerns in adulthood. Research indicates that adults with ADHD are more likely to engage in reckless driving behaviors, receive traffic violations, and be involved in motor vehicle accidents compared to their neurotypical peers (Biederman et al., 2006). Poor impulse control and risk-taking behaviors also contribute to an increased likelihood of legal involvement, including arrests for reckless conduct or related offences (Barkley, 2018).

Preventive interventions such as financial literacy training, harm reduction strategies for substance use, and targeted behavioral therapies can play a vital role in mitigating the long-term impacts of ADHD (Halperin et al., 2012; Seery et al., 2023; Sonuga-Barke et al., 2013). These interventions can promote safer decision-making, reduce impulsive behaviors, and improve overall well-being for adults with ADHD.

6.2.4 Co-Occurring Psychiatric Disorders and Mental Health Challenges

ADHD in adulthood is frequently accompanied by psychiatric comorbidities, which exacerbate functional impairments and reduce overall quality of life (Faraone et al., 2021). Elevated rates of anxiety and depression are particularly common among adults with ADHD, with studies indicating that 50–70% of adults with ADHD experience an anxiety disorder, and up to half develop major depressive disorder (MDD) during their lifetime (Asherson et al., 2016). Chronic stress stemming from occupational, financial, or interpersonal difficulties can further worsen mental health outcomes, making it more difficult for individuals to cope with the demands of daily life (Young et al., 2020).

Adults with ADHD are also at higher risk of suicidal ideation and self-harm. The combination of emotional dysregulation, impulsivity, and limited access to effective treatments can significantly increase vulnerability to these outcomes, particularly in individuals who lack adequate support or therapeutic interventions (Faraone et al., 2021).

Barriers to mental health treatment further complicate the clinical picture for adults with ADHD. Many individuals remain undiagnosed or misdiagnosed, delaying access to effective interventions such as pharmacological and behavioral treatments (Doyle, 2020). Stigma, financial constraints, and a shortage of ADHD-specialized clinicians also create substantial barriers to accessing mental health care, limiting opportunities for symptom management and functional improvement (Asherson et al., 2016).

Comprehensive ADHD management in adulthood should incorporate multimodal treatment strategies, including medication, psychotherapy, and workplace or academic accommodations. These integrated approaches are essential for improving long-term outcomes, promoting mental health, and enhancing quality of life for adults with ADHD.

6.3 Impact on Families and Caregivers

The impact of ADHD extends far beyond the affected individual, significantly influencing families and caregivers. Parents, siblings, and extended family members often experience emotional distress, financial strain, and disruptions to daily functioning due to the challenges associated with managing ADHD-related behaviors and securing necessary medical, educational, and psychological support (Johnston & Chronis-Tuscano, 2021; Faraone et al., 2021).

This section examines the burden of ADHD on families, emphasizing the caregiving responsibilities, financial costs, and emotional stressors that contribute to reduced family well-being and increased societal costs. Recognizing these challenges is essential for policymakers and healthcare providers in developing interventions that alleviate the caregiving burden and improve family outcomes.

6.3.1 Emotional and Financial Strain on Families

Families of children with ADHD face greater financial and psychological burdens compared to those with neurotypical children. The demand for specialized medical care, educational interventions, and behavioral support leads to increased household expenses and chronic stress (Biederman et al., 2006; Doshi et al., 2012). Increased healthcare expenditure is common among these families, as they often incur significantly higher medical costs, including expenses for psychiatric consultations, behavioral therapy, and pharmacological treatments (Faraone et al., 2021). Research suggests that annual healthcare costs for families managing ADHD are nearly double those of families without ADHD, with additional expenditures ranging from $2500 to $4000 per year (Doshi et al., 2012).

Educational expenses also contribute to the financial burden. Many children with ADHD require private tutoring, individualized education plans (IEPs), and specialized assessments, placing significant financial strain on families (Sayal et al., 2018). Parents frequently invest in behavioral therapy, executive function coaching, and ADHD-specific educational programs, further exacerbating financial challenges (Barkley, 2018).

Reduced workforce participation among parents is another critical concern. Caregiving responsibilities often compel parents, particularly mothers, to reduce their working hours or leave employment altogether, leading to lost income and long-term career consequences (Doshi et al., 2012). Studies estimate that families of children with ADHD experience significant productivity losses, amounting to billions in lost workdays and reduced earnings (Matza et al., 2005).

These financial and emotional burdens highlight the need for policy-driven solutions, including expanded insurance coverage for ADHD-related interventions, workplace accommodations for parents, and financial assistance programs to support affected families (Jalpa A. Doshi et al., 2012). Addressing these challenges is essential for improving family well-being and reducing the broader societal costs associated with ADHD (Doshi et al., 2012; Schein et al., 2022).

6.3.2 Parental Stress and Burnout from ADHD-Related Challenges

Parents of children with ADHD frequently report higher levels of stress, exhaustion, and mental health concerns compared to parents of neurotypical children (Johnston & Chronis-Tuscano, 2021; Theule et al., 2013). The persistent demands of managing impulsivity, emotional outbursts, academic struggles, and behavioral interventions contribute to parental burnout and increased vulnerability to anxiety and depression.

Heightened parental stress and anxiety are common experiences among caregivers of children with ADHD. Studies indicate that these parents experience significantly greater parenting stress than those caring for children with other neurodevelopmental conditions, including autism spectrum disorder (ASD) (Theule et al., 2013). Frequent conflicts over homework, behavioral management, and social interactions contribute to frustration, helplessness, and emotional exhaustion (Barkley, 2018).

Increased risk of parental depression and marital strain are also prevalent. Mothers of children with ADHD are at notably higher risk for anxiety and depressive disorders compared to mothers of neurotypical children (Johnston & Chronis-Tuscano, 2021). Differences in parenting approaches and disciplinary strategies can lead to marital discord, with research showing that couples raising a child with ADHD experience greater relationship distress and higher divorce rates (Biederman et al., 2006).

Limited social support and caregiver isolation further compound parental stress. Many parents feel isolated due to the stigma surrounding ADHD, which limits their ability to access social support networks and parenting resources (Matza et al., 2005). The demands of ADHD caregiving also restrict parental participation in social and recreational activities, further exacerbating stress and reducing overall well-being (Theule et al., 2013).

Parent training programs, family therapy, and peer support groups have consistently shown efficacy in reducing parental stress and improving coping mechanisms. For example, meta-analyses indicate that parent training programs significantly improve parenting skills and reduce child ADHD symptoms, with medium effect sizes (Hedges' $g \approx 0.50–0.60$) and corresponding reductions in parental stress (Chronis-Tuscano et al., 2017; Daley et al., 2014). Family-based interventions and parent-focused cognitive-behavioral therapies have also been associated with improvements in parental mental health and family functioning (Fabiano et al., 2009; van den Hoofdakker et al., 2007). Moreover, structured peer support and psychoeducation groups provide additional reductions in caregiver burden and enhanced coping, with reported improvements in parent-reported quality of life scores of up to 20–30% (Cordier et al., 2018). Healthcare policies should therefore prioritize caregiver mental health, as parental well-being is crucial for the effective management of ADHD and the long-term outcomes for children and families. Healthcare policies should prioritize caregiver mental health, as parental well-being is crucial for the effective management of ADHD and the long-term outcomes for children and families.

6.3.3 Emotional Impact on Siblings of Children with ADHD

The demands of ADHD caregiving often lead to an unequal distribution of parental attention, affecting the emotional well-being of siblings. Many neurotypical siblings experience feelings of neglect, resentment, and stress as parents focus on managing ADHD-related difficulties (Barkley, 2018). These dynamics can have long-term implications for sibling relationships and mental health.

Feelings of neglect and emotional distress are common among siblings of children with ADHD. Studies indicate that these siblings frequently feel less emotionally connected to their parents due to the disproportionate focus on ADHD-related challenges (Johnston & Chronis-Tuscano, 2021). Such experiences can contribute to lower self-esteem, anxiety, and emotional withdrawal in neurotypical siblings, potentially affecting their own development and well-being (Theule et al., 2013).

Increased sibling conflict and household tension also arise in families affected by ADHD. The impulsive and oppositional behaviors often associated with ADHD contribute to heightened sibling conflict, leading to frustration and resentment within the household (Barkley, 2018). Research suggests that families of children with ADHD experience greater sibling rivalry and disrupted household dynamics compared to families without ADHD (Sayal et al., 2018).

Additionally, siblings of children with ADHD are at higher risk of developing internalizing disorders such as anxiety and depression due to chronic household stress and perceived emotional neglect (Johnston & Chronis-Tuscano, 2021). Given the strong genetic and environmental influences of ADHD, some siblings may also exhibit ADHD-related traits, further complicating family interactions and support needs (Faraone et al., 2021).

Implementing family-based interventions and sibling support programs can help mitigate these effects, fostering healthier sibling relationships and overall family cohesion. Educators and healthcare providers should acknowledge the needs of siblings and ensure they receive equal emotional support to promote their mental health and well-being.

6.4 ADHD and Broader Social Consequences

Beyond its clinical symptoms, ADHD has extensive social consequences that affect interpersonal relationships, social integration, and interactions with societal systems such as the criminal justice and healthcare systems. The disorder influences multiple aspects of life, including peer relationships, risk of victimization, legal involvement, and substance use, all of which contribute to long-term social and economic burdens (Faraone et al., 2021; Young et al., 2020). Incorporating these broader contexts into policy considerations is essential for effective approaches that foster inclusion and mitigate adverse outcomes associated with ADHD.

This section explores the social impact of ADHD across the lifespan, examining how symptoms contribute to peer rejection, criminal justice involvement, and substance use. By considering these domains, we can better understand the complex ways ADHD affects social functioning and broader societal outcomes.

6.4.1 ADHD and Social Functioning

Social functioning is a key domain where individuals with ADHD can experience impairments resulting in peer rejection, social isolation, and increased vulnerability to bullying (Faraone et al., 2021; Barkley, 2018). These difficulties not only impact psychological well-being but also contribute to broader societal costs, such as higher rates of school dropout, workplace conflicts, and increased mental health service utilization (Young et al., 2020).

Difficulties forming and maintaining friendships are common among individuals with ADHD. Impairments in self-regulation, social perception, and conversational skills create challenges in building and sustaining relationships (Mikami, 2010; Bunford et al., 2018). Impulsivity and disruptive behaviors can strain friendships, as individuals with ADHD often interrupt conversations, struggle with turn-taking, or dominate discussions (Barkley, 2018). Emotional dysregulation can also lead to unpredictable emotional reactions, which may overwhelm peers and contribute to unstable friendships (Young et al., 2020).

Higher risk of social rejection is evident among children and adolescents with ADHD. Children with ADHD are significantly more likely to experience peer rejection due to difficulty following social norms, emotional reactivity, and disruptive behaviors (Bunford et al., 2018). This rejection in childhood is associated with long-term consequences, including increased risk of depression, anxiety, and social withdrawal in adolescence and adulthood (Shaw et al., 2014). Gender differences also emerge, with boys more frequently exhibiting externalizing behaviors such as aggression and impulsivity, while girls often experience more subtle social exclusion (Hinshaw, 2018).

Increased vulnerability to bullying in both school and online settings is another critical concern. Research indicates that students with ADHD are two to three times more likely to be bullied than their neurotypical peers. Cyberbullying presents additional risks, as individuals with ADHD are more likely to be harassed online due to social naïveté and poor risk assessment (Becker et al., 2017). Bullying is linked to increased anxiety, depression, and suicidal ideation, highlighting the urgent need for anti-bullying policies and social skills interventions (Faraone et al., 2021).

Promising interventions to address these include social-emotional learning (SEL) programs in schools (Hoza, 2007), peer mentoring initiatives (Haft et al., 2019), and strategies to raise ADHD awareness to reduce stigma and promote inclusion. Together, these approaches can foster supportive environments and enhance social integration for individuals with ADHD across the lifespan.

6.4.2 ADHD and the Criminal Justice System

Individuals with ADHD are overrepresented in the criminal justice system, highlighting systemic failures in early intervention, education, and healthcare access (Byrne & Guenter, 2023). ADHD is associated with higher rates of impulsive behavior, legal infractions, and incarceration, with many affected individuals remaining undiagnosed and untreated in correctional settings (Young et al., 2018; Mohr-Jensen & Steinhausen, 2016).

Elevated risk of legal issues and incarceration is a significant concern for individuals with ADHD. Research shows that people with ADHD are two to four times more likely to be arrested and convicted compared to those without ADHD (Mohr-Jensen & Steinhausen, 2016). The prevalence of ADHD among the prison populations is estimated at 25–45%, compared to 2–5% in the general population (Fazel et al., 2015). This stark disparity underscores the need for targeted interventions to address ADHD-related challenges in at-risk populations.

Higher rates of impulsive and aggressive crimes are also linked to ADHD. The disorder is strongly associated with impulsive offences, such as theft, reckless driving, and physical aggression (Barkley et al., 2004). Comorbid substance use further increases the likelihood of criminal involvement, contributing to a cycle of legal infractions and repeated incarceration (Young et al., 2018).

ADHD treatment in correctional settings remains limited, despite evidence that appropriate management can reduce recidivism rates by 30–40% (Young et al., 2018). Lack of resources for ADHD diagnosis and treatment in correctional facilities can exacerbate these challenges. Research suggests that incarcerated individuals with ADHD go undiagnosed, leading to misinterpretation of ADHD-related behaviors as defiance or deliberate misconduct (Fazel et al., 2015).

Early ADHD screening in correctional and juvenile justice settings (Byrne & Guenter, 2023), diversion programs based on the Sequential Intercept Model (Munetz & Griffin, 2006), and structured prison-based treatment initiatives (Byrne & Guenter, 2023) are promising strategies that can mitigate justice system disparities and reduce long-term societal costs. By implementing these interventions, the criminal justice system can better support individuals with ADHD and promote rehabilitation.

6.4.3 ADHD and Substance Use

Substance use disorders (SUDs) are a long-term consequence of ADHD, contributing to increased healthcare costs, reduced workforce productivity, and greater involvement with the legal system. Individuals with ADHD are significantly more likely to engage in substance use, with an earlier onset of drug experimentation and greater difficulty in addiction recovery than there neurotypical peers (Wilens et al., 2011; Faraone et al., 2021).

Increased likelihood of substance use as a coping mechanism is commonly observed among individuals with ADHD. Alcohol, nicotine, or illicit substance use is often used to self-medicate symptoms of impulsivity, inattention, and emotional distress (Kessler et al., 2005). This risk of addiction is further amplified by executive dysfunction and poor impulse control, which are core features of ADHD (Biederman et al., 2006).

Earlier onset of smoking, alcohol use, and drug experimentation is well-documented in adolescents with ADHD. Studies show that individuals with ADHD initiate substance use 1 to 3 years earlier than their neurotypical peers, significantly increasing their lifetime risk of addiction (Wilens et al., 2011). Nicotine dependence is disproportionately high, as smoking can temporarily improve focus and reduce hyperactivity, reinforcing addictive behaviors and complicating cessation efforts (Faraone et al., 2021).

Higher rates of addiction and challenges in recovery are also prevalent among individuals with ADHD. Traditional addiction treatments often have lower success rates in this population due to difficulties with impulse control and attention regulation (Asherson et al., 2016). However, specialized treatment approaches that integrate ADHD medication management and executive function training have been shown to improve long-term recovery outcomes (Wilens et al., 2011).

Expanding ADHD screening in addiction treatment settings and improving access to stimulant medications have been shown to reduce the risk of developing SUDs by 30–50% (Asherson et al., 2016).

6.5 The Economic Burden of ADHD

ADHD imposes a substantial economic burden on individuals, families, healthcare systems, educational institutions, and national economies. The disorder contributes to increased healthcare expenditures, higher education costs, lost workplace productivity, and significant public spending on welfare and criminal justice systems (Faraone et al., 2021; Doshi et al., 2012). These financial challenges extend beyond direct medical expenses, affecting long-term socioeconomic stability and workforce participation (Rietveld & Patel, 2019).

This section explores the primary drivers of ADHD-related economic costs, emphasizing the need for early intervention, cost-effective management strategies, and policy reforms to mitigate the broader financial burden of ADHD on society.

6.5.1 Healthcare Costs

The economic impact of ADHD on healthcare systems is considerable, driven by increased medical expenses, frequent healthcare utilization, and higher rates of comorbid conditions. Individuals with ADHD require more psychiatric care, emergency medical services, and long-term pharmacological treatment than their neurotypical peers, contributing to substantial direct and indirect healthcare costs (Doshi et al., 2012; Matza et al., 2005).

Higher medical expenses are common due to ADHD-related mental and physical health conditions. ADHD is associated with a high prevalence of comorbidities, including anxiety, depression, and substance use disorders, all of which require additional medical and psychological interventions (Faraone et al., 2021). In the United States, in 2012, it was estimated that individuals with ADHD incurred up to $2500–$4000 more per year in healthcare costs compared to those without ADHD (Doshi et al., 2012), potentially due to higher rates of comorbid mental and physical health conditions, greater use of healthcare services, injury-related care, and the need for long-term management. These increased costs may also reflect the long-term impacts of ADHD, including reduced educational attainment, lower workplace productivity, and greater reliance on social and disability services (Doshi et al., 2012).

Frequent doctor visits, medication costs, and therapy expenses further contribute to the economic burden. Children and adults with ADHD visit healthcare providers three to four times more often than the general population, leading to higher insurance claims and out-of-pocket expenses (Matza et al., 2005). In 2013, in the United States, ADHD medication costs, including stimulants (e.g., methylphenidate, amphetamines) and non-stimulants (e.g., atomoxetine, guanfacine), range from $1200 to $2500 annually per individual, placing a significant financial burden on families and healthcare systems (Shaw et al., 2014).

Increased emergency room visits and hospitalizations also escalate healthcare expenditures. Individuals with ADHD are twice as likely to visit emergency departments due to impulsivity-related accidents, injuries, and risk-taking behaviors (Biederman et al., 2006). Psychiatric hospitalizations for ADHD-related crises, such as self-harm and severe emotional dysregulation, further strain healthcare budgets (Wilens et al., 2011).

It is reasonable to predict that Early ADHD detection with comprehensive treatment strategies could significantly reduce long-term healthcare expenditures and improve patient outcomes, important components of cost-effective ADHD management.

6.5.2 Educational and Occupational Costs

As previously described, ADHD has enduring impacts on educational attainment and workforce productivity, contributing to long-term economic disadvantage. These effects are not confined to comorbid addiction but represent core functional impairments associated with ADHD itself. From childhood through adulthood, individuals with ADHD experience higher rates of grade retention, school dropout, and academic underachievement, leading to increased costs for special education services and remedial support (Faraone et al., 2021; Loe & Feldman, 2007). In adulthood, these early educational difficulties translate into elevated risks of unemployment, job instability, and substantially lower lifetime earnings, with some estimates indicating a reduction of 17–40% in income compared to non-ADHD peers (Doshi et al., 2012; Jangmo et al., 2021). Beyond lost earnings, ADHD is linked to increased rates of workplace accidents and absenteeism, which further exacerbate productivity losses at both individual and societal levels (Kessler et al., 2005; Schein et al., 2022). These challenges not only impact individuals and families but also impose substantial financial burdens on educational systems and employers (Schein et al., 2022).

Higher rates of academic failure and dropout are shown among individuals with ADHD. The disorder is associated with lower academic achievement, increased grade repetition, and reduced high school and college graduation, hindering long-term socioeconomic mobility (Biederman et al., 2006). In 2011, it was estimated that individuals with ADHD earned approximately $1.25 to $1.75 million less in their lifetime income than those without ADHD, primarily due to academic underachievement and employment difficulties (Doshi et al., 2012).

Increased costs for special education services and behavioral interventions also contribute to the economic burden. Students with ADHD are three times more likely to require special education services, significantly increasing public education expenditures (Shaw et al., 2014). Annual costs for ADHD-related special education services place substantial financial pressure on school systems. While older data (e.g., estimate of $2000–$6000 per student annually) have been widely cited, recent data show that the average public school spends over $13,000 per special education student, with local districts covering approximately $8160 out of pocket (Schein et al., 2022).

Lost productivity in the workforce and job retention contributes to unemployment, underemployed, or to frequently change jobs due to difficulties with executive functioning and workplace adaptation (Shaw et al., 2014). These employment challenges collectively translate into billions of dollars in annual productivity losses, driven by absenteeism, high turnover, and reduced work efficiency (Faraone et al., 2021).

Strategies to support educational outcomes, promote stable employment, and reduce long-term societal costs related to ADHD include, educational support programs, workplace accommodations, and vocational training initiatives tailored to individuals with ADHD.

6.5.3 *Societal Costs and Public Spending*

The societal costs of ADHD extend beyond health care and education, social assistance and services, to criminal justice systems, and overall economic productivity. Higher unemployment rates, increased reliance on social services, and legal system involvement contribute to billions in public spending annually (Faraone et al., 2021; Doshi et al., 2012). These costs affect both national economies and community-level resources, highlighting the need for comprehensive policy responses.

Increased burden on welfare and disability programs is a key concern. Individuals with ADHD are 50–80% more likely to rely on government assistance programs due to employment instability and reduced earning potential (Doshi et al., 2012). Many parents of children with ADHD reduce work hours or leave employment to manage caregiving responsibilities, further increasing reliance on public financial assistance and contributing to household economic strain (Matza et al., 2005).

Higher costs in the criminal justice system are also evident. ADHD places additional economic demands on the criminal justice system due to overrepresentation in prison populations and ADHD-related crimes increasing law enforcement expenditures, court costs, and incarceration expenses (Young et al., 2018).

Economic losses due to untreated ADHD are substantial. The total economic burden of ADHD exceeds US$100 billion annually in the United States alone, reflecting lost productivity, increased healthcare costs, and special education spending (Faraone et al., 2021). Workforce inefficiencies associated with ADHD contribute to substantial economic losses, with affected employees experiencing an estimated 15–20% reduction in work performance (Doshi et al., 2012).

Investing in a comprehensive intervention portfolio, including ADHD screening, treatment access, and workplace accommodations, could reduce public spending and enhance national economic sustainability. These investments would also improve individual outcomes and foster a more inclusive and productive society.

Summary

This chapter has explored the profound social and economic consequences of ADHD, emphasizing its impact on individuals, families, and society across the lifespan. The discussion highlighted key areas of concern, including social functioning, educational challenges, employment instability, criminal justice involvement, and financial burdens on health care and welfare systems.

The social impact of ADHD is significant, as individuals face persistent difficulties in social interactions, peer relationships, and emotional regulation. These challenges can lead to social rejection, bullying, and isolation, contributing to higher rates of anxiety, depression, and reduced quality of life (Faraone et al., 2021; Young et al., 2020).

ADHD also imposes a substantial economic burden on healthcare systems, educational institutions, and the workforce. Higher rates of emergency healthcare use, special education needs, and workplace absenteeism contribute to increased public spending and financial strain on families (Doshi et al., 2012; Matza et al., 2005).

People living with ADHD are overrepresented in the criminal justice system, related to increased risk of impulsive offenses and legal engagement. Lack of adequate ADHD screening and treatment in legal settings exacerbates these issues, leading to higher recidivism rates and additional costs for the criminal justice system (Fazel et al., 2015; Young et al., 2018).

In the workplace, many adults with ADHD experience difficulties maintaining stable employment, leading to lower lifetime earnings, career stagnation, and reliance on social welfare programs (Faraone et al., 2021; Shaw et al., 2014). Implementing workplace accommodations and ADHD-friendly employment policies can help mitigate these challenges and improve career trajectories.

Addressing the long-term impact of ADHD requires comprehensive, policy-driven interventions. Early diagnosis, accessible treatment, specialized educational support, and workplace accommodations are essential to reduce the economic and social burdens associated with ADHD. Targeted interventions across health care, education, and legal systems can enhance outcomes for individuals with ADHD and society at large.

By understanding the broad-reaching consequences of ADHD, policymakers, educators, healthcare providers, and employers can implement more effective solutions to support individuals with ADHD, improve their long-term well-being, and reduce the disorder's societal and economic burden.

References

Asherson, P., Buitelaar, J., Faraone, S. V., & Rohde, L. A. (2016). Adult attention-deficit hyperactivity disorder: Key conceptual issues. *Lancet Psychiatry, 3*(6), 568–578. https://doi.org/10.1016/s2215-0366(16)30032-3

Barkley, R. A. (2018). *Attention-deficit hyperactivity disorder: A handbook for diagnosis and treatment* (4th ed.). Guilford Press.

Barkley, R. A., et al. (2004). Young adult outcome of ADHD. *Journal of Abnormal Psychology, 113*(2), 279–289.

Becker, S. P., et al. (2017). Sluggish cognitive tempo in ADHD. *Journal of Child Psychology and Psychiatry, 58*(3), 231–244.

Biederman, J., et al. (2006). Functional impairments in adults with ADHD. *Journal of Clinical Psychiatry, 67*(4), 524–540.

Bunford, N., Evans, S. W., & Langberg, J. M. (2018). Emotion dysregulation and ADHD. *Clinical Child and Family Psychology Review, 21*(2), 155–176.

Byrne, C., & Guenter, D. (2023). Treatments for ADHD in adults in jails, prisons and correctional settings: A scoping review of the literature. *Health & Justice, 11*(1), 36. https://doi.org/10.1186/s40352-023-00234-9

Chronis-Tuscano, A., Clarke, T. L., O'Brien, K. A., Raggi, V. L., Diaz, Y., Mintz, A. D., Rooney, M. E., Knight, L. A., Seymour, K. E., Thomas, S. R., Seeley, J., Kosty, D., & Lewinsohn, P. (2013). Development and preliminary evaluation of an integrated treatment targeting parenting and depressive symptoms in mothers of children with attention-deficit/hyperactivity disorder. *Journal of Consulting and Clinical Psychology, 81*(5), 918–925. https://doi.org/10.1037/a0032112

Chronis-Tuscano, A., Wang, C. H., Woods, K. E., Strickland, J., & Stein, M. A. (2017). Parent ADHD and evidence-based treatment for their children: Review and directions for future research. *Journal of Abnormal Child Psychology, 45*(3), 501–517. https://doi.org/10.1007/s10802-016-0238-5

Cordier, R., Vilaysack, B., Doma, K., Wilkes-Gillan, S., & Speyer, R. (2018). Peer inclusion in interventions for children with ADHD: A systematic review and meta-analysis. *BioMed Research International, 2018*, 7693479. https://doi.org/10.1155/2018/7693479

Daley, D., van der Oord, S., Ferrin, M., Danckaerts, M., Doepfner, M., Cortese, S., & Sonuga-Barke, E. J. S. (2014). Behavioral interventions in attention-deficit/hyperactivity disorder: A meta-analysis of randomized controlled trials across multiple outcome domains. *Journal of the American Academy of Child & Adolescent Psychiatry, 53*(8), 835–847.e835. https://doi.org/10.1016/j.jaac.2014.05.013

Doshi, J. A., Hodgkins, P., Kahle, J., Sikirica, V., Cangelosi, M. J., Setyawan, J., Erder, M. H., & Neumann, P. J. (2012). Economic impact of childhood and adult attention-deficit/hyperactivity disorder in the United States. *Journal of the American Academy of Child & Adolescent Psychiatry, 51*(10), 990–1002.e1002. https://doi.org/10.1016/j.jaac.2012.07.008

Doyle, N. (2020). Neurodiversity at work: A biopsychosocial model and the impact on working adults. *British Medical Bulletin, 135*(1), 108–125.

DuPaul, G. J., & Stoner, G. (2014). *ADHD in the schools: Assessment and intervention strategies (3rd ed.)*. Guilford Press.

DuPaul, G. J., Weyandt, L. L., & Janusis, G. M. (2017). ADHD in the classroom: Effective intervention strategies. *Theory Into Practice, 56*(4), 285–292.

Evans, S. W., Owens, J. S., Wymbs, B. T., & Ray, A. R. (2018). Evidence-based psychosocial treatments for children and adolescents with attention deficit/hyperactivity disorder. *Journal of Clinical Child & Adolescent Psychology, 47*(2), 157–198. https://doi.org/10.1080/15374416.2017.1390757

Fabiano, G. A., Pelham, W. E., Coles, E. K., Gnagy, E. M., Chronis-Tuscano, A., & O'Connor, B. C. (2009). A meta-analysis of behavioral treatments for attention-deficit/hyperactivity disorder. *Clinical Psychology Review, 29*(2), 129–140. https://doi.org/10.1016/j.cpr.2008.11.001

Faraone, S. V., et al. (2021). The World Federation of ADHD International Consensus Statement: 208 evidence-based conclusions about the disorder. *Neuroscience & Biobehavioral Reviews, 128*, 789–818.

Fazel, S., et al. (2015). ADHD and risk of criminality. *JAMA Psychiatry, 72*(8), 827–834.

Haft, S. L., Chen, T., Leblanc, C., Tencza, F., & Hoeft, F. (2019). Impact of mentoring on socio-emotional and mental health outcomes of youth with learning disabilities and attention-deficit hyperactivity disorder. *Child and Adolescent Mental Health, 24*(4), 318–328. https://doi.org/10.1111/camh.12331

Halperin, J. M., Bédard, A.-C. V., & Curchack-Lichtin, J. T. (2012). Preventive interventions for ADHD: A neurodevelopmental perspective. *Neurotherapeutics, 9*(3), 531–541. https://doi.org/10.1007/s13311-012-0123-z

Hinshaw, S. P. (2018). Attention deficit hyperactivity disorder (ADHD): Controversy, developmental mechanisms, and multiple levels of analysis. *Annual Review of Clinical Psychology, 14*, 291–316.

Hoza, B. (2007). Peer functioning in children with ADHD. *Journal of Pediatric Psychology, 32*(6), 655–663. https://doi.org/10.1093/jpepsy/jsm024

Jangmo, A., Kuja-Halkola, R., Pérez-Vigil, A., Almqvist, C., Bulik, C. M., D'Onofrio, B., Lichtenstein, P., Ahnemark, E., Werner-Kiechle, T., & Larsson, H. (2021). Attention-deficit/hyperactivity disorder and occupational outcomes: The role of educational attainment, comorbid developmental disorders, and intellectual disability. *PLoS One, 16*(3), e0247724. https://doi.org/10.1371/journal.pone.0247724

Jensen-Doss, A., & Hawley, K. M. (2010). Understanding barriers to evidence-based assessment: Clinician attitudes toward standardized assessment tools. *Journal of Clinical Child & Adolescent Psychology, 39*(6), 885–896. https://doi.org/10.1080/15374416.2010.517169

Johnston, C., & Chronis-Tuscano, A. (2021). Families and ADHD. *Annual Review of Clinical Psychology, 17*, 291–316.

Katzman, M. A., Bilkey, T. S., Chokka, P. R., Fallu, A., & Klassen, L. J. (2017). Adult ADHD and comorbid disorders: Clinical implications of a dimensional approach. *BMC Psychiatry, 17*(1), 302. https://doi.org/10.1186/s12888-017-1463-3

Kessler, R. C., et al. (2005). The prevalence and correlates of adult ADHD in the United States. *American Journal of Psychiatry, 162*(4), 716–723.

Klein, R. G., et al. (2012). Clinical course of ADHD. *Journal of the American Academy of Child & Adolescent Psychiatry, 51*(6), 593–602.

Lawson, G. M., McKenzie, M. E., Becker, K. D., Selby, L., & Hoover, S. A. (2019). The Core components of evidence-based social emotional learning programs. *Prevention Science, 20*(4), 457–467. https://doi.org/10.1007/s11121-018-0953-y

Loe, I. M., & Feldman, H. M. (2007). Academic outcomes of ADHD. *Journal of Pediatric Psychology, 32*(6), 643–654.

Matza, L. S., et al. (2005). Quality of life in children with ADHD. *Journal of Attention Disorders, 9*(3), 501–508.

Miranda, A., Colomer, C., Berenguer, C., Roselló, R., & Roselló, B. (2016). Substance use in young adults with ADHD: Comorbidity and symptoms of inattention and hyperactivity/impulsivity. *International Journal of Clinical and Health Psychology, 16*(2), 157–165. https://doi.org/10.1016/j.ijchp.2015.09.001

Mikami, A. Y. (2010). The importance of friendship for youth with ADHD. *Clinical Child and Family Psychology Review, 13*(2), 181–198.

Mohr-Jensen, C., & Steinhausen, H.-C. (2016). Long-term outcomes of ADHD. *European Child & Adolescent Psychiatry, 25*(10), 1071–1082.

Mowlem, F. D., Rosenqvist, M. A., Martin, J., Lichtenstein, P., Asherson, P., & Larsson, H. (2019). Sex differences in predicting ADHD clinical diagnosis and pharmacological treatment. *European Child & Adolescent Psychiatry, 28*(4), 481–489. https://doi.org/10.1007/s00787-018-1211-3

Munetz, M. R., & Griffin, P. A. (2006). Use of the sequential intercept model as an approach to decriminalization of people with serious mental illness. *Psychiatric Services, 57*(4), 544–549. https://doi.org/10.1176/ps.2006.57.4.544

Power, T. J., Tresco, K. E., & Cassano, M. C. (2009). School-based interventions for students with attention-deficit/hyperactivity disorder. *Current Psychiatry Reports, 11*(5), 407–414. https://doi.org/10.1007/s11920-009-0061-6

Rietveld, C. A., & Patel, P. C. (2019). ADHD and later-life labor market outcomes in the United States. *The European Journal of Health Economics, 20*(7), 949–967. https://doi.org/10.1007/s10198-019-01055-0

Sayal, K., Prasad, V., Daley, D., Ford, T., & Coghill, D. (2018). ADHD in children and young people: Prevalence, care pathways, and service provision. *The Lancet Psychiatry, 5*(2), 175–186.

Schein, J., Adler, L. A., Childress, A., Cloutier, M., Gagnon-Sanschagrin, P., Davidson, M., Kinkead, F., Guerin, A., & Lefebvre, P. (2022). Economic burden of attention-deficit/hyperactivity disorder among children and adolescents in the United States: A societal perspective. *Journal of Medical Economics, 25*(1), 193–205. https://doi.org/10.1080/13696998.2022.2032097

Schein, J., Adler, L. A., Childress, A., Gagnon-Sanschagrin, P., Davidson, M., Kinkead, F., Cloutier, M., Guérin, A., & Lefebvre, P. (2022). Economic burden of attention-deficit/hyperactivity disorder among adults in the United States: A societal perspective. *Journal of Managed Care & Specialty Pharmacy, 28*(2), 168–179. https://doi.org/10.18553/jmcp.2021.21290

Seery, C., Leonard-Curtin, A., Naismith, L., King, N., Kilbride, K., Wrigley, M., Boyd, C., McHugh, L., & Bramham, J. (2023). The understanding and managing adult ADHD programme: A qualitative evaluation of online psychoeducation with acceptance and commitment therapy for adults with ADHD. *Journal of Contextual Behavioral Science, 29*, 254–263. https://doi.org/10.1016/j.jcbs.2023.08.005

Shaw, P., et al. (2014). Neurodevelopmental trajectories of ADHD. *Biological Psychiatry, 76*(8), 615–623.

Sonuga-Barke, E. J., Brandeis, D., Cortese, S., Daley, D., Ferrin, M., Holtmann, M., Stevenson, J., Danckaerts, M., van der Oord, S., Döpfner, M., Dittmann, R. W., Simonoff, E., Zuddas, A., Banaschewski, T., Buitelaar, J., Coghill, D., Hollis, C., Konofal, E., Lecendreux, M., et al. (2013). Nonpharmacological interventions for ADHD: Systematic review and meta-analyses of randomized controlled trials of dietary and psychological treatments. *The American Journal of Psychiatry, 170*(3), 275–289. https://doi.org/10.1176/appi.ajp.2012.12070991

Theule, J., et al. (2013). Parenting stress in families of children with ADHD. *Journal of Emotional and Behavioral Disorders, 21*(1), 3–17.

U.S. Department of Education. (2021). Students with disabilities preparing for postsecondary education: Know your rights and responsibilities.

van den Hoofdakker, B. J., van der Veen-Mulders, L., Sytema, S., Emmelkamp, P. M. G., Minderaa, R. B., & Nauta, M. H. (2007). Effectiveness of behavioral parent training for children with ADHD in routine clinical practice: A randomized controlled study. *Journal of the American Academy of Child and Adolescent Psychiatry, 46*(10), 1263–1271. https://doi.org/10.1097/chi.0b013e3181354bc2

Weyandt, L. L., & DuPaul, G. J. (2006). ADHD in college students. *Journal of Attention Disorders, 10*(1), 9–19.

Wilens, T. E., et al. (2011). Substance use disorders in ADHD. *Journal of Clinical Psychiatry, 72*(8), 1015–1023.

Young, S., et al. (2018). ADHD in adults: A review. *Psychological Medicine, 48*(3), 369–379.

Young, S., et al. (2020). Females with ADHD: An expert consensus statement. *BMC Psychiatry, 20*, 404.

Chapter 7
ADHD Across the Lifespan: Developmental Changes and Challenges

Abstract ADHD is a complex neurodevelopmental disorder that affects individuals across all stages of life. While traditionally associated with childhood, it is now widely recognized as a lifelong condition with varying manifestations and challenges in adolescence, adulthood, and older age. The evolving nature of ADHD means that symptoms such as inattention, impulsivity, and hyperactivity interact with different developmental transitions, shaping academic, occupational, and social experiences in distinct ways.

In this chapter, we examine how ADHD presents at different life stages, considering the impact of neurological maturation, environmental influences, and coping mechanisms. We explore how early intervention, tailored treatment approaches, and adaptive strategies can help individuals navigate these transitions successfully. Additionally, the chapter highlights the importance of recognizing ADHD in adulthood and later life, addressing misconceptions that ADHD diminishes over time.

By understanding the developmental trajectory of ADHD, we can better support individuals in maximizing their strengths, minimizing challenges, and improving long-term well-being.

7.1 Core Symptoms in Early Development

ADHD is a neurodevelopmental condition that typically emerges in early childhood, with symptoms often becoming evident before the age of 7 (American Psychiatric Association [APA], 2022). The disorder is characterized by persistent patterns of inattention, hyperactivity, and impulsivity, which significantly impact cognitive, emotional, and social development (Faraone et al., 2021). While the presentation of ADHD varies among individuals, the severity and expression of symptoms are influenced by genetic, neurobiological, and environmental factors (Shaw et al., 2014). Early identification and intervention are critical, as untreated ADHD can lead to persistent academic underperformance, social difficulties, and behavioral challenges—extending into adolescence and adulthood (French et al., 2024).

G. Ayano et al., *ADHD Across the Lifespan*, SpringerBriefs in Modern Perspectives on Disability Research,
https://doi.org/10.1007/978-981-95-8712-4_7

This section explores the core symptoms of ADHD in early childhood, focusing on inattention, hyperactivity, impulsivity, and the role of ADHD subtypes in symptom variability.

7.1.1 Inattention: Deficits in Focus, Organization, and Task Persistence

Children with untreated ADHD struggle with sustained attention, working memory, and task management, leading to academic and social difficulties. These challenges manifest in several ways. First, reduced ability to maintain focus in structured environments is common; children frequently lose concentration during tasks that require sustained mental effort, such as classroom lessons or reading (Faraone et al., 2021). External distractions—such as background noise, visual stimuli, or internal thoughts—further disrupt focus (Shaw et al., 2014). Second, children may have difficulty following instructions and completing multi-step tasks, often struggling to process and retain verbal instructions (Barkley, 2018). Misinterpretation of inattention as defiance is common, although working memory deficits often underlie these challenges. Finally, disorganization and forgetfulness in daily routines are hallmark features of ADHD; frequent misplacement of belongings and forgetfulness about tasks frustrate caregivers and educators alike (Shaw et al., 2014; Barkley, 2018).

7.1.2 Hyperactivity: Excessive Movement and Difficulty Regulating Activity Levels

Hyperactivity in early childhood is one of the most observable symptoms of ADHD. It often manifests as excessive motor activity and difficulty maintaining appropriate activity levels in structured settings. Core features include persistent restlessness and difficulty remaining seated; children may engage in excessive running or climbing even in inappropriate settings like classrooms (Shaw et al., 2014). Prolonged sitting, such as during meals or story time, is particularly challenging (Barkley, 2018). Constant fidgeting and inability to engage in quiet activities are also common; repetitive hand movements, tapping, and shifting positions frequently occur even during sedentary tasks (APA, 2022; Faraone et al., 2021). Additionally, excessive talking and difficulty modulating speech volume often manifest as rapid, intrusive speech patterns that can challenge social interactions (Barkley, 2018; Shaw et al., 2014). While hyperactivity often decreases with age, internal restlessness and difficulty sustaining attention can persist into adolescence and adulthood (Faraone et al., 2021).

7.1.3 *Impulsivity: Poor Self-Regulation and Risk-Prone Behaviors*

Impulsivity in ADHD is characterized by difficulty delaying gratification, regulating emotions, and considering consequences before acting. Children may interrupt conversations, blurt out answers, and struggle with turn-taking (Barkley, 2018). These behaviors can lead to social difficulties as peers perceive them as intrusive or domineering (Shaw et al., 2014). Emotional impulsivity also manifests in rapid mood shifts, heightened reactions, and difficulty calming down after frustration, contributing to conflicts with peers, teachers, and caregivers (Faraone et al., 2021). Risk-prone behaviors, such as running into traffic or climbing unsafe structures, highlight the tendency to act without considering long-term consequences (Shaw et al., 2014; Faraone et al., 2021).

7.1.4 *Symptom Variability: The Role of ADHD Subtypes*

ADHD is a heterogeneous disorder, with symptom expression varying by subtype as defined in the DSM-5-TR (APA, 2022). The Predominantly Inattentive Type (ADHD-I) is more common in girls and characterized by distractibility and poor organizational skills (Faraone et al., 2021). The Predominantly Hyperactive-Impulsive Type (ADHD-HI) is often diagnosed in younger children, with hyperactivity decreasing over time but impulsivity persisting (Barkley, 2018). Finally, the Combined Type (ADHD-C) involves both inattentive and hyperactive-impulsive symptoms, often associated with greater academic challenges, social difficulties, and emotional dysregulation (APA, 2022). Understanding these subtypes is essential for tailoring interventions to each child's unique needs.

7.2 Impact on Academic Performance

Untreated ADHD can have a profound impact on academic performance, with symptoms of inattention, hyperactivity, and impulsivity disrupting learning processes from early childhood (Faraone et al., 2021). These difficulties manifest as struggles with homework completion, test-taking, and classroom engagement, often resulting in lower academic achievement, increased disciplinary actions, and greater reliance on special education services (Barkley, 2018). Without targeted intervention, academic challenges persist into adolescence and adulthood, contributing to higher dropout rates, lower rates of college enrollment, and diminished career opportunities (Loe & Feldman, 2007).

7.2.1 *Struggles with Schoolwork, Homework Completion, and Test Performance*

Children with ADHD frequently experience significant difficulties in structured academic settings where sustained attention, executive function, and organizational skills are required. ADHD-related deficits in executive function often hinder task initiation and completion, leading to procrastination, incomplete assignments, and frequent errors (Faraone et al., 2021). Challenges with test-taking and working memory, including slow processing speed and susceptibility to distractions, further impair academic performance (Barkley, 2018; Loe & Feldman, 2007). Particular difficulties with mathematics, reading comprehension, and writing, where working memory, organization, and multi-step problem-solving are essential have been documented (Daley & Birchwood, 2010; Shaw et al., 2014). Without appropriate accommodations, these challenges contribute to chronic underachievement and school disengagement.

7.2.2 *Increased Likelihood of Disciplinary Actions Due to Classroom Behavior*

ADHD-related impulsivity and hyperactivity frequently result in behavioral challenges that interfere with classroom learning. Children with ADHD often talk excessively and disrupt the classroom, which are frequently misinterpreted by teachers as intentional misconduct (Barkley & Brown, 2008; French et al., 2024). Difficulties adhering to classroom rules and structured routines lead to frequent reprimands and removal from learning activities, reducing instructional time and further exacerbating academic struggles (Daley & Birchwood, 2010; Shaw et al., 2014). Negative teacher–student interactions and the lack of ADHD-specific training for educators contribute to low expectations and reduced engagement for students with ADHD (Biederman et al., 2006).

7.2.3 *Higher Likelihood of Grade Repetition and Special Education Placement*

Children with ADHD are at increased risk of grade retention, which is associated with decreased self-esteem, frustration, and higher school dropout rates (Barkley, 2018; Loe & Feldman, 2007). Many students qualify for Individualized Education Plans (IEPs) or Section 504 accommodations that provide supports such as extended test time and behavioral interventions (Daley & Birchwood, 2010). However, access to these services is inconsistent, and many children fail to receive the necessary supports for academic success (Shaw et al., 2014). The financial burden of

ADHD-related educational services is also substantial, with schools investing in one-on-one tutoring and behavioral support while families incur out-of-pocket costs for private interventions (Biederman et al., 2006; Faraone et al., 2021).

Impact of Treatment vs. No Treatment

Long-term outcomes vary dramatically between untreated and treated ADHD. A systematic review of long-term studies (2 years or more) revealed that 86% of untreated individuals exhibited significantly worse outcomes across multiple life domains, including academic achievement and social functioning. In contrast, 94% of treated individuals—whether pharmacologically, behaviorally, or through multimodal approaches—demonstrated improved or stabilized outcomes (Shaw et al., 2011). A focused analysis of 176 academic outcome studies found that 79% showed poorer achievement in untreated ADHD compared to controls—yet 100% of those treated with combined modalities improved in achievement tests, compared with just 75% for medication alone and 75% for non-pharmacological treatment (Arnold et al., 2015).

7.2.4 *Difficulties in Peer Relationships and Increased Risk of Social Rejection*

Beyond academic challenges, ADHD significantly affects social functioning in school settings. Children with ADHD often struggle with turn-taking, emotional regulation, and interpreting social cues, leading to difficulties forming positive peer relationships (Shaw et al., 2014; Mikami, 2010). These difficulties contribute to higher rates of bullying and victimization, as ADHD behaviors may be perceived as disruptive or irritating by peers (Becker et al., 2017). Social rejection in childhood can lead to increased risk of depression, substance use, and delinquency during adolescence (Barkley, 2018). Children with ADHD who experience peer rejection are also less likely to participate in extracurricular activities, limiting opportunities for positive social engagement and support (Faraone et al., 2021).

Social skills training and peer-mentoring programs are essential for improving interpersonal interactions and reducing the risk of social exclusion. Early intervention in academic and social domains is crucial for improving long-term educational and psychological outcomes for children with ADHD.

7.3 Family and Home Life Challenges

ADHD has far-reaching implications beyond the affected individual, profoundly shaping family dynamics, parental well-being, and sibling relationships (Johnston & Chronis-Tuscano, 2021). Managing a child with ADHD requires persistent supervision, structured routines, and adaptive parenting strategies, often leading to heightened parental stress, increased household conflicts, and disruptions in daily activities (Barkley, 2018). This section explores the multifaceted impact of ADHD on family life, emphasizing parental stress, difficulties in maintaining household routines, and the implications for sibling relationships. Effective interventions, including evidence-based parenting strategies, structured home environments, and family therapy, are essential in fostering resilience and mitigating long-term familial distress.

Parents of children with ADHD report significantly higher levels of stress, emotional exhaustion, and mental health difficulties compared to parents of neurotypical children (Theule et al., 2013). The persistent challenges associated with ADHD—including impulsivity, emotional dysregulation, and defiance—often result in chronic household tension and disagreements between caregivers. Elevated parental stress is common, with mothers frequently experiencing heightened rates of anxiety and depression attributable to the daily demands of managing ADHD-related behaviors (Johnston & Chronis-Tuscano, 2021). Parental burnout results from constant behavioral monitoring, repeated disciplinary interventions, and frequent school-related concerns (Barkley, 2018). Moreover, parents often differ in their approach to managing ADHD symptoms, leading to inconsistent discipline, confusion for the child, and further family discord (Theule et al., 2013). Financial and time burdens, such as costs for medication, behavioral therapy, and private tutoring, further strain family resources (Biederman et al., 2006). Some parents reduce work hours or leave the workforce to meet their child's needs, leading to additional financial instability (Johnston & Chronis-Tuscano, 2021). Parent training programs, mental health support, and consistent education on ADHD can mitigate these stressors by equipping parents with effective discipline strategies and coping mechanisms.

Children with ADHD often struggle with executive functioning skills, making it challenging to adhere to structured routines like morning preparations, homework, and bedtime. These difficulties disrupt family schedules and contribute to parental frustration. Inattentiveness results in forgetfulness around daily tasks, while distractibility and resistance to transitions can cause delays in school departures and missed appointments (Barkley, 2018). Procrastination and avoidance further complicate homework completion, often leading to parent–child conflicts (Johnston & Chronis-Tuscano, 2021). ADHD is also associated with sleep disturbances, including insomnia and difficulty settling at night, which in turn exacerbate morning irritability and inattention (Faraone et al., 2021; Shaw et al., 2014). Structured visual schedules, bedtime interventions, and breaking homework into manageable tasks can improve daily functioning and reduce conflicts at home (Hiscock et al., 2015; Thomas & Karuppali, 2022).

ADHD significantly affects sibling relationships, leading to heightened conflict, competition for parental attention, and emotional strain (Mikami, 2010). Siblings often feel overshadowed or neglected as parents focus on managing the ADHD child's needs, leading to resentment and decreased sibling bonding (Johnston & Chronis-Tuscano, 2021). ADHD-related impulsivity and frustration tolerance issues contribute to frequent physical and verbal conflicts (Barkley, 2018; Shaw et al.,

2014). Parents may experience guilt about uneven attention distribution, while non-ADHD siblings are at increased risk for anxiety, depression, and social isolation (Mikami, 2010; Johnston & Chronis-Tuscano, 2021). Providing dedicated one-on-one time for non-ADHD siblings, family counseling, and emotional regulation skills training can reduce household strain and promote healthier sibling relationships (Orm & Fjermestad, 2021).

7.4 Transition from Childhood to Adolescence

The transition from childhood to adolescence presents unique challenges for individuals with ADHD, as academic expectations, social pressures, and emotional regulation demands increase significantly (Faraone et al., 2021). While some ADHD symptoms, particularly hyperactivity, may decline, others, such as inattention, impulsivity, and emotional dysregulation, often persist, leading to difficulties in school, social relationships, and self-esteem (Barkley, 2018).

Adolescence is also a period of increased autonomy and responsibility, requiring greater self-regulation, executive function, and coping skills. For individuals with ADHD, these developmental shifts often exacerbate existing impairments, heightening the risk of academic underperformance, social rejection, and emotional distress. This section examines the evolving symptomatology of ADHD in adolescence, emphasizing its impact on academic functioning, emotional regulation, and social integration.

Although the core symptoms of ADHD—inattention, impulsivity, and hyperactivity—persist into adolescence, their presentation often changes, requiring tailored intervention strategies (Shaw et al., 2014). Overt hyperactivity often declines, but an internal sense of restlessness remains, manifesting as difficulty relaxing, maintaining focus, and sustaining attention during sedentary activities (Barkley, 2018; Faraone et al., 2021). Inattention becomes more impairing in academic and social contexts, as schoolwork grows more complex and requires increased sustained attention, task organization, and working memory. Adolescents with ADHD frequently struggle to track assignments, follow multi-step instructions, and manage deadlines, leading to academic underachievement (Biederman et al., 2006; Shaw et al., 2014). Impulsivity remains a prominent challenge, often leading to risky behaviors such as substance use, reckless driving, and unprotected sexual activity, which can pose significant health and social risks (Barkley, 2018).

Early intervention strategies that emphasize self-regulation training, executive function support, and structured academic accommodations are important at this life stage to address the evolving ADHD symptoms in adolescence.

The transition from elementary to secondary school brings a substantial increase in academic demands, including independent study, long-term assignments, and complex problem-solving. Adolescents with ADHD may struggle to meet these expectations due to deficits in executive function, time management, and organizational skills. Unlike elementary school, where teacher guidance is more consistent, middle and high-school settings require students to manage multi-step assignments independently. Adolescents with ADHD may procrastinate, mismanage deadlines, and struggle to break large tasks into smaller, manageable steps, leading to incomplete work and declining grades (Loe & Feldman, 2007; Daley & Birchwood, 2010). The increased reliance on self-regulation and independent learning compounds these challenges. High-school curricula emphasize independent study, requiring students to track assignments, prepare for exams, and manage their workload without continuous teacher supervision. Adolescents with ADHD often fail to use planners, underestimate the time needed for studying, and struggle with prioritization, increasing their risk of academic disengagement (Barkley, 2018). Persistent struggles with organization and performance can contribute to low self-esteem, school avoidance, and higher dropout rates. Without appropriate academic support, adolescents with ADHD are at greater risk of failing key subjects, repeating grades, or developing secondary mental health conditions such as anxiety and depression (Daley & Birchwood, 2010; Loe & Feldman, 2007).

To mitigate these impacts, enhance educational outcomes, and reduce academic burnout, tailored time management training, executive function coaching, and academic accommodations, and collaboration between parents and teachers are recommended.

Adolescence is also a critical period for emotional development, with increased social complexities, peer expectations, and identity formation. Individuals with ADHD can experience greater emotional reactivity, frustration intolerance, and heightened sensitivity to stress. Emotional impulsivity and frustration intolerance manifest as strong, rapidly shifting emotional responses that can lead to difficulties regulating anger, disappointment, or anxiety (Barkley, 2018). Even minor academic setbacks or social conflicts can provoke exaggerated emotional reactions, including outbursts, withdrawal, or oppositional behavior (Shaw et al., 2014). Rising academic and social pressures can exacerbate anxiety, perfectionism, and avoidance behaviors, leading to procrastination, incomplete schoolwork, or social withdrawal (Faraone et al., 2021). Adolescents with ADHD may resist constructive feedback or avoid challenging tasks due to fear of failure. Difficulties with social cues, impulse control, and turn-taking contribute to peer conflicts, social exclusion, and bullying (Mikami, 2010). These challenges can compound low self-esteem, depression, and engagement in risk-taking behaviors as maladaptive coping mechanisms (Biederman et al., 2006). Emotion regulation training, social skills development, and structured extracurricular activities are recommended to improve self-control, peer relationships, and overall well-being.

7.4.1 *Social and Peer Relationships*

Adolescence represents a critical period for social development, yet for individuals with ADHD, it is frequently characterized by peer rejection, increased engagement in risk-taking behaviors, and difficulties in romantic relationships (Mikami, 2010;

Barkley, 2018). Core ADHD-related challenges—including impulsivity, emotional dysregulation, and social reciprocity deficits—contribute to strained friendships, heightened vulnerability to negative peer influences, and difficulty managing intimate relationships (Beauchaine & Hinshaw, 2020). These social difficulties can affect self-esteem, mental health, and behavioral outcomes. Adolescents with ADHD often find it challenging to integrate into peer groups, establish reciprocal friendships, and engage in stable romantic relationships, increasing their risk of social isolation, bullying, delinquency, and emotional distress (Hoza, 2007). This section explores the key social challenges faced by adolescents with ADHD and discusses evidence-based interventions to promote social competence, improve peer relationships, and mitigate risk-taking behaviors.

Adolescents with ADHD often experience higher rates of peer rejection, difficulty forming lasting friendships, and social exclusion, largely due to deficits in impulse control, emotional regulation, and social cognition (Mikami, 2010; Hoza, 2007). Impulsivity and poor social reciprocity, such as interrupting conversations, dominating discussions, and difficulties interpreting nonverbal cues, humor, and sarcasm, lead to misunderstandings and awkward interactions that exacerbate social isolation (Beauchaine & Hinshaw, 2020; Mikami, 2010). Studies indicate that adolescents with ADHD are more likely to be disliked by peers, as their behaviors are often perceived as disruptive or immature, resulting in difficulties maintaining long-term friendships (Hoza, 2007; Barkley, 2018). This increased vulnerability to bullying and victimization can further undermine self-esteem and reinforce a cycle of rejection, social anxiety, and reluctance to engage in group activities (Becker et al., 2017; Mikami, 2010). Social skills training in context-specific settings (e.g., in vivo feedback) (Mikami et al., 2017) (Barkley et al., 2001), peer mentoring programs designed for students with learning disabilities or ADHD (Williams et al., 2024) (Williams et al., 2024), and school-based anti-bullying interventions shown to reduce victimization by approximately 15–25% (Gaffney et al., 2021) (Gaffney et al., 2021) have all demonstrated promise in improving social competence and fostering inclusive educational environments.

Adolescents with ADHD are also at heightened risk of engaging in impulsive and high-risk behaviors, including substance use, reckless driving, and delinquent activities (Wilens & Morrison, 2011; Barkley, 2018). ADHD-related deficits in impulse control and heightened sensation-seeking tendencies increase susceptibility to early substance use, with affected adolescents initiating smoking, drinking, or drug use at significantly younger ages than their neurotypical peers (Wilens & Morrison, 2011). These patterns can then escalate to binge drinking, illicit drug experimentation, and addiction (Sibley et al., 2014). ADHD symptoms also contribute to higher rates of reckless driving, traffic violations, and motor vehicle accidents due to impairments in hazard awareness, reaction time, and rule adherence (Barkley & Cox, 2007; Barkley, 2018). Furthermore, long-term planning and risk assessment difficulties increase the likelihood of impulsive criminal behaviors, including shoplifting, vandalism, and physical altercations, resulting in school suspensions or juvenile justice involvement (Sibley et al., 2014; Beauchaine & Hinshaw, 2020). Interventions focusing on impulse control (Barkley et al., 2001), risk-awareness

(Jensen et al., 2007), and structured extracurricular engagement (Fredricks & Eccles, 2006) may reduce risky behaviors and promote safer decision-making.

Adolescents with ADHD often experience intense but unstable romantic relationships, largely due to emotional impulsivity, communication Issues, and difficulties with emotional regulation (Barkley, 2018; Sibley et al., 2014). These challenges increase relationship dissatisfaction, emotional distress, and vulnerability to unhealthy relationship patterns (Beauchaine & Hinshaw, 2020). Emotional intensity and impulsive decision-making often manifest as overwhelming attachments, excessive jealousy, or difficulty coping with rejection, leading to intense emotional distress (Sibley et al., 2014; Barkley, 2018).

Communication difficulties, including poor active listening, difficulties remembering details, and emotional dysregulation, contribute to misunderstandings, conflict escalation, and reduced satisfaction in relationships (Beauchaine & Hinshaw, 2020). Low self-esteem and difficulty setting personal boundaries increase the likelihood of remaining in unhealthy or emotionally abusive relationships, while impulsivity may contribute to unprotected sexual behaviors, unintended pregnancies, and sexually transmitted infections (Barkley, 2018; Sibley et al., 2014). Interventions such as relationship coaching (Fleming & McMahon, 2012), social-emotional learning programs (Durlak et al., 2011), and parental guidance (Mikami et al., 2017) are therefore important to equip adolescents with ADHD with the skills and support needed for healthy and fulfilling romantic relationships.

7.4.2 Comorbidities and Mental Health Risks

Co-occurring psychiatric conditions in adolescence can compound the challenges of living with ADHD, intensifying functional impairments and elevating the risk of self-harm, suicidal ideation, and long-term emotional distress (SUDs) (Barkley, 2018; Faraone et al., 2021) (Beauchaine & Hinshaw, 2020). The onset and severity of these comorbidities are shaped by an interplay between neurobiological vulnerabilities and environmental stressors, including peer rejection, academic challenges, and family conflict. Failure to identify and address these comorbidities significantly worsens prognosis, increasing the risk of chronic mental illness, social dysfunction, and poor life outcomes (Pliszka, 2003). This section examines the most prevalent mental health risks associated with ADHD in adolescence, emphasizing the need for early identification, integrated treatment, and targeted interventions to mitigate long-term adverse outcomes.

Adolescents with ADHD have a substantially increased likelihood of developing internalizing disorders, such as depression and generalized anxiety disorder, as well as externalizing disorders, including ODD and conduct disorder (CD) (Biederman et al., 2006; Nigg et al., 2020). Approximately 30–50% of adolescents with ADHD develop major depressive disorder, driven by chronic academic failure, peer rejection, and parental criticism, which foster low self-esteem, social withdrawal, and persistent negative self-perception (Meinzer et al., 2014; Barkley, 2018; Seymour et al., 2021). Adolescents with comorbid ADHD and depression also exhibit higher rates of suicidal ideation and self-harm than those with ADHD alone (Beauchaine & Hinshaw, 2020). Additionally, ADHD is associated with a two- to threefold increased risk of anxiety disorders, including GAD, social anxiety, and panic disorder (Nigg et al., 2020; Seymour et al., 2021). Anxiety symptoms often exacerbate inattention and avoidance behaviors, resulting in academic underachievement and school refusal (Biederman et al., 2006). Adolescents with ADHD and comorbid anxiety frequently struggle with task initiation, perfectionism, and performance-related stress, which can complicate transitions to higher education (Meinzer et al., 2014). Externalizing disorders are also common, with approximately 40–50% of adolescents developing ODD, marked by chronic defiance, argumentativeness, and emotional outbursts, and 25–30% developing CD, significantly increasing the risk of delinquency, aggression, and legal involvement (Barkley, 2018; Faraone et al., 2021; Seymour et al., 2021).

Adolescents with ADHD face significantly increased risks of self-harm and suicide, often driven by impulsivity, emotion dysregulation, and social stressors (Hinshaw et al., 2012). Research indicates that these adolescents are three to five times more likely to attempt suicide than their non-ADHD peers, with females at even higher risk, particularly when depression and social struggles co-occur (Meinzer et al., 2014; Hinshaw et al., 2012; Seymour et al., 2021). Impulsivity further contributes to higher rates of non-suicidal self-injury, such as cutting or burning, as a maladaptive coping mechanism for emotional distress. Poor impulse control increases the likelihood of rash, unplanned suicide attempts, often triggered by interpersonal conflicts or acute emotional distress (Beauchaine & Hinshaw, 2020). Social isolation, academic difficulties, and family conflicts intensify feelings of loneliness and hopelessness, driving self-harm behaviors (Seymour et al., 2021). Experiences of bullying further elevate the risk of suicidal behavior, underscoring the importance of peer support and anti-bullying interventions (Barkley, 2018).

Substance use disorders are among the most prevalent and dangerous comorbidities in adolescents with ADHD, fueled by impulsivity, risk-seeking behaviors, and difficulty delaying gratification (Wilens & Morrison, 2011; Sibley et al., 2014). These adolescents are twice as likely to begin using substances before age 14, increasing their risk of long-term addiction (Wilens & Morrison, 2011). Nicotine and cannabis use are particularly common, as adolescents with ADHD self-medicate symptoms of inattention and anxiety (Sibley et al., 2014). The risk of developing SUDs is two to three times higher than in the general population, with deficits in impulse control and emotional regulation complicating efforts to quit or moderate use (Barkley, 2018). Additionally, ADHD is associated with higher rates of polysubstance use, leading to increased risks of overdose, accidents, and legal consequences (Sibley et al., 2014). Unstructured peer environments, low parental supervision, and sensation-seeking tendencies further exacerbate these risks (Beauchaine & Hinshaw, 2020).

Adolescence introduces significant hormonal and neurobiological changes—such as surges in sex hormones and ongoing prefrontal cortex development—that create a period of heightened vulnerability for individuals with ADHD. Pubertal fluctuations in estrogen and testosterone can further disrupt dopamine and norepinephrine pathways, potentially exacerbating symptoms of inattention, emotional dysregulation, and impulsivity (Luo et al., 2024). At the same time, adolescents must navigate increasing academic pressures, evolving peer group dynamics, and greater autonomy, all while their regulatory brain circuits remain under construction—leading to greater difficulty in managing emotions and behavior (Kumar & Jha, 2025). This confluence of biological and psychosocial stressors not only aggravates core ADHD symptoms but also elevates the risk of co-occurring mental health problems, such as mood disorders and substance use, making adolescence an especially critical period for monitoring and early intervention.

7.5 Evolution of Symptoms in Adults

ADHD is now widely recognized as a lifelong neurodevelopmental disorder, with 60–80% of individuals diagnosed in childhood continuing to experience symptoms into adulthood (Faraone et al., 2021; Barkley, 2018). However, the manifestation of ADHD symptoms evolve over time, reflecting both neurological maturation and compensatory adaptations that individuals develop as they navigate different life stages (Kooij et al., 2019). While overt hyperactivity often diminishes, adults with ADHD continue to experience significant challenges with inattention, impulsivity, emotional dysregulation, and executive function. These persistent symptoms affect professional performance, financial stability, relationship maintenance, and daily life management. This section explores the evolution of ADHD symptoms in adulthood, emphasizing their functional implications across key domains.

In adulthood, hyperactivity typically transitions from externalized physical restlessness to a subjective sense of inner agitation. During childhood, hyperactivity often manifests as overt behaviors like excessive running, climbing, and difficulty remaining seated (APA, 2013). However, in adults, these symptoms transform into a persistent sensation of being "on edge," with difficulty relaxing and unwinding (Faraone et al., 2021). Adults with ADHD frequently report feeling driven by an internal motor, experiencing chronic impatience, and struggling to remain still, particularly in professional settings such as meetings or long conferences (Kooij et al., 2019). This internal restlessness can contribute to stress-related disorders, anxiety, and even workaholic tendencies, as individuals may seek constant stimulation to manage feelings of agitation (Barkley, 2018). Many adults with ADHD also report low frustration tolerance and impatience, often struggling to wait in lines, endure slow conversations, or navigate bureaucratic processes, leading to irritability and impulsive frustration.

While hyperactivity may decrease, inattention and executive dysfunction can persist as significant barriers to productivity and independent living in adulthood. Adults with ADHD often struggle with chronic forgetfulness, disorganization, and poor time management, which impact workplace performance, household responsibilities, and overall life organization (Kooij et al., 2019). Forgetting appointments, misplacing important items, and failing to recall conversation details can lead to poor professional reliability, financial mismanagement, and interpersonal strain (Barkley, 2018). Difficulties with task prioritization, time estimation, and meeting deadlines often result in chronic lateness, last-minute work rushes, and persistent feelings of being overwhelmed (Faraone et al., 2021; Kooij et al., 2019). Additionally, adults with ADHD frequently struggle to maintain structured environments, contributing to cluttered workspaces, incomplete projects, and erratic scheduling, all of which can exacerbate job instability, financial insecurity, and relationship challenges.

Impulsivity remains a core ADHD symptom in adulthood, often manifesting as poor decision-making, difficulty with self-regulation, and interpersonal struggles. Financial management is a common area of concern, with many adults engaging in impulsive spending, poor budgeting, and erratic financial planning, which increases the risk of credit card debt, overspending, and economic instability (Barkley, 2018). These impulsive tendencies often extend to workplace behaviors, where adults with ADHD may interrupt colleagues, make rash decisions without evaluating consequences, or frequently change jobs due to boredom or frustration (Kooij et al., 2019). Adapting to workplace hierarchies and maintaining long-term productivity can also be challenging, leading to career instability and inconsistent income. Interpersonal relationships often suffer due to impulsive conversational habits—such as interrupting, blurting out unfiltered thoughts, or overreacting emotionally—creating strain in romantic partnerships and social circles (Barkley, 2018). Forgetfulness and inconsistent emotional availability can further challenge long-term relationship maintenance (Faraone et al., 2021).

7.5.1 Workplace and Career Challenges

ADHD presents persistent challenges in professional environments, affecting career stability, job performance, and workplace relationships. Adults with ADHD often experience higher job turnover, difficulties with task prioritization, and an increased risk of workplace conflicts and burnout (Barkley, 2018; Faraone et al., 2021). Core executive function deficits, including poor time management, impulsivity, and difficulty with organization, can compromise productivity, limit career advancement, and increase stress. Addressing these challenges requires targeted workplace accommodations, structured career planning, and evidence-based interventions to optimize job performance and professional success.

Adults with ADHD experience greater job instability, often characterized by frequent job changes, difficulties maintaining consistent employment, and challenges in career progression (Biederman et al., 2006; Kessler et al., 2005). Research indicates that adults with ADHD are significantly more likely to be dismissed from jobs due to missed deadlines, impulsive decision-making, or conflicts with supervisors

(Faraone et al., 2021). Many report difficulty finding fulfilling roles, leading to repeated job changes and career instability. Boredom intolerance, impulsivity, and low frustration tolerance make it challenging for adults with ADHD to remain engaged in routine or repetitive tasks, often prompting them to switch jobs in search of more stimulating work, which can disrupt long-term career growth and financial security (Barkley, 2018; Kooij et al., 2019). Unstable employment patterns may lead to irregular income, difficulty saving money, and increased financial stress, while limited workplace accommodations can further hinder career advancement and long-term earnings (Biederman et al., 2006; Faraone et al., 2021).

Executive function impairments can also interfere with an individual's ability to manage multiple tasks, prioritize responsibilities, and meet deadlines. Adults with ADHD may experience "time blindness," underestimating how long tasks will take and postponing work until the last minute, which results in missed deadlines, frequent extensions, and rushed, lower-quality work (Kooij et al., 2019; Barkley, 2018). Multitasking is another significant challenge as many jobs require juggling multiple projects and individuals with ADHD struggle to shift focus between tasks, increasing errors and incomplete work. This frequent task switching can become overwhelming, leading to reduced efficiency and mental fatigue (Faraone et al., 2021). Disorganized workspaces, misplaced files, and erratic scheduling contribute to inconsistent performance, difficulties following instructions, and frustration among colleagues and supervisors (Barkley, 2018; Kooij et al., 2019).

Social difficulties, impulsivity, and emotional dysregulation often contribute to workplace misunderstandings, conflicts with colleagues, and challenges in maintaining professional relationships (Faraone et al., 2021). Adults with ADHD may interrupt conversations, struggle with turn-taking in meetings, or speak impulsively, leading to tension with supervisors and colleagues (Kooij et al., 2019). Impulsive decision-making can result in hasty project execution, overlooked details, and miscommunications in team settings. Individuals with ADHD can be sensitive to negative feedback, making constructive criticism feel overwhelming, which can lead to defensive reactions, strained workplace relationships, and reduced job satisfaction (Barkley, 2018; Faraone et al., 2021). Chronic struggles with work performance and perfectionism contribute to occupational burnout, as adults with ADHD are prone to overcommitting, struggle with work–life balance, and thus experience chronic stress. Perfectionism and overcompensation for ADHD-related challenges can result in exhaustion, demotivation, and mental fatigue over time (Biederman et al., 2006).

A comprehensive multifaceted approach is recommended to address these workplace challenges requires, with promising targeted interventions supporting executive functioning (Barkley & Murphy, 2010), structured time management strategies (Solanto, 2011), and career coaching to identify ADHD-friendly job roles (Nadeau, 2005). Workplace accommodations, such as flexible schedules, structured workflows, and ADHD-specific communication training, may enhance job stability and professional growth (Advokat et al., 2011). Prioritizing the development of emotional regulation and stress management skills can also reduce the risk of burnout and improve workplace relationships (Priebe et al., 2011), ultimately fostering long-term professional success for adults with ADHD.

7.5.2 Relationships and Family Life

ADHD profoundly impacts romantic relationships, parenting, and household management, often leading to relationship instability, challenges in raising children, and difficulties with daily organization (Barkley, 2018; Faraone et al., 2021). These difficulties may stem from impulsivity, emotional dysregulation, forgetfulness, and executive function deficits, which can strain partnerships and create tension within families (Kooij et al., 2019). Adults with ADHD experience higher rates of marital dissatisfaction, relationship conflict, and divorce, primarily due to communication difficulties, impulsivity, emotional dysregulation, and inconsistent follow-through on commitments (Biederman et al., 2006; Barkley, 2018). Married adults with ADHD are nearly twice as likely to divorce compared to neurotypical individuals, with emotional outbursts, inattentiveness, and inconsistency in household responsibilities contributing to frustration and resentment among partners (Faraone et al., 2021). Difficulties maintaining emotional intimacy and trust can also arise, as adults with ADHD often struggle with emotional impulsivity, mood swings, and difficulty expressing emotions, making it harder to maintain deep emotional connections. Forgetfulness and poor time management can lead to missed anniversaries, forgotten commitments, or perceived lack of effort, further straining relationships (Kooij et al., 2019). Impulsivity can escalate arguments, as individuals may blurt out hurtful comments, interrupt discussions, or struggle with patience (Barkley, 2018). Partners without ADHD may feel burdened with a disproportionate share of responsibilities, leading to burnout and emotional withdrawal. Couples therapy with ADHD-informed therapists to develop effective communication strategies and emotional regulation techniques, as well as structured conflict-resolution methods and shared accountability systems can assist in addressing these relationship issues.

Parenting is inherently demanding, but raising children while managing ADHD symptoms presents unique difficulties. Parents with ADHD often struggle with consistent discipline, routine-setting, and managing their child's emotional needs (Chronis-Tuscano et al., 2020). When both the parent and child have ADHD, challenges are amplified by executive function deficits, emotional intensity, and impulsivity (Barkley, 2018). Inconsistent parenting due to executive function difficulties may result in unpredictable discipline and challenges in managing child behavior (Chronis-Tuscano et al., 2020). Forgetfulness and distraction can lead to missed school meetings, irregular bedtime routines, and disorganized households, causing children to feel uncertain about expectations (Biederman et al., 2006). ADHD-related low frustration tolerance makes it harder for parents to remain patient during tantrums, sibling conflicts, or homework struggles, often leading to frequent outbursts and self-doubt about parenting effectiveness (Faraone et al., 2021;

Chronis-Tuscano et al., 2020). Given the strong genetic component of ADHD, children of parents with ADHD have a higher risk of developing the disorder themselves, amplifying challenges with daily routines, emotional regulation, and conflict resolution (Barkley, 2018; Chronis-Tuscano et al., 2020). Parent training programs, mindfulness, and external support mechanisms (e.g., co-parenting arrangements, ADHD coaching) can provide structure, consistency, and improved parent–child interactions (Lee et al., 2022).

Adults with ADHD also often experience difficulties with household management due to executive function deficits, affecting daily tasks, financial responsibilities, and long-term planning. Forgetfulness and disorganization frequently lead to missed payments, misplaced financial documents, and difficulty with budgeting, resulting in financial instability (Kooij et al., 2019). Impulsive spending habits can further exacerbate credit card debt, inconsistent savings, and overall financial stress (Biederman et al., 2006). Many adults struggle to maintain an organized home and feel overwhelmed by clutter and unfinished household projects. Challenges with task initiation and completion can lead to inconsistent home maintenance and frustration among partners (Barkley, 2018). ADHD-related time-blindness and difficulty prioritizing make it challenging to plan for home maintenance, retirement savings, and even meal preparation, contributing to a sense of always "catching up" rather than proactively managing responsibilities (Faraone et al., 2021; Kooij et al., 2019). Automated financial systems, dividing household tasks into manageable steps, and accountability systems with partner support can help reduce financial stress and maintain organization, ultimately improving overall family functioning.

7.5.3 ADHD and Mental Health in Adulthood

ADHD in adulthood is strongly associated with persistent emotional dysregulation, mood instability, anxiety, depression, and substance use disorders (Faraone et al., 2021; Barkley, 2018). Beyond executive dysfunction and attention deficits, adults with ADHD often face impulsive financial decisions, legal difficulties, and chronic addiction disorders, compounding the functional impairments already present (Kooij et al., 2019). Neurological vulnerabilities interact with environmental stressors, including occupational instability, social rejection, and chronic self-doubt, which together exacerbate the risk of psychiatric comorbidities. Understanding and addressing these mental health risks is critical for developing prevention and management strategies that enhance long-term well-being.

Emotional dysregulation remains a core feature of ADHD in adults, contributing to mood swings, frustration intolerance, and impulsive emotional reactions to stress (Barkley, 2018). Many adults experience rapid shifts in mood, transitioning from enthusiasm to frustration or sadness within minutes, reflecting difficulties in regulating emotions. This hypersensitivity can lead to overreactions to minor stressors and prolonged emotional distress, which in turn affect interpersonal relationships, professional functioning, and self-esteem (Kooij et al., 2019). Rejection Sensitivity Dysphoria (RSD)—an extreme emotional response to perceived criticism, failure, or social rejection—often intensifies these challenges (Barkley, 2018). Even minor setbacks, such as negative feedback at work or misunderstandings in relationships, can trigger severe distress, withdrawal, or avoidance behaviors (Faraone et al., 2021). Poor stress management further exacerbates tensions in the workplace, family conflicts, and personal setbacks, leading to chronic overwhelm and avoidance. High daily stress levels are also linked to an increased risk of anxiety, depression, and maladaptive coping mechanisms, including substance use or social withdrawal (Kooij et al., 2019).

Adults with ADHD have higher rates of psychiatric comorbidities, particularly generalized anxiety disorder (GAD), major depressive disorder (MDD), and substance use disorders (SUDs) (Biederman et al., 2006; Faraone et al., 2021). Up to half of adults with ADHD meet criteria for GAD, social anxiety disorder, or panic disorder (Kessler et al., 2006), with anxiety often stemming from executive dysfunction, fear of failure, and difficulties managing everyday responsibilities. Depression is also common, with adults with ADHD three to five times more likely to develop MDD compared to neurotypical individuals (Barkley, 2018). Chronic underachievement, career instability, and relational conflicts contribute to feelings of worthlessness, guilt, and hopelessness, reinforcing cycles of mental health difficulties (Faraone et al., 2021). SUDs are prevalent among adults with ADHD, as many individuals turn to alcohol, nicotine, cannabis, or stimulants to self-medicate symptoms of inattention, impulsivity, or emotional distress (Wilens & Morrison, 2011). Approximately 30–50% of adults with ADHD struggle with substance dependence, and relapse rates are higher than among those without ADHD (Biederman et al., 2006).

Impulsivity also contributes to financial instability, legal troubles, and risk-taking behaviors (Barkley, 2018). Adults with ADHD are more likely to overspend, accumulate debt, and struggle with budgeting, often resulting in chronic financial stress (Faraone et al., 2021). Poor money management skills can strain relationships, impede career advancement, and create long-term economic insecurity (Kooij et al., 2019). Legal issues also arise from ADHD-related impulsivity, including traffic violations, excessive gambling, and other reckless behaviors. Poor impulse control increases the likelihood of legal consequences, such as drug-related offences or aggressive outbursts (Barkley, 2018). Additionally, adults with ADHD frequently use substances to manage stress, boredom, or emotional dysregulation, which may lead to cycles of addiction that are difficult to break (Wilens & Morrison, 2011). Higher impulsivity and poor distress tolerance further complicate recovery efforts, highlighting the need for specialized addiction treatment (Faraone et al., 2021).

Effective management strategies must integrate multimodal approaches that combine medication, cognitive-behavioral therapy (CBT), and ADHD-specific interventions (Corbisiero et al., 2018). Financial coaching, structured routines, and social support networks can mitigate impulsive financial behaviors and reduce stress. Legal education and self-regulation training can help decrease risk-taking behaviors and prevent criminal involvement. Specialized addiction treatment that integrates ADHD medication management, executive function coaching, and therapy is essential to improving recovery outcomes and reducing relapse rates (Wilens & Morrison, 2011). Addressing these mental health challenges holistically is critical to enhancing quality of life and functional success for adults with ADHD.

7.6 ADHD in Late Adulthood

The historical perception of ADHD as a childhood disorder has resulted in significant underdiagnosis among older adults (Kooij et al., 2019; Torgersen et al., 2022). Many individuals with undiagnosed ADHD reach late adulthood without formal recognition, attributing lifelong struggles with attention, impulsivity, and executive function deficits to personality traits, stress, or age-related cognitive decline. This lack of awareness means that ADHD often goes unrecognized by both patients and clinicians, with many older adults internalizing their difficulties as personal failings rather than identifying them as symptoms of a neurodevelopmental condition.

ADHD symptoms persist into late adulthood, manifesting as cognitive difficulties, emotional, and impairments in daily functioning, financial independence, and social relationships (Michielsen et al., 2012). Despite this, ADHD in older adults remains widely overlooked due to overlapping symptoms with neurodegenerative disorders, frequent misdiagnosis, and limited clinical awareness (Torgersen et al., 2022). For instance, memory problems and concentration difficulties, which are hallmark features of ADHD, can be misattributed to mild cognitive impairment (MCI) or dementia rather than recognized as longstanding attention-related challenges. Unlike Alzheimer's disease, ADHD-related memory issues stem from inattention and poor information encoding rather than neurodegenerative processes (Kooij et al., 2019).

Emotional dysregulation also remains a significant concern, often leading to misdiagnoses of depression or anxiety. Many older adults with ADHD experience heightened rates of depression and anxiety, frequently rooted in lifelong struggles with productivity, social relationships, and self-regulation (Michielsen et al., 2012). This can result in treatment that addresses only mood symptoms without recognizing the underlying ADHD, leaving executive function impairments unaddressed (Torgersen et al., 2022). Similarly, symptoms such as restlessness, impulsivity, and fatigue can be misinterpreted as stress-related conditions or late-onset bipolar disorder. Differentiating ADHD from these conditions requires careful clinical evaluation, including neuropsychological testing and ADHD-specific screening tools for older adults (Müller et al., 2007).

ADHD-related executive function deficits continue to impact daily living in older adults, particularly in financial management, household organization, and long-term planning (Kooij et al., 2019). Difficulties in budgeting, timely paying of bills, and making impulsive financial contribute to economic vulnerability during retirement (Torgersen et al., 2022). Research indicates that older adults with ADHD are more likely to experience debt, impulsive spending, and challenges with saving, further compounding financial stress. Additionally, maintaining household routines and organizing daily responsibilities can be especially challenging, leading to missed medical appointments, unpaid bills, and disorganized living environments (Michielsen et al., 2012). These challenges can increase reliance on caregivers and contribute to frustration and decreased quality of life (Kooij et al., 2019).

Adapting to major life transitions, such as retirement, can also by difficult for older adults with ADHD. The loss of structured daily routines and increased social isolation can heighten emotional distress and reduce overall life satisfaction (Torgersen et al., 2022). Moreover, impulsivity and disorganization can complicate long-term health planning, increasing the risk of medical complications and decreasing independence.

Educating clinicians about ADHD in older adults, to improve recognition and diagnosis, is important to address these challenges, Routine ADHD screening in late adulthood, particularly for those with lifelong cognitive difficulties, can enhance detection rates (Torgersen et al., 2016). Reducing stigma and raising awareness about ADHD's persistence can encourage older adults to seek diagnosis and treatment, fostering better health outcomes. Additionally, interventions such as executive function coaching, financial literacy programs, and structured daily routines can help older adults manage their symptoms, maintain independence, and improve their overall quality of life (Rapport et al., 2001).

7.6.1 Impact on Health and Well-Being

ADHD in late adulthood is associated with increased physical health risks, financial instability, and emotional distress, largely related to the consequences of lifelong impulsivity, executive dysfunction, and difficulties with self-regulation (Torgersen et al., 2022). Many older adults with ADHD grapple with chronic health conditions, economic struggles, and psychological challenges that collectively contribute to reduced independence and quality of life (Michielsen et al., 2012). Many older adults with ADHD report difficulties with meal planning, emotional eating, and inconsistent medication adherence, contributing to obesity, diabetes, and cardiovascular diseases (Kooij et al., 2019). The disorder also predisposes individuals to higher rates of smoking and substance use, with adults with ADHD being twice as likely to use cigarettes, alcohol, or illicit drugs compared to the general population (Torgersen et al., 2022). Low levels of physical activity and inconsistent self-care further exacerbate health vulnerabilities, leading to increased emergency healthcare visits and higher mortality risk (Jakicic, 2024). Structured lifestyle interventions, including supervised exercise programs (Lindvall et al., 2023), guided meal planning (Pinto et al., 2022), and behavioral coaching (Vasiliadis et al., 2024), are recommended to promote healthier habits and improve chronic disease management in older adults with ADHD.

Financial instability is another significant concern, as impulsivity and disorganization frequently undermine economic well-being in late adulthood (Kooij et al., 2019). Many older adults with ADHD report difficulty saving money, adhering to budgets, and planning for retirement, resulting in inadequate retirement savings and greater dependence on financial assistance programs (Michielsen et al., 2012). Overspending, risky investments, and challenges with tax obligations contribute to higher rates of debt and legal disputes (Torgersen et al., 2022). Furthermore, older adults with ADHD are particularly vulnerable to financial scams and fraudulent advisors, which heightens their risk of economic exploitation and long-term financial instability (Beach et al., 2020).

Financial literacy programs, ADHD-informed money management coaching, and the use of automated bill payment systems and digital tracking tools can enhance budgeting skills, reduce impulsive spending, and protect against fraud (Frees et al., 2024).

Emotional well-being in older adults with ADHD is often marked by distress related to past impulsive decisions, career instability, relationship difficulties, and unfulfilled life goals. Many individuals experience feelings of regret, self-criticism, and disappointment over missed opportunities, which can evolve into chronic rumination, low self-esteem, and persistent emotional distress (Kooij et al., 2019; Michielsen et al., 2012). These challenges are compounded by social isolation, as inconsistent social engagement and difficulties in maintaining relationships often lead to loneliness and estrangement from family and friends (Torgersen et al., 2022). This isolation is linked to worsened mental health, cognitive decline, and reduced life satisfaction. Moreover, higher rates of late-onset depression and anxiety have been observed among older adults with ADHD, often driven by unresolved life stressors and challenges adjusting to the realities of aging (Torgersen et al., 2022). Targeted interventions such as cognitive-behavioral therapy (CBT) and acceptance and commitment therapy (ACT) are recommended to address self-criticism, build resilience, and improve emotional regulation. Social engagement programs and ADHD peer support groups can help combat isolation, while education on ADHD and self-compassion strategies can assist older adults in reframing past experiences more positively and maintaining a sense of purpose in later life (Othman et al., 2025).

7.6.2 *The Need for Late-Life ADHD Support*

Despite increasing recognition that ADHD persists into late adulthood, there remains a significant gap in clinical guidelines, research, and tailored interventions to effectively manage ADHD in older adults (Kooij et al., 2019). Many individuals reach late adulthood without a formal diagnosis, resulting in functional impairments, emotional distress, and reduced quality of life (Torgersen et al., 2022).

Addressing this unmet need requires the development of evidence-based strategies, cognitive interventions, and carefully monitored medication management to enhance independence, daily functioning, and long-term well-being.

A critical challenge is the lack of clinical guidelines specifically designed for diagnosing and managing ADHD in older adults. Most ADHD research and diagnostic frameworks focus on children and younger adults, with a gap in age-specific protocols that account for the unique presentations of ADHD in aging populations (Michielsen et al., 2012). Many healthcare providers are not adequately trained to screen for ADHD in older adults, often attributing symptoms to age-related cognitive decline, depression, or anxiety (Adler et al., 2019). The DSM-5 criteria, for instance, were developed primarily for younger individuals and are often difficult to apply to aging populations with overlapping symptoms from other conditions (Sharma et al., 2021). This under- and misdiagnosis perpetuate stigma and impede appropriate care. Moreover, the absence of standardized treatment guidelines leads to inconsistent management, particularly regarding medication dosing (Goodman & Mattingly, 2023), therapy selection (Goodman & Mattingly, 2023), and cognitive rehabilitation strategies (Sibley, 2021). To address this, experts recommend the development of age-specific diagnostic criteria and screening tools, increased training for clinicians on ADHD in older adults, and expanded research efforts to establish evidence-based clinical guidelines (Sibley, 2021).

Structured cognitive interventions and environmental supports can play a crucial role in mitigating the impact of ADHD on daily life in late adulthood (Torgersen et al., 2022). Cognitive-behavioral therapy (CBT) for ADHD has demonstrated efficacy in improving time management, problem-solving, and emotional regulation, while memory training programs can enhance attention and support daily task completion (Michielsen et al., 2012). Routine-building strategies, such as daily planners, visual schedules, and digital reminders, can help older adults to organize their activities, reduce cognitive overload, and increase task completion (Baric et al., 2019). Simplifying home environments and creating designated spaces for essential items also promotes daily functioning and reduce disorganization (Kooij et al., 2019). Behavioral coaching can provide personalized strategies for adaptive coping and organization, while peer support groups can reduce isolation and offer emotional validation and shared coping techniques. Integrating CBT, executive function coaching, and structured daily routines with community-based ADHD support groups can improve daily functioning and social engagement (Chacko et al., 2024).

Medication management in late adulthood requires careful monitoring due to age-related changes in metabolism, increased cardiovascular risks, and potential drug interactions (Kooij et al., 2019). Although stimulant medications such as methylphenidate and amphetamines remain the first-line treatment for ADHD, their use in older adults must be approached with caution. Lower starting doses and gradual titration are recommended to minimize side effects and assess tolerance, particularly in those with cardiovascular concerns (Michielsen et al., 2012). Non-stimulant medications, including atomoxetine, guanfacine, and bupropion, may be safer alternatives for individuals with heart disease, hypertension, or co-occurring anxiety disorders (Torgersen et al., 2022). Atomoxetine, for instance, has shown efficacy in improving attention and impulse control with fewer cardiovascular side effects than traditional stimulants (Kooij et al., 2019). Importantly, psychotherapy remains a cornerstone of ADHD management in older adults, especially for those who cannot tolerate medications or prefer non-pharmacological approaches. CBT can help older adults develop structured routines, manage emotional dysregulation, and process past regrets or self-criticism (Torgersen et al., 2022). Implementing individualized medication plans with cardiovascular monitoring, integrating non-stimulant options, and combining therapy with medication management can maximize treatment benefits and improve long-term outcomes for older adults with ADHD.

Summary
Chapter 7 examined ADHD as a lifelong condition, highlighting the evolving nature of symptoms and challenges from early childhood to late adulthood. It described how core symptoms like inattention, hyperactivity, and impulsivity persist and transform over time, contributing to difficulties in academic, social, and occupational functioning. The chapter emphasized the compounding risks of psychiatric comorbidities, emotional dysregulation, and executive function deficits across the lifespan. It also addressed the often-overlooked presentation of ADHD in older adults, noting that many remain undiagnosed or misdiagnosed due to symptom overlap with cognitive aging and limited clinical awareness. The chapter concluded by underscoring the need for age-appropriate interventions—such as structured routines, executive function coaching, targeted therapy, and carefully monitored medication—to support individuals with ADHD at every stage of life.

References

Adler, L. A., Farahbakhshian, S., Romero, B., Flood, E., & Doll, H. (2019). Healthcare provider perspectives on diagnosing and treating adults with attention-deficit/hyperactivity disorder. *Postgraduate Medicine, 131*(7), 461–472.

Advokat, C., Lane, S. M., & Luo, C. (2011). College students with and without ADHD: Comparison of self-report of medication usage, study habits, and academic achievement. *Journal of Attention Disorders, 15*(8), 656–666. https://doi.org/10.1177/1087054710371168

American Psychiatric Association. (2022). Diagnostic and Statistical Manual of Mental Disorders (5th ed., text rev.; DSM-5-TR).

APA. (2013). Diagnostic and statistical manual of mental disorders. *American Psychiatric Association, 21*(21), 591–643.

Arnold, L. E., Hodgkins, P., Kahle, J., Madhoo, M., & Kewley, G. (2015). Long-term outcomes of ADHD: Academic achievement and performance. *Journal of Attention Disorders, 24*(1), 73–85. https://doi.org/10.1177/1087054714566076

Baric, V., Andreassen, M., Öhman, A., & Hemmingsson, H. (2019). Using an interactive digital calendar with mobile phone reminders by senior people – A focus group study. *BMC Geriatrics, 19*(1), 116. https://doi.org/10.1186/s12877-019-1128-9

Barkley, R. A. (2018). *Attention-deficit hyperactivity disorder: A handbook for diagnosis and treatment (4th ed.)*. Guilford Press.

Barkley, R. A., & Brown, T. E. (2008). Unrecognized attention-deficit/hyperactivity disorder in adults presenting with other psychiatric disorders. *CNS Spectrums, 13*(11), 977–984. https://doi.org/10.1017/S1092852900014036

Barkley, R. A., & Cox, D. (2007). A review of driving risks and impairments associated with ADHD. *Journal of Safety Research, 38*(1), 113–128.

Barkley, R. A., Edwards, G., Laneri, M., Fletcher, K., & Metevia, L. (2001). Executive functioning, temporal discounting, and sense of time in adolescents with attention deficit hyperactivity disorder (ADHD) and oppositional defiant disorder (ODD). *Journal of Abnormal Child Psychology, 29*(6), 541–556. https://doi.org/10.1023/A:1012233310098

Barkley, R. A., & Murphy, K. R. (2010). Impairment in occupational functioning and adult ADHD: The predictive utility of executive function (EF) ratings versus EF tests. *Archives of Clinical Neuropsychology, 25*(3), 157–173. https://doi.org/10.1093/arclin/acq014

Beach, S., Czaja, S., Schulz, R., Loewenstein, D., & Lichtenberg, P. (2020). Vulnerability to financial scams among older adults: Cognitive and psychosocial factors. *Innovation in Aging, 4*(Supplement_1), 447–447. https://doi.org/10.1093/geroni/igaa057.1447

Beauchaine, T. P., & Hinshaw, S, P. (2020). RDoC and Psychopathology among Youth: Misplaced Assumptions and an Agenda for Future Research. *Journal of Clinical Child & Adolescent Psychology, 49*(3), 322–340. https://doi.org/10.1080/15374416.2020.1750022. PMID: 32525746; PMCID: PMC7495028.

Becker, S. P., et al. (2017). Sluggish cognitive tempo in ADHD. *Journal of Child Psychology and Psychiatry, 58*(3), 231–244.

Biederman, J., et al. (2006). Functional impairments in adults with ADHD. *Journal of Clinical Psychiatry, 67*(4), 524–540.

Chacko, A., Merrill, B. M., Kofler, M. J., & Fabiano, G. A. (2024). Improving the efficacy and effectiveness of evidence-based psychosocial interventions for attention-deficit/hyperactivity disorder (ADHD) in children and adolescents. *Translational Psychiatry, 14*(1), 244. https://doi.org/10.1038/s41398-024-02890-3

Corbisiero, S., Bitto, H., Newark, P., Abt-Mörstedt, B., Elsässer, M., Buchli-Kammermann, J., Künne, S., Nyberg, E., Hofecker-Fallahpour, M., & Stieglitz, R. D. (2018). A comparison of cognitive-Behavioral therapy and pharmacotherapy vs. pharmacotherapy alone in adults with attention-deficit/hyperactivity disorder (ADHD)-a randomized controlled trial. *Frontiers in Psychiatry, 9*, 571. https://doi.org/10.3389/fpsyt.2018.00571

Daley, D., & Birchwood, J. (2010). ADHD and academic performance: why does ADHD impact on academic performance and what can be done to support ADHD children in the classroom? *Child Care Health Development, 36*(4), 455–64. https://doi.org/10.1111/j.1365-2214.2009.01046.x. Epub 2010 Jan 13. PMID: 20074251.

Durlak, J. A., Weissberg, R. P., Dymnicki, A. B., Taylor, R. D., & Schellinger, K. B. (2011). The impact of enhancing students' social and emotional learning: A meta-analysis of school-based universal interventions. *Child Development, 82*(1), 405–432. https://doi.org/10.1111/j.1467-8624.2010.01564.x

Faraone, S. V., et al. (2021). The World Federation of ADHD International Consensus Statement: 208 evidence based conclusions about the disorder. *Neuroscience & Biobehavioral Reviews*, 128, 789–818.

Fleming, A. P., & McMahon, R. J. (2012). Developmental context and treatment principles for ADHD among college students. *Clinical Child and Family Psychology Review, 15*(4), 303–329. https://doi.org/10.1007/s10567-012-0121-z

Fredricks, J. A., & Eccles, J. S. (2006). Is extracurricular participation associated with beneficial outcomes? Concurrent and longitudinal relations. *Developmental Psychology, 42*(4), 698–713. https://doi.org/10.1037/0012-1649.42.4.698

Frees, D., Gangal, A., & Shaviro, C. (2024). Quantifying the causal effect of financial literacy courses on financial health. *arXiv preprint arXiv:2405.01789.*

French, B., Nalbant, G., Wright, H., Sayal, K., Daley, D., Groom, M. J., Cassidy, S., & Hall, C. L. (2024). The impacts associated with having ADHD: An umbrella review. *Frontiers in Psychiatry, 15*, 1343314. https://doi.org/10.3389/fpsyt.2024.1343314

Gaffney, H., Ttofi, M. M., & Farrington, D. P. (2021). Effectiveness of school-based programs to reduce bullying perpetration and victimization: An updated systematic review and meta-analysis. *Campbell Systematic Reviews, 17*(2), e1143. https://doi.org/10.1002/cl2.1143

Goodman, D. W., & Mattingly, G. (2023). Practice guidelines development: The APSARD United States guidelines for the diagnosis and treatment of ADHD in adults. *Psychiatric Annals, 53*(10), 449–454.

Hinshaw, S. P., Owens, E. B., Zalecki, C., Huggins, S. P., Montenegro-Nevado, A. J., Schrodek, E., & Swanson, E. N. (2012). Prospective follow-up of girls with attention-deficit/hyperactivity disorder into early adulthood: Continuing impairment includes elevated risk for suicide attempts and self-injury. *Journal of Consulting and Clinical Psychology, 80*(6), 1041–1051. https://doi.org/10.1037/a0029451. Epub 2012 Aug 13. PMID: 22889337; PMCID: PMC3543865.

Hiscock, H., Sciberras, E., Mensah, F., Gerner, B., Efron, D., Khano, S., & Oberklaid, F. (2015). Impact of a behavioural sleep intervention on symptoms and sleep in children with attention deficit hyperactivity disorder, and parental mental health: Randomised controlled trial. *BMJ, 350*, h68. https://doi.org/10.1136/bmj.h68

Hoza, B. (2007). Peer functioning in children with ADHD. *Journal of Pediatric Psychology, 32*(6), 655–663.

Jakicic, J. M. (2024). Physical activity and reduced mortality regardless of age—Considerations for public health. *JAMA Network Open, 7*(11), e2446811–e2446811. https://doi.org/10.1001/jamanetworkopen.2024.46811

Jensen, P. S., Youngstrom, E. A., Steiner, H., Findling, R. L., Meyer, R. E., Malone, R. P., Carlson, G. A., Coccaro, E. F., Aman, M. G., Blair, J., Dougherty, D., Ferris, C., Flynn, L., Green, E., Hoagwood, K., Hutchinson, J., Laughren, T., Leve, L. D., Novins, D. K., & Vitiello, B. (2007). Consensus report on impulsive aggression as a symptom across diagnostic categories in child psychiatry: Implications for medication studies. *Journal of the American Academy of Child and Adolescent Psychiatry, 46*(3), 309–322. https://doi.org/10.1097/chi.0b013e31802f1454

Johnston, C., & Chronis-Tuscano, A. (2021). Families and ADHD. *Annual Review of Clinical Psychology, 17*, 291–316.

Kessler, R. C., et al. (2005). The prevalence and correlates of adult ADHD in the United States. *American Journal of Psychiatry, 162*(4), 716–723.

Kooij, J. J. S., Bijlenga, D., Salerno, L., Jaeschke, R., Bitter, I., Balázs, J., Thome, J., Dom, G., Kasper, S., Nunes Filipe, C., Stes, S., Mohr, P., Leppämäki, S., Casas, M., Bobes, J., Mccarthy, J. M., Richarte, V., Kjems Philipsen, A., Pehlivanidis, A., . . . Asherson, P. (2019). Updated European Consensus Statement on diagnosis and treatment of adult ADHD. *European Psychiatry, 56*, 14–34. https://doi.org/10.1016/j.eurpsy.2018.11.001.

Kumar, M., & Jha, A. K. (2025). Adolescent brain development: Limbic system and emotions. In T. Shackelford (Ed.), *Encyclopedia of religious psychology and behavior* (pp. 1–10). Springer Nature Switzerland. https://doi.org/10.1007/978-3-031-38971-9_10-1

Lee, C. S. C., Ng, K.-H., Chan, P. C. K., & Peng, X. (2022). Effectiveness of mindfulness parent training on parenting stress and children's ADHD-related behaviors: A systematic review and meta-analysis. *Hong Kong Journal of Occupational Therapy, 35*(1), 3–24. https://doi.org/10.1177/15691861211073826

Lindvall, M. A., Holmqvist, K. L., Svedell, L. A., Philipson, A., Cao, Y., & Msghina, M. (2023). START—Physical exercise and person-centred cognitive skills training as treatment for adult

ADHD: Protocol for a randomized controlled trial. *BMC Psychiatry, 23*(1), 697. https://doi.org/10.1186/s12888-023-05181-1
Loe, I. M., & Feldman, H. M. (2007). Academic and educational outcomes of children with ADHD. *Journal of Pediatric Psychology, 32*(6), 643–654.
Luo, D., Dashti, S. G., Sawyer, S. M., & Vijayakumar, N. (2024). Pubertal hormones and mental health problems in children and adolescents: A systematic review of population-based studies. *EClinicalMedicine, 76*, 102828. https://doi.org/10.1016/j.eclinm.2024.102828
Meinzer, M. C., Pettit, J. W., & Viswesvaran, C. (2014). The co-occurrence of attention-deficit/hyperactivity disorder and unipolar depression in children and adolescents: A meta-analytic review. *Clinical Psychology Review, 34*(8), 595–607. https://doi.org/10.1016/j.cpr.2014.10.002. Epub 2014 Oct 13. PMID: 25455624.
Michielsen, M., et al. (2012). Prevalence of ADHD in older adults. *British Journal of Psychiatry, 201*(4), 298–305.
Mikami, A. Y. (2010). The importance of friendship for youth with ADHD. *Clinical Child and Family Psychology Review, 13*(2), 181–198.
Mikami, A. Y., Smit, S., & Khalis, A. (2017). Social skills training and ADHD-what works? *Current Psychiatry Reports, 19*(12), 93. https://doi.org/10.1007/s11920-017-0850-2
Müller, B. W., Gimbel, K., Keller-Pliessnig, A., Sartory, G., Gastpar, M., & Davids, E. (2007). Neuropsychological assessment of adult patients with attention-deficit/hyperactivity disorder. *European Archives of Psychiatry and Clinical Neuroscience, 257*(2), 112–119. https://doi.org/10.1007/s00406-006-0688-9
Nadeau, K. G. (2005). Career choices and workplace challenges for individuals with ADHD. *Journal of Clinical Psychology, 61*(5), 549–563. https://doi.org/10.1002/jclp.20119
Nigg, J. T., Sibley, M. H., Thapar, A., & Karalunas, S. L. (2020). Development of ADHD: Etiology, Heterogeneity, and Early Life Course. *Annual Review of Developmental Psychology, 2*(1), 559–583. https://doi.org/10.1146/annurev-devpsych-060320-093413. Epub 2020 Oct 23. PMID: 34368774; PMCID: PMC8336725.
Orm, S., & Fjermestad, K. (2021). A scoping review of psychosocial adjustment in siblings of children with attention-deficit/hyperactivity disorder. *Advances in Neurodevelopmental Disorders, 5*(4), 381–395. https://doi.org/10.1007/s41252-021-00222-w
Othman, S., Steen, M., & Abdelnasser, N. (2025). Self-compassion education for older adults' mental health and wellbeing: A mixed methods systematic review. *Aging & Mental Health, 29*(7), 1166–1178. https://doi.org/10.1080/13607863.2025.2476653
Pinto, S., Correia-de-Sá, T., Sampaio-Maia, B., Vasconcelos, C., Moreira, P., & Ferreira-Gomes, J. (2022). Eating patterns and dietary interventions in ADHD: A narrative review. *Nutrients, 14*(20), 4332. https://doi.org/10.3390/nu14204332
Pliszka, S. R. (2003). Psychiatric comorbidities in children with attention deficit hyperactivity disorder: Implications for management. *Paediatric Drugs, 5*(11), 741–750. https://doi.org/10.2165/00148581-200305110-00003
Priebe, S., Dimic, S., Wildgrube, C., Jankovic, J., Cushing, A., & McCabe, R. (2011). Good communication in psychiatry—A conceptual review. *European Psychiatry, 26*(7), 403–407. https://doi.org/10.1016/j.eurpsy.2010.07.010
Rapport, L. J., Van Voorhis, A., Tzelepis, A., & Friedman, S. R. (2001). Executive functioning in adult attention-deficit hyperactivity disorder. *The Clinical Neuropsychologist, 15*(4), 479–491. https://doi.org/10.1076/clin.15.4.479.1878
Retz, W., Ginsberg, Y., Turner, D., Barra, S., Retz-Junginger, P., Larsson, H., & Asherson, P. (2021). Attention-Deficit/Hyperactivity Disorder (ADHD), antisociality and delinquent behavior over the lifespan. *Neuroscience and BioBehavioral Reviews, 120*, 236–248. https://doi.org/10.1016/j.neubiorev.2020.11.025. Epub 2020 Nov 30. PMID: 33271164.
Seymour, K. E., Chronis-Tuscano, A., Iwamoto, D. K., Kurdziel, G., & Macpherson, L. (2014). Emotion regulation mediates the association between ADHD and depressive symptoms in a community sample of youth. *Journal of Abnormal Child Psychology, 42*(4), 611–21. https://doi.org/10.1007/s10802-013-9799-8. PMID: 24221724; PMCID: PMC4207628.

Sharma, M. J., Lavoie, S., & Callahan, B. L. (2021). A call for research on the validity of the age-of-onset criterion application in older adults being evaluated for ADHD: A review of the literature in clinical and cognitive psychology. *The American Journal of Geriatric Psychiatry, 29*(7), 669–678. https://doi.org/10.1016/j.jagp.2020.10.016

Shaw, M., Caci, H., Hodgkins, P., Kahle, J., Callamaras, N., & Woods, A. (2011). Review of studies of ADHD: Long-term outcomes with and without treatment. *European Psychiatry, 26*(S2), 579–579. https://doi.org/10.1016/S0924-9338(11)72286-6

Shaw, P., et al. (2014). Neurodevelopmental trajectories of the human cerebral cortex. *Biological Psychiatry, 76*(8), 615–623.

Sibley, M. H. (2021). Diagnosing ADHD in older adults: Critical next steps for research. *The American Journal of Geriatric Psychiatry, 29*(7), 679–681. https://doi.org/10.1016/j.jagp.2020.11.012

Sibley, M. H., et al. (2014). Defining ADHD persistence in adulthood. *Journal of the American Academy of Child & Adolescent Psychiatry, 53*(3), 299–308.

Solanto, M. V. (2011). *Cognitive-behavioral therapy for adult ADHD: Targeting executive dysfunction*. The Guilford Press.

Theule, J., et al. (2013). Parenting stress in families of children with ADHD. *Journal of Emotional and Behavioral Disorders, 21*(1), 3–17.

Thomas, N., & Karuppali, S. (2022). The efficacy of visual activity schedule intervention in reducing problem behaviors in children with attention-deficit/hyperactivity disorder between the age of 5 and 12 years: A systematic review. *Soa Chongsonyon Chongsin Uihak, 33*(1), 2–15. https://doi.org/10.5765/jkacap.210021

Torgersen, K., Rahman, Z., Bahrami, S., Hindley, G. F. L., Parker, N., Frei, O., Shadrin, A., O'Connell, K. S., Tesli, M., Smeland, O. B., Munkhaugen, J. Djurovic, S., Dammen, T., & Andreassen, O. A. (2022). Shared genetic loci between depression and cardiometabolic traits Solanto MV. The efficacy of cognitive-behavioral therapy for adults with ADHD. *World Psychiatry, 24*(3), 378–379. https://doi.org/10.1002/wps.21349. PMID: 40948055; PMCID: PMC12434339.

Torgersen, T., Gjervan, B., Lensing, M. B., & Rasmussen, K. (2016). Optimal management of ADHD in older adults. *Neuropsychiatric Disease and Treatment, 12*, 79–87. https://doi.org/10.2147/ndt.S59271

Vasiliadis, H.-M., Lunghi, C., Rahme, E., Rochette, L., Gignac, M., Massamba, V., Diallo, F. B., Fansi, A., Cortese, S., & Lesage, A. (2024). ADHD medications use and risk of mortality and unintentional injuries: A population-based cohort study. *Translational Psychiatry, 14*(1), 128. https://doi.org/10.1038/s41398-024-02825-y

Wilens, T. E., & Morrison, N. R. (2011). The intersection of attention-deficit/hyperactivity disorder and substance abuse. *Current Opinion in Psychiatry, 24*(4), 280–5. https://doi.org/10.1097/YCO.0b013e328345c956. PMID: 21483267; PMCID: PMC3435098.

Williams, C. J., Chen, J. M., Quirion, A., & Hoeft, F. (2024). Peer mentoring for students with learning disabilities: The importance of shared experience on students' social and emotional development. In *Frontiers in Education* (Vol. 9, p. 1292717). Frontiers Media SA.

Chapter 8
Intersectionality in ADHD: Gender, Race, and Socioeconomic Status

Abstract This chapter explores the complex interplay of gender, race, and socioeconomic status (SES) in ADHD, emphasizing how structural inequalities, implicit biases, and healthcare disparities shape diagnosis, treatment, and outcomes. ADHD is often viewed through a universal clinical lens, yet growing evidence suggests that sociocultural factors profoundly influence its recognition and management.

Many individuals with ADHD face barriers to diagnosis and appropriate intervention, particularly those from historically marginalized backgrounds. Gender differences contribute to misdiagnosis or delayed identification, with females often presenting with inattentive symptoms that are overlooked, while males are more frequently diagnosed due to externalizing behaviors. Racial and ethnic disparities further complicate ADHD care, with overdiagnosis in some populations and underdiagnosis in others, often influenced by clinician bias and systemic inequities. Additionally, socioeconomic status plays a critical role in ADHD outcomes, affecting access to health care, educational support, and long-term stability.

Research highlights the urgent need for an intersectional approach in ADHD diagnosis and treatment, moving beyond traditional frameworks to consider how multiple social identities intersect to shape an individual's ADHD experience. This chapter examines the latest evidence on gender-based differences in ADHD presentation and their impact on clinical identification; racial disparities in ADHD diagnosis and treatment, including the influence of clinician bias; and the role of socioeconomic status in ADHD management, particularly access to health care and educational accommodations. By understanding the intersectionality of ADHD, practitioners, researchers, and policymakers can work toward more equitable diagnostic frameworks, targeted interventions, and inclusive support systems, ultimately improving ADHD outcomes for diverse populations.

G. Ayano et al., *ADHD Across the Lifespan*, SpringerBriefs in Modern Perspectives on Disability Research,
https://doi.org/10.1007/978-981-95-8712-4_8

8.1 Gender Disparities in ADHD Diagnosis

ADHD has long been perceived as a predominantly male condition, a misconception stemming from historical biases in clinical research and diagnostic frameworks that have largely emphasized male presentations of the disorder (Rucklidge, 2010; Quinn & Madhoo, 2014). Early ADHD studies focused heavily on males, shaping diagnostic criteria and treatment approaches that prioritize externalizing behaviors, such as hyperactivity and impulsivity, which are more commonly exhibited by males. As a result, females with ADHD are frequently underdiagnosed or misdiagnosed, often initially treated for anxiety or depression before their ADHD is recognized (Hinshaw et al., 2022). Gender-based disparities in ADHD diagnosis stem not only from biological differences but also from variations in symptom presentation and societal expectations. Boys are more likely to display overt externalizing behaviors that attract clinical attention, while girls often present with internalizing symptoms such as inattention, emotional dysregulation, and anxiety, which tend to be less disruptive and therefore are more easily overlooked by teachers, parents, and clinicians (Quinn & Madhoo, 2014; Gershon, 2002). These diagnostic challenges contribute to delayed diagnoses and limited access to appropriate interventions for females, increasing their risk of academic struggles, emotional distress, and long-term mental health complications.

ADHD is diagnosed more frequently in males, with epidemiological data showing a male-to-female ratio of approximately 2:1 to 3:1 (Rucklidge, 2010; Hinshaw et al., 2022). Recent research indicates that this disparity likely reflects diagnostic biases rather than true differences in prevalence (Nussbaum, 2011). Community studies suggest that ADHD is more evenly distributed across genders, yet boys are significantly more likely to receive a formal diagnosis (Gershon, 2002). This pattern emerges because teachers, parents, and clinicians are quicker to recognize externalizing behaviors, leading to earlier referrals and diagnoses for boys (Quinn & Madhoo, 2014). Girls with ADHD are often diagnosed 5–10 years later than boys, if at all, because their symptoms are more subtle (Hinshaw et al., 2022). Many girls first receive diagnoses for anxiety or depression, which delays appropriate ADHD treatment (Rucklidge, 2010).

Gender differences in ADHD symptom presentation further complicate accurate diagnosis. Boys typically display externalizing behaviors such as hyperactivity, impulsivity, and behavioral disruptions, which lead to higher rates of disciplinary action and earlier ADHD identification (Gershon, 2002). Boys with ADHD also engage in risk-taking behaviors and impulsive decision-making, making their symptoms more visible in both school and social settings (Hinshaw et al., 2022). In contrast, girls often exhibit internalizing symptoms, including inattention, emotional dysregulation, and social withdrawal, which do not align with the traditional hyperactive-impulsive ADHD profile (Quinn & Madhoo, 2014). Low self-esteem, perfectionism, and anxiety are also common among females with ADHD, making it harder to differentiate from generalized anxiety disorder or depression (Rucklidge, 2010). Moreover, many girls develop masking and compensatory behaviors—such as perfectionism, people-pleasing, and overcompensation—to hide their executive function difficulties (Quinn & Madhoo, 2014). These strategies may initially help them function in academic or social settings but often lead to late-life burnout, internal distress, and a higher likelihood of developing comorbid mental health conditions (Hinshaw et al., 2022).

The consequences of delayed or missed ADHD diagnoses for females are substantial. Females with ADHD are at increased risk of depression and anxiety, with late-diagnosed women more likely to internalize their struggles and experience higher rates of emotional dysregulation in adulthood (Rucklidge, 2010). Undiagnosed ADHD is also linked to higher rates of suicidal ideation, eating disorders, and self-harm, particularly in adolescent and young adult women, highlighting the importance of creating opportunities for regular social engagement to reduce isolation (Hinshaw et al., 2022). Academically and professionally, girls with ADHD often go unnoticed in school, making them less likely to receive necessary accommodations and contributing to chronic self-doubt and reduced career opportunities (Quinn & Madhoo, 2014). Adult women with ADHD report higher rates of underemployment, workplace conflicts, and career dissatisfaction due to persistent executive function challenges, difficulties with organization, and time management struggles (Gershon, 2002). In their personal lives, emotional dysregulation and impulsivity can contribute to unstable friendships, romantic conflicts, and higher divorce rates among women with ADHD (Hinshaw et al., 2022). Many women with ADHD also experience social rejection and feelings of isolation, particularly if their symptoms remain unrecognized and untreated (Rucklidge, 2010).

Addressing these gender disparities in ADHD diagnosis requires targeted strategies. Specific clinician training is required to improve awareness and recognition of ADHD in females and to differentiate it from anxiety or depression (Nussbaum, 2011). Screening guidelines must account for gender differences in symptom presentation, masking behaviors, and social expectations to ensure early and accurate diagnosis. Tailored intervention and gender-sensitive treatment plans are essential to provide appropriate support for both males and females with ADHD. Finally, encouraging self-advocacy and fostering peer support networks can empower girls and women with ADHD, facilitating greater self-understanding and access to appropriate care.

8.2 Treatment Disparities Between Genders

Gender differences in ADHD extend beyond diagnostic rates, affecting treatment access, medication use, and mental health outcomes. Research consistently shows that boys are more likely to receive ADHD treatment, while girls are frequently misdiagnosed with anxiety or depression, which delays access to effective ADHD interventions (Hinshaw et al., 2022; Quinn & Madhoo, 2014). This disparity is rooted in both clinician bias and differences in symptom presentation, with girls often exhibiting inattentive-type ADHD, which tends to be less disruptive in school and social settings and therefore more easily overlooked. Females with ADHD also experience higher rates of emotional distress, self-harm, and eating disorders, yet research focusing on ADHD in females remains underdeveloped. Additionally, hormonal fluctuations across puberty, pregnancy, and menopause can exacerbate ADHD symptoms, but these changes are poorly understood within current clinical treatment frameworks (Gershon, 2002). This section explores these gender-based disparities, highlighting issues related to medication use, misdiagnosis trends, mental health risks, and the impact of hormonal changes on ADHD symptoms.

Boys are consistently more likely to receive ADHD medication than girls, even when symptom severity is comparable. Studies show that boys with ADHD are prescribed stimulant medications at significantly higher rates than girls, with males being two to three times more likely to receive stimulants such as methylphenidate or amphetamines (Quinn & Madhoo, 2014). This discrepancy is partly due to the externalizing nature of ADHD symptoms in boys, which are more disruptive and noticeable in school and social environments, prompting earlier recognition and treatment (Hinshaw et al., 2022). In contrast, girls often present with inattentive-type symptoms, contributing to delays in diagnosis and lower treatment rates. Clinician biases also play a role, as healthcare providers may perceive girls' symptoms as less severe or more manageable than boys' (Gershon, 2002). Parental concerns about potential side effects of medication—such as appetite suppression, sleep disturbances, or social stigma—further contribute to underprescription in girls.

Girls with ADHD are frequently misdiagnosed with depression or anxiety instead of ADHD, given their higher rates of internalizing symptoms. Emotional dysregulation and social struggles—common in ADHD—are often mistakenly attributed to personality traits or psychological distress rather than neurodevelopmental differences (Quinn & Madhoo, 2014). Many girls first receive diagnoses of generalized anxiety disorder (GAD) or major depressive disorder (MDD), delaying appropriate ADHD treatment (Hinshaw et al., 2022). These misdiagnoses lead to the prescription of antidepressants or anti-anxiety medications rather than ADHD treatments, failing to address core executive dysfunctions, attention deficits, or impulsivity (Gershon, 2002). Consequently, women with undiagnosed ADHD face a significantly higher risk of developing severe depression, anxiety, and chronic emotional distress in adulthood.

The delayed recognition and treatment of ADHD in females also significantly increase their risk for self-harm, eating disorders, and suicidal ideation. Research indicates that women with ADHD are up to five times more likely to attempt suicide than their neurotypical counterparts (Quinn & Madhoo, 2014), and self-harm behaviors such as cutting, burning, or scratching are far more common in females with ADHD compared to males (Hinshaw et al., 2022). Moreover, ADHD is strongly associated with bulimia nervosa and binge-eating disorder (BED), particularly in females. Impulsivity and emotional dysregulation contribute to binge-eating cycles, purging behaviors, and unhealthy weight control habits in adolescent and adult women with ADHD (Gershon, 2002). Emotional hypersensitivity and relationship struggles are also common, with women reporting extreme mood swings, heightened sensitivity to criticism, and emotional overreactivity, all of which contribute to relationship instability and social isolation (Rucklidge, 2010). Rejection Sensitivity Dysphoria (RSD), characterized by intense emotional responses to perceived social rejection or criticism, is particularly pronounced in females with ADHD, increasing distress in friendships and romantic relationships (Quinn & Madhoo, 2014).

Hormonal fluctuations—including those during puberty, pregnancy, and menopause—can further exacerbate ADHD symptoms in females, yet research on these interactions remains limited. During puberty and adolescence, rising estrogen levels increase dopamine receptor sensitivity, leading to fluctuating ADHD symptoms (Hinshaw et al., 2022). Adolescent girls often experience worsening mood swings, emotional dysregulation, and cognitive difficulties that are dismissed as typical "teenage behavior" rather than ADHD-related issues (Quinn & Madhoo, 2014). During pregnancy, high estrogen levels may temporarily improve ADHD symptoms, but the postpartum hormonal drop can result in severe cognitive and emotional difficulties, often misdiagnosed as postpartum depression (PPD) (Gershon, 2002). Menopause brings a sharp decline in estrogen levels, increasing attention deficits, brain fog, and executive dysfunction. Many women receive ADHD diagnoses for the first time during menopause, as their symptoms become more disruptive and harder to manage (Quinn & Madhoo, 2014).

Addressing gender-based ADHD treatment disparities requires multifaceted interventions. Clinician education on gender differences in ADHD symptom presentation is an important strategy to reduce misdiagnosis and improve treatment access. ADHD treatment guidelines that account for hormonal fluctuations across puberty, pregnancy, and menopause are also needed (Kooij et al., 2025). Expanding research on ADHD gender differences to explore what would improve treatment personalization and long-term outcomes is recommended. Finally, screening for ADHD in women diagnosed with anxiety, depression, or eating disorders could help ensure proper identification and comprehensive treatment.

8.3 Gender and ADHD Outcomes

Gender differences in ADHD extend beyond diagnosis and treatment to impact long-term life outcomes, including criminal justice involvement, mental health, relationships, education, and career stability. Research indicates that males with ADHD are more likely to engage in criminal behavior and substance use, while females with ADHD experience greater struggles with self-esteem, relationships, and internalizing disorders (Quinn & Madhoo, 2014; Hinshaw et al., 2022). Additionally, late-diagnosed women with ADHD report greater educational and professional setbacks, largely due to untreated executive dysfunction, emotional dysregulation, and societal expectations that obscure or minimize their struggles

(Gershon, 2002). These disparities highlight the urgent need for ADHD interventions that address the unique risks and challenges faced by males and females.

Males with ADHD face higher rates of criminal justice involvement and substance use disorders than their female counterparts. Studies show that 25–40% of incarcerated males have ADHD, compared to just 5–7% in the general population (Young et al., 2015). ADHD-related impulsivity, poor emotional regulation, and risk-taking behaviors often increase the likelihood of engaging in aggression, theft, reckless driving, and other criminal activities (Barkley et al., 2004). Males with ADHD are more likely to misuse alcohol, nicotine, and illicit drugs, often as a form of self-medication for impulsivity and emotional distress (Wilens et al., 2011). Male Adolescents and young adults with ADHD are at a two- to three-fold higher risk for developing substance use disorders, with earlier initiation of smoking, alcohol, and drug use compared to their neurotypical peers (May et al., 2023). Despite this high prevalence, ADHD remains significantly underdiagnosed and undertreated in correctional facilities, with few incarcerated individuals receiving proper ADHD evaluation or management (Young et al., 2015). Without appropriate interventions, individuals—particularly males—with ADHD are at increased risk of recidivism and poor rehabilitation outcomes (Barkley et al., 2004).

In contrast, females with ADHD are more likely to internalize their difficulties, leading to greater struggles with relationships, self-esteem, and internalizing disorders. Girls and women with ADHD frequently experience social rejection, misunderstandings, and difficulties forming lasting friendships (Hinshaw et al., 2022). Emotional dysregulation and intense mood swings contribute to higher rates of relationship conflicts, breakups, and divorce (Gershon, 2002). Up to half of females with ADHD develop generalized anxiety disorder (GAD) or major depressive disorder (MDD) at some point in life. Rejection Sensitivity Dysphoria (RSD)—an extreme emotional reaction to perceived rejection or criticism—is particularly severe in females with ADHD, making them vulnerable to social withdrawal and chronic self-doubt (Quinn & Madhoo, 2014). Late-diagnosed women with ADHD often report chronic self-criticism, perfectionism, and feelings of failure, particularly if they struggled academically or professionally (Gershon, 2002). Females with ADHD engage in self-harming behaviors (such as cutting, burning, or scratching) at significantly higher rates than neurotypical females, largely due to emotional dysregulation and untreated mental health conditions (Hinshaw et al., 2022).

Because ADHD in females is often overlooked until adulthood, these women can experience significant setbacks in education, employment, and career progression (Quinn & Madhoo, 2014). Executive function deficits, such as chronic procrastination, poor organization, and difficulties with sustained attention, may lead to lower academic achievement, with many girls dropping out of high school or college, limiting their future career prospects (Gershon, 2002; Hinshaw et al., 2022). Women with ADHD report higher rates of job dissatisfaction, frequent job changes, and difficulties maintaining long-term employment, largely due to challenges with disorganization, forgetfulness, and workplace dynamics (Quinn & Madhoo, 2014). Executive function difficulties also make it challenging to meet deadlines, complete projects, and maintain workplace efficiency, leading to lower income levels and fewer opportunities for career advancement. Many late-diagnosed women with ADHD experience career burnout, driven by chronic stress, overcommitment, and difficulties balancing multiple responsibilities (Gershon, 2002). Financial instability is also common, particularly for those who struggle with budgeting, time management, or impulsive decision-making (Hinshaw et al., 2022).

Addressing these gender-based ADHD outcome disparities requires expanding access to ADHD screening in at-risk populations, including in juvenile detention settings and female psychiatric clinics, to improve early diagnosis and intervention (Dimitri et al., 2025). Treatment tailored to gender-specific needs is warranted, ensuring females with ADHD receive support for emotional dysregulation, self-esteem challenges, and executive function deficits. Workplace coaching and executive function training can improve job retention, career advancement, and financial independence (Chan & Langberg, 2024). Targeted mental health interventions for females with ADHD are essential to reduce self-harm risks, relationship struggles, and internalized distress.

8.4 ADHD Diagnosis Across Different Racial and Ethnic Groups

Although ADHD occurs at similar rates across all racial and ethnic groups, Black, Hispanic, and Indigenous children are significantly less likely to be diagnosed with ADHD compared to White children (Coker et al., 2016; Morgan et al., 2014). This disparity stems from a combination of structural inequalities, cultural stigma, implicit bias in health care, and barriers to accessing mental health services, often leading to underdiagnosis, misdiagnosis, and unequal treatment. Understanding the factors that contribute to these diagnostic inequities is essential to ensure that all children receive timely and appropriate care.

Research consistently shows that Black, Hispanic, and Indigenous children face significantly lower rates of ADHD diagnosis, even after controlling for socioeconomic status and symptom severity (Morgan et al., 2014). In 2016, U.S. data from the National Survey of Children's Health found that White children were diagnosed with ADHD at nearly twice the rate of Black and Hispanic children, despite exhibiting comparable levels of ADHD symptoms (Coker et al., 2016). Indigenous children also experience disproportionately low rates of ADHD diagnosis, despite facing substantial ADHD-related challenges in educational settings. These disparities often lead to delayed or missed diagnoses in minority populations, with Black and Hispanic children receiving ADHD diagnoses an average of 13–21 months later than their White peers, delaying critical early interventions (Morgan et al., 2014). Without proper diagnosis, children of color frequently experience increased academic struggles, behavioral conflicts, and higher dropout rates (Coker et al., 2016).

Cultural stigma and systemic biases further compound these disparities by contributing to the misinterpretation of ADHD symptoms as conduct problems rather than as signs of a neurodevelopmental disorder. Within Black, Hispanic, and Indigenous communities, ADHD is often viewed as a discipline issue rather than a medical condition, reducing the likelihood that families will seek mental health evaluations (Morgan et al., 2014). Many families also worry that an ADHD diagnosis will lead to negative labeling, segregation into special education programs, or disciplinary action. Educators and clinicians frequently misread ADHD symptoms—such as impulsivity, restlessness, and difficulty following instructions—as defiance or oppositional behavior, particularly in Black and Indigenous boys (Coker et al., 2016). This misinterpretation increases the likelihood that children of color will be disciplined rather than referred for appropriate mental health evaluation and support (Morgan et al., 2014).

Implicit biases within the healthcare system also contribute to the underdiagnosis of ADHD and the overdiagnosis of oppositional defiant disorder (ODD) and conduct disorder (CD) in children of color. Black and Hispanic children are disproportionately diagnosed with ODD or CD, especially when presenting with hyperactivity or impulsivity (Morgan et al., 2014). Clinicians' biases may lead them to interpret ADHD-related behaviors as aggression or antisocial tendencies rather than as symptoms of neurodevelopmental differences (Coker et al., 2016). Even when children of color are accurately diagnosed with ADHD, they are significantly less likely to receive stimulant medications compared to their White peers, even after controlling for symptom severity and socioeconomic situation (Morgan et al., 2014). Furthermore, mistrust in the healthcare system, rooted in historical and systemic inequities, contributes to lower adherence to ADHD treatment plans among many families of color.

Addressing these disparities requires culturally competent interventions. Clinicians and educators should receive training in cultural competency to reduce diagnostic bias and improve ADHD identification in minority populations. Community-based mental health education programs can increase awareness and reduce stigma surrounding ADHD in Black, Hispanic, and Indigenous communities (Yau et al., 2024). Equitable access to ADHD evaluations and early intervention is essential to ensure timely diagnosis and to prevent academic and social setbacks. Additionally, policy reforms are needed to address racial disparities in school discipline, prioritizing supportive interventions over punitive responses to ADHD-related behaviors.

8.5 Treatment Inequities and Access Barriers

Racial disparities in ADHD treatment persist across healthcare systems, with Black, Hispanic, and Indigenous children significantly less likely to receive medication or behavioral therapy compared to White children, even when diagnosed with ADHD

(Coker et al., 2016; Morgan et al., 2014). These disparities result from systemic healthcare inequities, medical mistrust, and structural barriers that limit access to appropriate ADHD treatment and reduce treatment adherence among minority populations. Understanding these inequities is essential to designing interventions that ensure equitable access to care.

Despite comparable ADHD symptom prevalence, children of color are significantly less likely than White children to receive evidence-based treatments, such as stimulant medications and behavioral therapy (Coker et al., 2016). Studies show that White children with ADHD are nearly twice as likely to receive stimulant medication compared to Black and Hispanic children, even after adjusting for symptom severity, insurance status, and SES (Morgan et al., 2014). Only 36% of Black children and 30% of Hispanic children with ADHD receive stimulant medication, compared to 65% of White children (Coker et al., 2016). Indigenous children also experience lower medication rates, with many families preferring traditional healing practices over Western pharmacological interventions. Behavioral therapy utilization is similarly underrepresented in minority communities, where Black and Hispanic children with ADHD are significantly less likely to access school-based or outpatient counseling services (Coker et al., 2016). Limited availability of ADHD specialists and behavioral health services exacerbates the treatment gap in these populations (Morgan et al., 2014).

Historical injustices and systemic discrimination have contributed to medical mistrust among many communities of color, affecting both treatment-seeking behaviors and adherence to ADHD interventions. Black communities report heightened mistrust due to historical trauma, such as in the Tuskegee Syphilis Study, and ongoing disparities in healthcare outcomes (Coker et al., 2016). Indigenous populations also share deep-rooted mistrust rooted in past forced medical interventions and neglect in healthcare systems. Families of color often perceive ADHD diagnoses as a labels used to control or marginalize their children's behavior in educational settings (Morgan et al., 2014), and stimulant medications carry stigma in many communities, with concerns about addiction, side effects, and potential impacts on brain development (Coker et al., 2016). Parents of color frequently report negative healthcare experiences, including feeling dismissed, judged, or pressured into treatment. This mistrust contributes to lower engagement in ADHD care and increases the risk of discontinuing treatment (Coker et al., 2016).

Structural barriers compound these disparities, including language barriers, limited provider diversity, and geographic disparities that hinder access to ADHD services in marginalized communities. Many minority families live in healthcare deserts with few pediatric psychiatrists, school psychologists, or ADHD specialists (Morgan et al., 2014), resulting in long wait times, fewer treatment options, and delays in intervention (Coker et al., 2016). Hispanic families frequently report difficulties accessing Spanish-speaking ADHD providers, leading to miscommunication and lower treatment adherence. A lack of culturally competent clinicians also contributes to misunderstandings of cultural norms, impacting diagnosis and treatment acceptance (Morgan et al., 2014). Financial barriers, such as high out-of-pocket costs, transportation challenges, and inflexible work schedules, further complicate access to consistent care. Families of color are more likely to rely on public health insurance, such as Medicaid, yet children on Medicaid are less likely to receive specialist ADHD care—only about 25% see a specialist compared to nearly 50% of those with private insurance—and are also more likely to experience gaps in treatment follow-ups (CDC, 2024; Hu et al., 2023).

Addressing ADHD treatment disparities requires multifaceted solutions. Training more diverse clinicians and offering multilingual ADHD services can improve cultural competence and accessibility (Dong et al., 2020). Expanding community-based education programs can reduce stigma and increase awareness of ADHD in marginalized populations. Enhancing Medicaid and insurance coverage for ADHD services would make evaluations, medications, and therapy more affordable (Danielson et al., 2024). Finally, implementing school-based ADHD programs in underserved areas can provide early screening, counseling, and behavioral interventions to bridge the treatment gap (Larson et al., 2025).

8.6 Long-Term Consequences of Racial Disparities

Racial disparities in ADHD diagnosis and treatment have profound and lasting consequences for children of color, affecting their academic success, risk of legal system involvement, and overall mental health (Morgan et al., 2014). Minority children with undiagnosed or untreated ADHD face higher rates of school disciplinary actions, increased interactions with the juvenile justice system, and worsening psychological outcomes due to stigma, lack of access to care, and systemic barriers (Coker et al., 2016). Understanding these long-term effects is critical to developing interventions that mitigate racial disparities and improve health outcomes for children of color.

Children of color—especially Black, Hispanic, and Indigenous students—are disproportionately disciplined in school settings, often for behaviors linked to undiagnosed ADHD (Morgan et al., 2014). Studies show that Black children with ADHD symptoms are more likely to be suspended or expelled than White children, even when engaging in similar behaviors. Hispanic and Indigenous students with ADHD also face higher rates of punitive discipline rather than receiving behavioral interventions, leading to worsened academic performance and increased dropout rates (Coker et al., 2016). Many educators misinterpret hyperactivity and impulsivity as intentional defiance, resulting in disciplinary actions rather than mental health referrals (Morgan et al., 2014). Consequently, children of color with undiagnosed ADHD are often funneled into special education programs, alternative schools, or disciplinary tracks instead of receiving ADHD-appropriate support. This dynamic contributes to the "school-to-prison pipeline," as Black and Indigenous students who are suspended or expelled face significantly higher risks of subsequent justice system involvement (Coker et al., 2016). The failure to recognize and treat ADHD early perpetuates cumulative disadvantages that limit future educational and career opportunities (Morgan et al., 2014).

The intersection of racial disparities and untreated ADHD significantly increases the risk of justice system involvement for minority youth in the United States. Black and Indigenous adolescents with ADHD are disproportionately represented in U.S. juvenile detention facilities, often due to behavioral issues that were left untreated in early childhood (Morgan et al., 2014). Failure to diagnose and manage ADHD symptoms early results in impulsive decision-making, difficulty following rules, and increased conflict with authority figures, which can escalate into arrests and legal trouble (Coker et al., 2016). Youth of color with ADHD are more likely to be perceived as "troublemakers" rather than as individuals needing mental health support. Unlike White youth, who are more often referred to mental health programs, Black and Indigenous adolescents with ADHD are frequently placed in detention centers rather than receiving rehabilitative services (Morgan et al., 2014). Research indicates that juvenile offenders with untreated ADHD are more likely to reoffend, particularly when ADHD is left untreated while incarcerated (Coker et al., 2016). The absence of ADHD screening and intervention within the juvenile justice system prevents affected youth from accessing effective coping strategies and rehabilitation programs.

Stigma and lack of mental health awareness within Black, Hispanic, and Indigenous communities in the US contribute to delayed ADHD diagnoses and worsening long-term mental health challenges. In many communities of color, mental health conditions—including ADHD—are stigmatized, leading families to avoid seeking professional evaluation or treatment (Morgan et al., 2014). Parents may interpret ADHD symptoms as discipline issues, believing that strict parenting or punishment is the appropriate response rather than seeking medical or behavioral intervention (Coker et al., 2016). Additionally, many Black and Hispanic families report that mental health professionals do not fully understand their cultural perspectives on ADHD, leading to miscommunication and mistrust. The underrepresentation of minority mental health providers further discourages families from seeking treatment, as they feel their concerns are not taken seriously by predominantly White clinicians (Coker et al., 2016). Research shows that children of color with untreated ADHD are more likely to develop secondary mental health conditions, including anxiety disorders, depression, and post-traumatic stress disorder (PTSD) (Morgan et al., 2014). The combination of racial discrimination, socioeconomic stress, and untreated ADHD symptoms creates compounded mental health burdens for minority children.

Addressing these long-term disparities requires the implementation of school-based ADHD screening programs in racially diverse and underserved communities to ensure early detection and intervention (Coghill et al., 2022). Reducing school disciplinary disparities through ADHD-informed teacher training and behavioral support programs can help replace punitive measures with supportive interventions (Ward et al., 2022). Expanding culturally competent mental health services by increasing the representation of Black, Hispanic, and Indigenous ADHD specialists would help build trust and engagement with affected families (Stubbe, 2020). Finally, integrating ADHD screening into juvenile justice systems can ensure that youth offenders receive appropriate mental health interventions rather than incarceration without treatment (Tedeschi et al., 2024).

8.7 ADHD Diagnosis and Socioeconomic Status

Socioeconomic status plays a pivotal role in shaping ADHD diagnosis and treatment pathways, with children from socioeconomically disadvantaged backgrounds facing significant barriers to obtaining timely and appropriate care. These barriers result in delayed diagnoses, untreated symptoms, and poorer long-term outcomes (Russell et al., 2014; Larson et al., 2011). Key factors contributing to these disparities include limited access to health care, financial constraints, and heightened exposure to environmental stressors. Conversely, children from high-income families benefit from private healthcare access, earlier diagnoses, and comprehensive intervention plans, highlighting the broader influence of socioeconomic status on ADHD recognition, treatment adherence, and developmental trajectories (Sayal et al., 2018).

Children from lower-income households are disproportionately affected by delayed ADHD diagnoses due to systemic healthcare limitations (Russell et al., 2014). Public healthcare systems, on which many low-SES families rely, frequently have extended wait times, limited availability of child psychiatrists, and a shortage of ADHD-trained specialists. These systemic gaps result in reduced rates of formal ADHD assessments, leaving symptoms unaddressed during critical developmental periods (Larson et al., 2011). Moreover, geographic inequities in healthcare provision further exacerbate these challenges, as rural and low-income urban areas often experience a dearth of ADHD specialists, increasing the burden of travel and financial strain on affected families (Sayal et al., 2018). Transportation limitations and inflexible employment schedules can obstruct consistent access to care, compounding the problem (Russell et al., 2014). Additionally, school systems in lower-income areas often serve as the primary route for ADHD detection; however, resource constraints undermine the effectiveness of these screenings, contributing to diagnostic delays and suboptimal support services (Larson et al., 2011).

In contrast, children from high-income families experience expedited ADHD diagnoses and more robust treatment access due to systemic advantages (Sayal et al., 2018). These families often bypass public healthcare bottlenecks by securing private neuropsychological assessments, enabling timely diagnosis (Russell et al., 2014). Early identification facilitates timely interventions and improved developmental outcomes. These families also have greater access to behavioral therapies and specialist services, including CBT, ADHD coaching, and parent training, which enhance symptom management (Larson et al., 2011). In contrast, families with financial constraints may rely primarily on pharmacological interventions, with limited access to supplementary behavioral therapies (Sayal et al., 2018). Furthermore, parents from high-socioeconomic backgrounds typically possess enhanced knowledge about ADHD and are more adept at navigating complex healthcare systems (Russell et al., 2014). Lower income caregivers often lack access to educational resources, contributing to diagnostic delays and reduced advocacy for their children.

Socioeconomic stressors further exacerbate ADHD symptomatology and complicate treatment adherence (Russell et al., 2014). Poverty-associated factors—such as food insecurity, unstable housing, and community violence—are linked to heightened inattention, impulsivity, and emotional dysregulation in children. Chronic exposure to toxic stress impairs neurodevelopmental pathways, aggravating ADHD-related cognitive and behavioral challenges (Larson et al., 2011). Parental psychosocial stress, including elevated rates of depression, anxiety, and chronic stress in low socioeconomic caregivers, can impair their capacity to consistently implement ADHD management strategies (Russell et al., 2014). High-stress household environments can contribute to the intensification of ADHD symptoms in children (Sayal et al., 2018). Financial obstacles, lack of insurance coverage, and logistical challenges—such as transportation and inflexible work hours—further limit consistent access to medication and follow-up care. These systemic barriers often result in fragmented treatment trajectories and suboptimal symptom control (Larson et al., 2011).

To address socioeconomic-related inequities in ADHD diagnosis and treatment, expanded public insurance coverage to encompassing ADHD assessments, pharmacological treatments, and evidence-based behavioral therapy is recommended (Sayal et al., 2010). Implementing school-based ADHD screening and intervention programs in socioeconomically disadvantaged communities can help identify cases early (Froehlich et al., 2007). Developing subsidized ADHD care options, including low-cost therapy and executive function coaching, would support underserved populations (Devoe et al., 2007). Enhancing parental education initiatives to improve health literacy and empower caregivers to advocate for early ADHD evaluation is also vital. Additionally, Increasing investment in community-based ADHD services—particularly by leveraging telehealth platforms for screening, diagnosis, treatment, and care coordination—can help bridge geographic and resource gaps, ensuring more equitable access to ADHD care for underserved populations (Myers et al., 2015).

8.8 Barriers to Treatment for Low-Income Families

Children from low-income families encounter multiple barriers to accessing ADHD treatment, including financial hardship, geographic limitations, and educational inequity (Russell et al., 2014; Sayal et al., 2018). The cumulative effect of these challenges results in lower treatment rates, delayed interventions, and poorer long-term outcomes compared to children from higher-income households. Financial barriers are a significant obstacle for families with limited resources. The cost of comprehensive ADHD evaluations in the United States, including neuropsychological testing, can range from $500 to $2500 out-of-pocket (Sayal et al., 2018). Public healthcare systems often have long waitlists for ADHD assessments, delaying timely diagnosis and access to interventions. Once diagnosed, monthly costs for stimulant medications can range from $100 to $300 without insurance, creating affordability issues for underinsured families (Russell et al., 2014). Even with Medicaid and private insurance in the United States, restrictive co-pays, prior authorization policies, and refill limits reduce medication adherence (Larson et al., 2011). The cost of evidence-based behavioral therapies, such as CBT and ADHD coaching, is often inaccessible due to out-of-pocket costs ranging from $100 to $200 per session. Parent training programs, essential for effective symptom management at home, are similarly unaffordable or unavailable in many underserved communities (Sayal et al., 2018). Financial priorities like housing, food, and utilities often take precedence over healthcare expenses, resulting in inconsistent ADHD treatment (Russell et al., 2014).

Geographic disparities and limited access to ADHD specialists further hinder treatment for children in rural and low-income urban areas (Larson et al., 2011). While telemedicine has expanded ADHD service delivery, many low-income households lack broadband access, appropriate devices, or private spaces for virtual care (Russell et al., 2014). Public insurance plans do not always reimburse telehealth-based ADHD services, restricting remote care options.

Educational inequities also play a critical role in ADHD treatment barriers. Schools are central to managing ADHD, yet under-resourced districts often lack the capacity to provide adequate interventions (Sayal et al., 2018). Wealthier schools are more likely to provide Individualized Education Programs (IEPs), 504 plans, and in-class behavioral supports, while low-income schools struggle with insufficient funding and staffing. Teachers in underfunded districts often lack training on ADHD identification and management, leading to misinterpretation of symptoms as disruptive behavior (Sayal et al., 2018). Parents in low-income families may work multiple jobs, limiting their ability to attend school meetings or advocate for accommodations. Language barriers and unfamiliarity with special education rights can further reduce parental engagement with the school system (Russell et al., 2014).

To address these barriers, experts recommend expanding Medicaid and public insurance coverage to fully include ADHD diagnosis, pharmacotherapy, and behavioral interventions (Myers & Cain, 2008). Ultimately, addressing upstream divers of inequality is the solution, to ensure a livable minimum incomes and adequate welfare, affordable housing, education and universal health care and social assistance (Hilty et al., 2013) Increasing funding for school-based ADHD programs in underserved districts can improve early identification and in-school support. Developing mobile ADHD clinics and telehealth services tailored to rural and low-income communities can bridge geographic gaps (Hilty et al., 2013). Strengthening investments in special education and ADHD-specific teacher training would also improve outcomes. Additionally, providing free or subsidized parent training programs and caregiver support resources can empower families to better manage ADHD symptoms at home.

8.9 ADHD and Long-Term Economic Impacts

Untreated or inadequately managed ADHD has significant economic consequences, particularly for individuals from socioeconomically disadvantaged backgrounds. The disorder contributes to lifelong challenges, including educational underachievement, employment instability, reliance on social welfare, and disproportionate involvement in the criminal justice system (Russell et al., 2014). These challenges often begin with academic difficulties during childhood. Adolescents with untreated ADHD are two to three times more likely to leave school early than their peers, a risk that is magnified in under-resourced educational settings (Sayal et al., 2018). Students from disadvantaged backgrounds are less likely to receive timely ADHD accommodations, compounding academic disengagement and limiting educational attainment. Reduced educational attainment correlates with limited job prospects, underemployment, and lower wages (Russell et al., 2014). Adults with ADHD often experience job turnover, workplace conflicts, and challenges related to executive function deficits that undermine job performance and stability. Lifetime earnings are substantially lower for adults with a history of childhood ADHD—projected to earn $1.27 million less over the course of their lives compared to their non-ADHD peers (Pelham et al., 2020). Poor financial management and impulsivity further contribute to economic insecurity, making it difficult for individuals to achieve financial stability.

Persistent employment difficulties lead many adults with ADHD—especially those from low-income backgrounds—to rely on public assistance programs (Sayal et al., 2018). ADHD-related impairments often contribute to higher reliance on income support, food assistance, and housing subsidies. Workforce participation barriers, such as executive dysfunction and difficulties adhering to traditional work structures, limit job retention and advancement opportunities (Sayal et al., 2018). The cumulative costs of lost productivity, increased social service utilization, and unmet mental health needs result in substantial economic losses at the societal level (Russell et al., 2014).

Moreover, children and adolescents with ADHD, particularly in low-income settings, are at elevated risk for exclusionary discipline and subsequent involvement with the justice system, further perpetuating economic disadvantage (Eme, 2021). Students with ADHD are more likely to face suspensions and expulsions, especially in schools lacking adequate behavioral supports (Russell et al., 2014). Black and Indigenous youth with ADHD experience heightened rates of punitive measures compared to their White peers, reflecting both systemic bias and the intersection of socioeconomic and racial disparities (Eme, 2021). The prevalence of ADHD is disproportionately high among detained youth, many of whom were never diagnosed or treated during childhood (Sayal et al., 2018). Once incarcerated, individuals with ADHD often lack access to evidence-based treatments, which increases recidivism rates and perpetuates economic marginalization.

To mitigate these ADHD-related economic disadvantages, experts recommend scaling up school-based ADHD prevention and intervention programs to reduce academic failure and dropout (Moore et al., 2019). Expanding employment support initiatives—including ADHD-sensitive job coaching and workplace accommodations—can improve job retention and career outcomes. Integrating ADHD screening and treatment into juvenile justice and adult correctional systems ensures that individuals receive appropriate mental health interventions rather than punitive responses. Advocating for ADHD-inclusive workplace policies and financial literacy initiatives can further empower individuals with ADHD to achieve financial stability (Froehlich et al., 2007). Finally, enhancing welfare-to-work programs that are tailored for ADHD-related challenges can support sustained employment and economic independence.

Summary

Chapter 8 underscores the profound impact of gender, race, and socioeconomic status (SES) on the ADHD experience, emphasizing that ADHD cannot be fully understood or effectively managed without considering these intersecting factors. Historically, ADHD research and diagnostic frameworks have prioritized male-typical presentations of the disorder, leading to underdiagnosis and misdiagnosis in females who often present with inattentive and internalizing symptoms. This diagnostic bias results in delays in treatment and greater risk of comorbid mental health issues, including depression, anxiety, self-harm, and eating disorders.

Racial and ethnic disparities further exacerbate inequities in ADHD diagnosis and treatment. Black, Hispanic, and Indigenous children are less likely to be diagnosed with ADHD compared to White peers, despite comparable symptom severity. This underdiagnosis stems from clinician bias, cultural stigma, and systemic barriers in health care and education. These children are also less likely to receive evidence-based treatments such as stimulant medications and behavioral therapies, contributing to higher rates of school disciplinary actions, academic failure, and subsequent involvement with the justice system.

Socioeconomic factors also shape ADHD trajectories. Children from low-income families often face substantial barriers to timely diagnosis and effective treatment, including financial constraints, limited access to specialists, and under-resourced schools. These challenges lead to delayed interventions, lower educational attainment, and poorer long-term outcomes, perpetuating cycles of disadvantage.

Addressing these disparities requires a concerted effort to implement culturally competent and gender-sensitive ADHD assessments, enhance training for educators and healthcare providers, and expand access to comprehensive interventions. School-based programs, community education, and policy reforms are essential to ensure equitable access to ADHD care and support services. By integrating intersectionality into ADHD research, diagnosis, and treatment, clinicians, educators, and policymakers can better meet the needs of all individuals affected by ADHD, fostering more equitable outcomes across the lifespan.

References

Barkley, R. A., Fischer, M., Smallish, L., & Fletcher, K. (2004). Young adult outcome of hyperactive children: Adaptive functioning in major life activities. *Journal of the American Academy of Child & Adolescent Psychiatry, 43*(1), 77–85. https://doi.org/10.1097/00004583-200401000-00012

CDC. (2024). Centers for Disease Control and Prevention. (2024). Data and Statistics on ADHD. Retrieved from CDC.govcdc.gov https://www.cdc.gov/adhd/data/index.html?utm_source=chatgpt.com

Chan, E. S. M., & Langberg, J. M. (2024). Predicting occupational outcomes for individuals with ADHD: The role of hyperactivity/impulsivity and executive functioning. *Journal of Occupational Rehabilitation, 36*(1), 223–233. https://doi.org/10.1007/s10926-024-10259-y

Coker, T. R., Elliott, M. N., Toomey, S. L., Schwebel, D. C., Cuccaro, P., Davies, S. L., Visser, S. N., & Schuster, M. A. (2016). *Racial and ethnic disparities in ADHD diagnosis and treatment. Pediatrics, 138*(3), e20160407. https://doi.org/10.1542/peds.2016-0407

Coghill, D., Du, Y., Jiang, W., Xian Lu, D., Qian, Y., Mulraney, M., & Su, L. (2022). A novel school-based approach to screening for attention deficit hyperactivity disorder. *European Child & Adolescent Psychiatry, 31*(6), 909–917. https://doi.org/10.1007/s00787-021-01721-w

Danielson, M. L., Claussen, A. H., Arifkhanova, A., Gonzalez, M. G., & Surman, C. (2024). Who provides outpatient clinical care for adults with ADHD? Analysis of healthcare claims by types of providers among private insurance and medicaid enrollees, 2021. *Journal of Attention Disorders, 28*(8), 1225–1235.

Devoe, J. E., Baez, A., Angier, H., Krois, L., Edlund, C., & Carney, P. A. (2007). Insurance + access not equal to health care: Typology of barriers to health care access for low-income families. *Annals of Family Medicine, 5*(6), 511–518. https://doi.org/10.1370/afm.748

Dimitri, D., Delia, G., Cavallo, F., Varini, M., & Fioretto, F. (2025). Sex differences in children and adolescents with attention-deficit/hyperactivity disorder: A literature review. *Frontiers in Child and Adolescent Psychiatry, 4*, 1582502.

Dong, Q., Garcia, B., Pham, A. V., & Cumming, M. (2020). Culturally responsive approaches for addressing ADHD within multi-tiered systems of support. *Current Psychiatry Reports, 22*(6), 27.

Froehlich, T. E., Lanphear, B. P., Epstein, J. N., Barbaresi, W. J., Katusic, S. K., & Kahn, R. S. (2007). Prevalence, recognition, and treatment of attention-deficit/hyperactivity disorder in a national sample of US children. *Archives of Pediatrics & Adolescent Medicine, 161*(9), 857–864. https://doi.org/10.1001/archpedi.161.9.857

Gershon, J. (2002). A meta-analytic review of gender differences in ADHD. *Journal of Attention Disorders, 5*(3), 143–154. https://doi.org/10.1177/108705470200500302

Hilty, D. M., Ferrer, D. C., Parish, M. B., Johnston, B., Callahan, E. J., & Yellowlees, P. M. (2013). The effectiveness of telemental health: A 2013 review. *Telemedicine Journal and E-Health, 19*(6), 444–454. https://doi.org/10.1089/tmj.2013.0075

Hinshaw, S. P., Nguyen, P. T., O'Grady, S. M., & Rosenthal, E. A. (2022). Annual research review: Attention-deficit/ hyperactivity disorder in girls and women: Underrepresentation, longitudinal processes, and key directions. *Journal of Child Psychology and Psychiatry, 63*(4), 484–496. https://doi.org/10.1111/jcpp.13480

Hu, J.-C., Cummings, J. R., Ji, X., & Wilk, A. S. (2023). State-level variation in medicaid managed care enrollment and specialty care for publicly insured children. *JAMA Network Open, 6*(10), e2336415–e2336415. https://doi.org/10.1001/jamanetworkopen.2023.36415

Kooij, J. J. S., de Jong, M., Agnew-Blais, J., Amoretti, S., Bang Madsen, K., Barclay, I., Bölte, S., Borg Skoglund, C., Broughton, T., Carucci, S., van Dijken, D. K. E., Ernst, J., French, B., Frick, M. A., Galera, C., Groenman, A. P., Kopp Kallner, H., Kerner Auch Koerner, J., Kittel-Schneider, S., et al. (2025). Research advances and future directions in female ADHD: The lifelong interplay of hormonal fluctuations with mood, cognition, and disease. *Frontiers in Global Women's Health, 6*, 1613628. https://doi.org/10.3389/fgwh.2025.1613628

Larson, J. M., Gregus, S., Ali, E., McGill, S. K., Blackhurst, Z., Sensenbaugh, J., & Klaus, N. (2025). Preliminary outcomes from an after-school treatment program for children with ADHD. *Evidence-Based Practice in Child and Adolescent Mental Health, 10*(2), 285–298.

Larson, K., Russ, S. A., Kahn, R. S., & Halfon, N. (2011). Patterns of comorbidity, functioning, and service use for US children with ADHD. *Pediatrics, 127*(3), 462–470. https://doi.org/10.1542/peds.2010-0165

May, T., Birch, E., Chaves, K., Cranswick, N., Culnane, E., Delaney, J., Derrick, M., Eapen, V., Edlington, C., Efron, D., Ewais, T., Garner, I., Gathercole, M., Jagadheesan, K., Jobson, L., Kramer, J., Mack, M., Misso, M., Murrup-Stewart, C., et al. (2023). The Australian evidence-based clinical practice guideline for attention deficit hyperactivity disorder. *The Australian and New Zealand Journal of Psychiatry, 57*(8), 1101–1116. https://doi.org/10.1177/00048674231166329

Moore, D. A., Richardson, M., Gwernan-Jones, R., Thompson-Coon, J., Stein, K., Rogers, M., Garside, R., Logan, S., & Ford, T. J. (2019). Non-pharmacological interventions for ADHD in school settings: An overarching synthesis of systematic reviews. *Journal of Attention Disorders, 23*(3), 220–233. https://doi.org/10.1177/1087054715573994

Morgan, C., Lappin, J., Heslin, M., Donoghue, K., Lomas, B., Reininghaus, U., Onyejiaka, A., Croudace, T., Jones, P. B., Murray, R. M., Fearon, P., Doody, G. A., & Dazzan, P. (2014). Reappraising the long-term course and outcome of psychotic disorders: The AESOP-10 study. *Psychological Medicine, 44*(13), 2713–2726. https://doi.org/10.1017/S0033291714000282

Myers, K., & Cain, S. (2008). Practice parameter for telepsychiatry with children and adolescents. *Journal of the American Academy of Child and Adolescent Psychiatry, 47*(12), 1468–1483. https://doi.org/10.1097/CHI.0b013e31818b4e13

Myers, K., Vander Stoep, A., Zhou, C., McCarty, C. A., & Katon, W. (2015). Effectiveness of a telehealth service delivery model for treating attention-deficit/hyperactivity disorder: A community-based randomized controlled trial. *Journal of the American Academy of Child and Adolescent Psychiatry, 54*(4), 263–274. https://doi.org/10.1016/j.jaac.2015.01.009

Nussbaum, N. L. (2011). ADHD and female specific concerns: A review of the literature and clinical implications. *Journal of Attention Disorders, 16*(2), 87–100. https://doi.org/10.1177/1087054711416909

Pelham, W. E., Page, T. F., Altszuler, A. R., Gnagy, E. M., Molina, B. S. G., & Pelham, W. E. (2020). The long-term financial outcome of children diagnosed with ADHD. *Journal of Consulting and Clinical Psychology, 88*(2), 160–171. https://doi.org/10.1037/ccp0000461

Quinn, P. O., & Madhoo, M. (2014). A review of attention-deficit/hyperactivity disorder in women and girls: Uncovering this hidden diagnosis. *The Primary Care Companion for CNS Disorders, 16*(3), PCC.13r01596. https://doi.org/10.4088/PCC.13r01596

Rucklidge, J. J. (2010). Gender differences in attention-deficit/hyperactivity disorder. *Psychiatric Clinics of NorthAmerica, 33*(2), 357–373. https://doi.org/10.1016/j.psc.2010.01.006

Russell, G., Ford, T., Rosenberg, R., & Kelly, S. (2014). The association of attention-deficit/ hyperactivity disorder with socioeconomic disadvantage: Alternative explanations and evidence. *Journal of Child Psychology and Psychiatry, 55*(5), 436–445. https://doi.org/10.1111/jcpp.12170

Sayal, K., Owen, V., White, K., Merrell, C., Tymms, P., & Taylor, E. (2010). Impact of early school-based screening and intervention programs for ADHD on children's outcomes and access to services: Follow-up of a school-based trial at age 10 years. *Archives of Pediatrics & Adolescent Medicine, 164*(5), 462–469. https://doi.org/10.1001/archpediatrics.2010.40

Sayal, K., Prasad, V., Daley, D., Ford, T., & Coghill, D. (2018). ADHD in children and young people: Prevalence, care pathways, and service provision. *The Lancet Psychiatry, 5*(2), 175–186. https://doi.org/10.1016/S2215-0366(17)30167-0

Stubbe, D. E. (2020). Practicing cultural competence and cultural humility in the care of diverse patients. *Focus (American Psychiatric Publishing), 18*(1), 49–51. https://doi.org/10.1176/appi.focus.20190041

Tedeschi, F., Horwitz, S. M., Surko, M., Weinberger, E., Bart, A., Baetz, C., Guo, F., Alexander, A., & Havens, J. F. (2024). Mental health service referral and treatment following screening and assessment in juvenile detention. *The Journal of the American Academy of Psychiatry and the Law, 52*(4), 460–469. https://doi.org/10.29158/jaapl.240082-24

Ward, R. J., Bristow, S. J., Kovshoff, H., Cortese, S., & Kreppner, J. (2022). The effects of ADHD teacher training programs on teachers and pupils: A systematic review and meta-analysis. *Journal of Attention Disorders, 26*(2), 225–244. https://doi.org/10.1177/1087054720972801

Wilens, T. E., Martelon, M., Joshi, G., Bateman, C., Fried, R., Petty, C., & Biederman, J. (2011). Does attention-deficit/hyperactivity disorder predict substance-use disorders? A 10-year follow-up study of young adults with ADHD. *Journal of the American Academy of Child & Adolescent Psychiatry, 50*(6), 543–553. https://doi.org/10.1016/j.jaac.2011.01.021

Yau, M. Y., Baltrushes, N., Cooper, T. J., Lee, R. J., Michalska, K., Kim, M., Nguyen, C., & Ahmed, N. (2024). 5.32 promoting ADHD awareness in diverse communities using community-based participatory research. *Journal of the American Academy of Child & Adolescent Psychiatry, 63*(10), S265–S266. https://doi.org/10.1016/j.jaac.2024.08.353

Young, S., Moss, D., Sedgwick, O., Fridman, M., & Hodgkins, P. (2015). A meta-analysis of the prevalence of attention-deficit/hyperactivity disorder in incarcerated populations. *Psychological Medicine, 45*(2), 247–258. https://doi.org/10.1017/S0033291714000762

Chapter 9
Interventions and Treatments for ADHD Across the Lifespan

Abstract This chapter offers a comprehensive overview of interventions and treatments for Attention-Deficit/Hyperactivity Disorder (ADHD) across the lifespan. Recognizing that ADHD symptoms and associated impairments shift as individuals transition from childhood through adolescence and into adulthood, an adaptive, lifespan approach to management is essential. The chapter outlines evidence-based treatment strategies, incorporating both pharmacological and non-pharmacological interventions. These include medications, behavioral therapies, and lifestyle modifications, all of which are tailored to the individual's developmental stage, symptom severity, and co-occurring conditions. Ensuring optimal outcomes requires a collaborative and person-centered approach, where healthcare professionals, educators, families, and individuals with ADHD work in partnership to promote well-being and functional recovery at every life stage.

9.1 Comprehensive Management of ADHD Across the Lifespan

The management of ADHD requires a comprehensive, integrated, and multidisciplinary approach, drawing on both pharmacological and non-pharmacological interventions. Effective treatment involves identifying an individual's strengths and challenges and tailoring support to enhance functioning across the lifespan. Clinicians must develop individualized treatment plans in collaboration with the patient and, where appropriate, their families or caregivers. Such plans aim to capitalize on strengths while addressing areas of difficulty through targeted interventions.

A successful ADHD management plan often includes a combination of medications, psychological therapies, school or workplace interventions, and lifestyle modifications, designed to evolve alongside the individual's developmental and psychosocial needs. Importantly, an integrated model fosters collaboration among healthcare providers, educators, and families to ensure continuity of care.

G. Ayano et al., *ADHD Across the Lifespan*, SpringerBriefs in Modern Perspectives on Disability Research,
https://doi.org/10.1007/978-981-95-8712-4_9

9.1.1 Pharmacological Treatments for ADHD

Pharmacological treatments remain a key component of ADHD management, with stimulant and non-stimulant medications serving as primary therapeutic options. While medications are commonly used across all age groups, their specific application and monitoring differ depending on developmental stage.

9.1.1.1 Medications for Childhood and Adolescence

In children and adolescents, stimulant medications such as methylphenidate (e.g., Ritalin, Concerta) and amphetamines (e.g., Adderall, Vyvanse) are frequently prescribed. These agents work by increasing dopamine and norepinephrine levels, thereby improving attention, impulse control, and reducing hyperactivity (Faraone et al., 2021). Stimulants are highly effective, showing benefits in 70–80% of young patients and contributing to improvements in academic and social functioning (Storebø et al., 2015). Despite their effectiveness, these medications may cause side effects such as appetite suppression, sleep disturbances, emotional lability, and cardiovascular changes, requiring regular monitoring (Banaschewski et al., 2016).

Non-stimulant options, including atomoxetine (Strattera) and alpha-2 adrenergic agonists such as guanfacine (Intuniv) and clonidine (Kapvay), are also used (Cortese et al., 2018; Mechler et al., 2022). These medications are particularly valuable for children with comorbid conditions such as anxiety or tic disorders, offering symptom control with a lower potential for abuse (Molina et al., 2019; Stevenson et al., 2014). Non-stimulants typically have a slower onset of action but can be effective for those who experience intolerable side effects from stimulants (Cortese et al., 2018).

9.1.1.2 Medications for Adults with ADHD

In adults, stimulants remain a first-line treatment but require careful monitoring due to an increased risk of misuse and cardiovascular side effects (Knouse et al., 2017). Extended-release formulations and non-stimulants such as atomoxetine are commonly used to enhance adherence and reduce rebound symptoms (Faraone et al., 2021). Adult patients often benefit from medication plans that address both ADHD symptoms and comorbid conditions, including mood and anxiety disorders.

Additionally, some clinicians use off-label medications, including bupropion (Wellbutrin) and modafinil (Provigil), to improve focus and executive functioning. Medication adherence is generally lower in adults compared to children, underscoring the need for integrated treatment plans that include behavioral and psychosocial supports (Molina et al., 2019).

9.1.1.3 ADHD Medication in Older Adults

While research on ADHD treatment in older adults is limited, available evidence suggests that symptoms often persist into later life (Vysniauske et al., 2020). Stimulants can help manage executive dysfunction in this population, though heightened cardiovascular risks necessitate close monitoring (Banaschewski et al., 2016).

Non-stimulant medications may be favored to avoid potential drug interactions with medications for other age-related conditions, such as hypertension and diabetes (Stevenson et al., 2014). There is a pressing need for further research to develop age-appropriate guidelines for ADHD treatment in aging populations.

9.2 Non-pharmacological Interventions for ADHD

Non-pharmacological interventions target the cognitive, emotional, and behavioral challenges associated with ADHD. These therapies play a pivotal role, either as standalone treatments or in combination with pharmacotherapy, and can reduce symptom severity, improve functioning, and enhance quality of life (Cortese et al., 2018).

Behavioral and psychological therapies, psychoeducation, lifestyle modifications, and school- or workplace-based interventions are commonly employed to improve executive function, emotional regulation, and social functioning (David Daley et al., 2014). These interventions are especially critical for individuals who experience side effects from medication or who prefer non-pharmacological strategies.

9.2.1 Behavioral and Psychological Therapies

Cognitive Behavioral Therapy (CBT) is particularly effective for adolescents and adults with ADHD. It focuses on addressing deficits in executive functioning, emotional regulation, and impulse control while equipping individuals with structured routines and coping strategies (Knouse et al., 2017; Molina et al., 2019).

Parent training programs, such as Behavioral Parent Training (BPT) and Parent–Child Interaction Therapy (PCIT), are well-established interventions that empower caregivers to manage disruptive behaviors and foster positive habits in children (Chronis-Tuscano et al., 2017; Faraone et al., 2021).

Social skills training is another valuable approach for children and adolescents, enhancing peer relationships through targeted instruction on emotional regulation, conflict resolution, and effective communication (Banaschewski et al., 2016; Vysniauske et al., 2020).

9.3 Integrating Treatment Approaches Across the Lifespan

Integrated treatment approaches adapt to the unique developmental needs of individuals with ADHD across childhood, adolescence, adulthood, and older adulthood. The dynamic nature of ADHD symptoms across the lifespan necessitates flexible and tailored interventions.

9.3.1 Childhood and Adolescence

For children and adolescents, multimodal treatment—combining pharmacotherapy with behavioral therapies, parent training, and school-based interventions—is most effective (Faraone et al., 2021). Parental involvement is essential to promoting adherence and fostering positive behavioral changes (David Daley et al., 2014). Early intervention improves long-term academic and social outcomes and helps prevent secondary difficulties, such as low self-esteem and social withdrawal (Chronis-Tuscano et al., 2017).

9.3.2 Adulthood

In adulthood, stimulant medications and non-stimulants are often paired with CBT, coaching, and workplace accommodations to address executive functioning challenges and occupational impairments (Knouse et al., 2017; Molina et al., 2019). Adults with ADHD frequently experience comorbid conditions, including anxiety, depression, and substance use disorders, requiring individualized and comprehensive treatment plans.

9.3.3 Older Adults

For older adults, ADHD diagnosis is often complicated by overlapping symptoms with cognitive decline (Vysniauske et al., 2020). Non-pharmacological interventions, such as CBT and the establishment of structured routines, are effective strategies to manage executive dysfunction (Daley et al., 2014). Additionally, addressing comorbid health conditions, including cardiovascular disease and mood disorders, is essential to safe and effective ADHD management in this population (Faraone et al., 2021).

Summary

ADHD is a lifelong neurodevelopmental disorder requiring multimodal management that evolves across developmental stages. Evidence supports the integration of pharmacological treatments—primarily stimulants and nonstimulants—with behavioral therapies, such as cognitive behavioral therapy (CBT), parent training, and social skills interventions. Early interventions in childhood focus on parent-mediated strategies and school-based support, while adult care emphasizes CBT, coaching, and workplace accommodations.

Despite therapeutic advances, critical gaps persist, particularly in the recognition and treatment of ADHD among older adults, where research remains limited. Addressing these gaps is essential to delivering equitable and age-appropriate care. The dynamic nature of ADHD across the lifespan underscores the need for continuous refinement of integrated treatment strategies.

References

Banaschewski, T., Coghill, D., Santosh, P., Zuddas, A., Asherson, P., Buitelaar, J., Danckaerts, M., Döpfner, M., Faraone, S. V., Rothenberger, A., Sergeant, J., Steinhausen, H. C., Sonuga-Barke, E. J., & Taylor, E. (2016). Long-acting medications for attention-deficit/hyperactivity disorder: A systematic review and European treatment guideline. *European Child & Adolescent Psychiatry, 25*(6), 637–655. https://doi.org/10.1007/s00787-015-0709-7

Chronis-Tuscano, A., Wang, C. H., Woods, K. E., Strickland, J., & Stein, M. A. (2017). Parent ADHD and evidence-based treatment for their children: Review and directions for future research. *Journal of Abnormal Child Psychology, 45*(3), 501–517. https://doi.org/10.1007/s10802-016-0238-5

Cortese, S., Adamo, N., Del Giovane, C., Mohr-Jensen, C., Hayes, A. J., Carucci, S., Atkinson, L. Z., Tessari, L., Banaschewski, T., Coghill, D., Hollis, C., Simonoff, E., Zuddas, A., Barbui, C., Purgato, M., Steinhausen, H. C., Shokraneh, F., Xia, J., & Cipriani, A. (2018). Comparative efficacy and tolerability of medications for attention-deficit hyperactivity disorder in children, adolescents, and adults: A systematic review and network meta-analysis. *Lancet Psychiatry, 5*(9), 727–738. https://doi.org/10.1016/s2215-0366(18)30269-4

Faraone, S. V., Banaschewski, T., Coghill, D., Zheng, Y., Biederman, J., Bellgrove, M. A., Newcorn, J. H., Gignac, M., Al Saud, N. M., Manor, I., Rohde, L. A., Cortese, S., Almagor, D., Stein, M. A., Albatti, T. H., Aljoudi, H. F., Alqahtani, M. M. J., Asherson, P., Atwoli, L., … Wang, Y. (2021). The World Federation of ADHD International Consensus Statement: 208 evidence-based conclusions about the disorder. *Neuroscience & Biobehavioral Reviews, 128*, 789–818. https://doi.org/10.1016/j.neubiorev.2021.01.022

Daley, D., van der Oord, S., Ferrin, M., Danckaerts, M., Doepfner, M., Cortese, S., & Sonuga-Barke, E. J. S. (2014). Behavioral interventions in attention-deficit/hyperactivity disorder: A meta-analysis of randomized controlled trials across multiple outcome domains. *Journal of the American Academy of Child & Adolescent Psychiatry, 53*(8), 835–847.e835. https://doi.org/10.1016/j.jaac.2014.05.013

Knouse, L. E., Teller, J., & Brooks, M. A. (2017). Meta-analysis of cognitive-behavioral treatments for adult ADHD. *Journal of Consulting and Clinical Psychology, 85*(7), 737–750. https://doi.org/10.1037/ccp0000216

Mechler, K., Banaschewski, T., Hohmann, S., & Häge, A. (2022). Evidence-based pharmacological treatment options for ADHD in children and adolescents. *Pharmacology & Therapeutics, 230*, 107940. https://doi.org/10.1016/j.pharmthera.2021.107940

Molina, B. S. G., Arnold, L. E., Swanson, J. M., Pelham, W. E., Hechtman, L., Hoza, B., Epstein, J. N., Vitiello, B., Jensen, P. S., Hinshaw, S. P., Abikoff, H. B., Elliott, G. R., Greenhill, L. L., Newcorn, J. H., Wells, K. C., Wigal, T., Gibbons, R. D., Hur, K., Houck, P. R., & MTA Cooperative Group. (2019). Adolescent substance use in the Multimodal Treatment Study of ADHD (MTA). *Journal of the American Academy of Child & Adolescent Psychiatry, 58*(3), 267–276. https://doi.org/10.1016/j.jaac.2018.06.024

Stevenson, J., Buitelaar, J., Cortese, S., Ferrin, M., Konofal, E., Lecendreux, M., Simonoff, E., Wong, I. C. K., Sonuga-Barke, E., & European ADHD Guidelines Group. (2014). Research review: The role of diet in the treatment of attention-deficit/hyperactivity disorder. *Journal of Child Psychology and Psychiatry, 55*(5), 416–427. https://doi.org/10.1111/jcpp.12145

Storebø, O. J., Ramstad, E., Krogh, H. B., Nilausen, T. D., Skoog, M., Holmskov, M., Rosendal, S., Groth, C., Magnusson, F. L., Moreira-Maia, C. R., Gillies, D., Buch Rasmussen, K., Gauci, D., Zwi, M., Kirubakaran, R., Forsbøl, B., Simonsen, E., & Gluud, C. (2015). Methylphenidate for attention deficit hyperactivity disorder (ADHD) in children and adolescents. *Cochrane Database of Systematic Reviews, (11)*, CD009885. https://doi.org/10.1002/14651858.CD009885.pub2

Vysniauske, R., Verburgh, L., Oosterlaan, J., & Molendijk, M. L. (2020). The effects of physical exercise on functional outcomes in the treatment of ADHD: A meta-analysis. *Journal of Attention Disorders, 24*(5), 644–654. https://doi.org/10.1177/1087054715627489

Chapter 10
ADHD in Global and National Health Frameworks

Abstract This chapter provides a critical examination of the positioning of Attention-Deficit/Hyperactivity Disorder (ADHD) within global and national health frameworks. ADHD is formally recognized as a neurodevelopmental disorder by the World Health Organization (WHO) in the International Classification of Diseases (ICD-11) and by the American Psychiatric Association (APA) in the Diagnostic and Statistical Manual of Mental Disorders (DSM-5). Yet, despite this recognition, ADHD remains underrepresented in public health agendas worldwide. This underrepresentation contributes to fragmented policies, inconsistent service delivery, and stark disparities in diagnosis and treatment across diverse health systems.

The chapter explores variations in ADHD-related policies and practices between high-income countries and low- and middle-income countries (LMICs). It examines how differing health priorities, constrained resources, and cultural perceptions influence the identification, management, and treatment pathways of ADHD globally. Finally, the chapter encourages readers to reflect on the broader challenges and opportunities for embedding ADHD more firmly within public health strategies, with a view to reducing inequities and enhancing outcomes for affected individuals across varying socio-political and economic contexts.

10.1 ADHD Recognition and Policy in Global and National Frameworks

Although ADHD has gained formal recognition within leading diagnostic systems—including the World Health Organization's International Classification of Diseases (ICD-11) and the American Psychiatric Association's Diagnostic and Statistical Manual of Mental Disorders (DSM-5)—it remains largely underrepresented in global and national health agendas. This limited prioritization has contributed to fragmented and inconsistent policy landscapes across countries, leading to significant disparities in the diagnosis, treatment, and support of individuals with ADHD. While some high-income countries have enacted legal frameworks and

G. Ayano et al., *ADHD Across the Lifespan*, SpringerBriefs in Modern Perspectives on Disability Research,
https://doi.org/10.1007/978-981-95-8712-4_10

clinical guidelines to address ADHD, many low- and middle-income countries (LMICs) continue to face considerable challenges, including inadequate public health initiatives, limited access to trained specialists, and pervasive cultural stigma. These issues underscore the need for coordinated global efforts to enhance ADHD recognition, standardize care, and address inequities across diverse populations. This section critically examines the positioning of ADHD within international health classifications and outlines the varied national approaches to its management.

10.1.1 ADHD Recognition in Global Health Frameworks

The World Health Organization's ICD-11 identifies ADHD as a neurodevelopmental disorder marked by persistent impairments in cognitive, academic, and social functioning (WHO, 2021). Despite this formal classification, ADHD remains absent from any global public health strategy endorsed by the WHO, leaving national governments without clear direction for policy development or service implementation. Consequently, ADHD management falls outside the scope of national mental health priorities, particularly in LMICs where competing health challenges and limited resources prevail. Similarly, the American Psychiatric Association's DSM-5 provides widely accepted diagnostic criteria for ADHD, distinguishing between inattentive, hyperactive-impulsive, and combined presentations (APA, 2013). Although the DSM-5 has significantly shaped diagnostic practices worldwide, its adoption is uneven, contributing to variability in ADHD recognition and treatment protocols across different countries and regions.

10.1.2 Variability in National ADHD Policies

National ADHD policies vary widely, reflecting differences in healthcare systems, resource allocation, and public awareness. In the United States, ADHD is integrated into key disability and public health frameworks, including the Individuals with Disabilities Education Act (IDEA) and the Americans with Disabilities Act (ADA), which ensure access to educational accommodations and protection against discrimination (Sonuga-Barke et al., 2013; Visser et al., 2016). National agencies, such as the Centers for Disease Control and Prevention (CDC), have supported programs aimed at raising awareness and promoting early intervention (Cortese et al., 2018). Despite these advances, disparities in treatment access remain, particularly among socioeconomically disadvantaged populations. In the United Kingdom, the National Health Service (NHS) offers ADHD-related services guided by the National Institute for Health and Care Excellence (NICE) recommendations (NICE, 2018). However, implementation is inconsistent, and patients often face lengthy wait times and regional variability in service availability. Across the European Union, countries such as Sweden and Denmark have established robust, publicly funded ADHD services, including accessible medication coverage and specialized clinics (Y. Ginsberg et al., 2014). In contrast, several Southern and Eastern European nations lack formal ADHD policies, leading to pronounced disparities in service provision across the region (French et al., 2019). In Australia, ADHD is acknowledged under the Disability Discrimination Act (DDA), but its recognition as a disability is typically restricted to severe cases. Public ADHD services are unevenly distributed, and access to specialist care varies significantly across states and territories, reflecting broader systemic challenges (French et al., 2019).

10.1.3 ADHD in Low- and Middle-Income Countries (LMICs)

In many LMICs, ADHD remains marginalized within public health priorities, resulting in a substantial proportion of undiagnosed and untreated cases. Contributing barriers include a critical shortage of trained mental health professionals, limited access to medications, and entrenched social stigma. For instance, in several African countries, it is estimated that fewer than 10% of children with ADHD receive a formal diagnosis (Mukherjee et al., 2021). Cultural beliefs frequently frame ADHD symptoms as behavioral or disciplinary issues, further obstructing clinical recognition and intervention. In Latin America, while awareness of ADHD is gradually increasing, treatment largely remains confined to private healthcare sectors—making services financially inaccessible for many families within public systems (Polanczyk et al., 2008). These disparities suggest there is a specific need for culturally tailored policies, strengthened health system capacity, and targeted public awareness campaigns to improve ADHD care and reduce inequities globally.

To address these barriers, experts recommend expanding Medicaid and public insurance coverage to fully include ADHD diagnosis, pharmacotherapy, and behavioral interventions. Ultimately, addressing upstream drivers of inequality—such as income insecurity, inadequate housing, limited educational opportunities, and gaps in universal health and social assistance—is essential, as these social determinants directly influence timely ADHD identification, access to evidence-based treatment, and long-term functional outcomes (Danielson et al., 2018; Froehlich et al., 2007).

10.1.4 Gaps in ADHD Policy and Healthcare Systems

Despite the growing recognition of ADHD as a neurodevelopmental disorder, many healthcare systems worldwide lack dedicated policies and sufficient resources to adequately support individuals with ADHD. Underfunding, extended wait times for diagnosis, limited training for healthcare providers, and a general lack of workplace accommodations contribute to significant barriers in accessing appropriate care (Young et al., 2021). Additionally, the high cost of ADHD medications and therapies further limits treatment access, particularly for uninsured and socioeconomically disadvantaged populations (Hinshaw & Arnold, 2022). These systemic challenges highlight the urgent need for comprehensive policies and investment to address ADHD as a public health priority.

A major gap in ADHD policy is the limited public funding allocated for ADHD research, diagnosis, and treatment services. Compared to other neurodevelopmental and mental health conditions, such as autism and depression in children and young people, ADHD receives substantially less attention in public health budgets. This underinvestment in research impedes the development of innovative treatments and effective early intervention strategies, while the lack of national-level epidemiological studies creates knowledge gaps regarding ADHD prevalence patterns and treatment outcomes (Faraone et al., 2021). Furthermore, ADHD is seldom included in national mental health programs or campaigns, leaving policymakers and the general public with limited awareness of the disorder's impact. Many public health systems are constrained by underfunded diagnostic and treatment services, resulting in overburdened clinics and long waitlists. School-based ADHD support programs also remain under-resourced, limiting the implementation of essential behavioral interventions and staff training.

Long wait times for ADHD diagnosis represent another critical barrier, delaying early intervention during important developmental periods. In some countries, diagnostic wait times can exceed 12–24 months. ADHD often receives lower prioritization than severe psychiatric disorders, leading to insufficient availability of specialists such as child psychiatrists, clinical psychologists, and ADHD-trained providers. These delays have serious consequences, including increased risk of academic failure, behavioral problems, and comorbid mental health issues (Faraone et al., 2021). For adults with ADHD, the situation is even more complex, as many health systems continue to focus diagnostic services on children and adolescents. In some countries, adult ADHD assessments are not covered under public insurance schemes, creating additional financial barriers to care.

Training deficits among primary care providers and educators exacerbate underdiagnosis and misdiagnosis of ADHD. General practitioners (GPs) and teachers receive little formal training on ADHD diagnosis or management (Brinkman et al., 2020). ADHD symptoms often overlap with anxiety, mood disorders, and learning difficulties, complicating diagnostic accuracy for clinicians without specialized expertise (Faraone et al., 2021). Some providers may also fail to recognize ADHD as a valid adult diagnosis. Inconsistent referral pathways for ADHD further delay access to appropriate care, as some primary care settings lack clear protocols for referring patients to specialized ADHD services. Teachers play a critical role in identifying early ADHD signs, but many lack training on the disorder, resulting in inconsistent responses ranging from supportive accommodations to punitive disciplinary actions (Hinshaw & Arnold, 2022).

Adults with ADHD also face inadequate workplace accommodations and legal protections, which undermine occupational functioning and economic stability. Despite ADHD's significant impact on work performance, many countries lack formal recognition of ADHD as a disability under employment law (Brinkman et al., 2020). Even where ADHD is legally protected—such as under the Americans with

Disabilities Act (ADA) in the United States—awareness and enforcement are inconsistent, leaving many employees without effective support. Workplace stigma and discrimination remain significant concerns, discouraging individuals from disclosing their diagnosis due to fears of negative perceptions and reduced productivity. Employers often lack education about ADHD, contributing to misunderstandings and insufficient accommodations for executive function challenges. Few workplaces offer practical adjustments such as flexible scheduling, task prioritization support, or noise-reducing environments, which could substantially improve work performance and job retention for employees with ADHD.

Finally, the high costs of ADHD medications and therapy pose substantial financial burdens, particularly for uninsured populations. Stimulant medications like methylphenidate and amphetamines can cost between $100 and $300 per month without insurance (Faraone et al., 2021). Even in publicly funded healthcare systems, ADHD medications are not always fully subsidized, leaving families with out-of-pocket expenses. Coverage for evidence-based therapies, such as cognitive-behavioral therapy (CBT) and ADHD coaching, is often limited, forcing many individuals to rely solely on medication. For low-income families, the cumulative costs of assessments, prescriptions, and therapies can lead to inconsistent treatment adherence, and families with multiple children diagnosed with ADHD face even greater financial strain. When ADHD remains untreated, individuals face higher risks of academic underachievement, occupational instability, relationship breakdowns, substance misuse, and criminal justice involvement (Jensen, 2009; Shaw et al., 2012; Sikirica et al., 2015) By contrast, timely and comprehensive treatment—combining medication, behavioral therapy, and educational supports—has been shown to improve academic and work performance, enhance social functioning, and reduce associated health and social risks (Daley & Birchwood, 2010; Faraone et al., 2021).

10.2 ADHD Advocacy and Awareness Initiatives

Advocacy organizations play a pivotal role in shaping ADHD-related policies, promoting public awareness, and expanding access to essential resources for individuals with ADHD and their families. They also advocate for evidence-based guidelines on the safe and timely initiation of treatment, with most clinical recommendations supporting diagnosis and, where appropriate, pharmacological intervention from the age of 6, complemented by behavioral strategies in younger children when symptoms cause significant functional impairment (Health & Excellence, 2018; Wolraich et al., 2019). These organizations are critical in reducing stigma, influencing public health policy, providing educational tools, and establishing networks of support at both national and international levels (Brady et al., 2021). Through their efforts, these groups help bridge the gap between clinical research, service provision, and everyday experiences of those living with ADHD, making them an indispensable component of ADHD care ecosystems globally (Health & Excellence, 2018).

One of the leading ADHD advocacy organizations in the United States is Children and Adults with Attention-Deficit/Hyperactivity Disorder (CHADD), which has made significant strides in providing educational resources, webinars, and training programs for parents, educators, and clinicians. CHADD also actively engages with policymakers to shape ADHD-related legislation, such as provisions under the Individuals with Disabilities Education Act (IDEA), and advocates for expanded insurance coverage to support comprehensive ADHD diagnosis and treatment services. In the United Kingdom, the ADHD Foundation plays a similar role, working to reduce stigma and enhance support for individuals with ADHD across schools, workplaces, and healthcare systems (Young et al., 2021). The foundation collaborates with key stakeholders to promote ADHD accommodations and lobbies for national initiatives, including expanded services within the National Health Service (NHS). Annual ADHD Awareness Month campaigns, led by the foundation, have significantly contributed to public education and destigmatization efforts in the United Kingdom.

Beyond these prominent organizations, influential platforms such as ADDitude Magazine and various online advocacy communities have become vital sources of information, peer support, and practical tools for navigating ADHD-related challenges. These independent voices shape media discourse and provide accessible resources to individuals and families affected by ADHD, filling gaps left by traditional healthcare systems. Additionally, grassroots organizations—including local parent support groups and neurodiversity movements—play a crucial role at the community level. These groups provide peer-led education, advocacy training, and direct support while working closely with local schools and governments to promote inclusive practices and challenge prevailing misconceptions about ADHD.

Advocacy organizations make multifaceted contributions to both policy development and public understanding of ADHD. Many groups collaborate with governmental bodies and health agencies to integrate ADHD into national education, employment, and healthcare policies, aiming to expand insurance coverage, secure research funding, and strengthen ADHD representation within disability frameworks. Annual campaigns, such as ADHD Awareness Month in October, are instrumental in dispelling myths and promoting ADHD as a legitimate neurodevelopmental condition rather than a purely behavioral issue. Social media and public engagement initiatives led by these organizations have proven effective in reducing stigma and broadening societal understanding of ADHD.

Educational resource development is another cornerstone of advocacy organizations' work. Many produce practical guides for schools and workplaces, offering ADHD-friendly classroom strategies, accommodations, and parenting advice. Training sessions for teachers and employers help foster more supportive and inclusive environments for individuals with ADHD. Furthermore, advocacy groups provide critical community support and peer networks that reduce isolation and empower families to navigate complex healthcare systems, educational services, and legal processes. Through webinars, online forums, and community workshops, these organizations empower families and individuals with ADHD to advocate for their needs and access appropriate care.

10.2.1 Public Awareness Campaigns

Public awareness campaigns can be instrumental in reducing stigma, increasing ADHD literacy, and encouraging early diagnosis and intervention (McKenna et al., 2025). Persistent misconceptions—such as viewing ADHD as a result of poor parenting or a lack of self-discipline—continue to hinder timely diagnosis and treatment, perpetuating discrimination in educational and workplace settings (Brady et al., 2021). These campaigns employ diverse strategies to change societal perceptions, improve diagnosis rates, and enhance service access, making them a crucial component of comprehensive ADHD advocacy.

Digital media and social platforms have significantly expanded the reach of ADHD awareness efforts globally. Campaigns such as ADHD Awareness Month—coordinated by organizations including CHADD (U.S.), the ADHD Foundation (UK), and CADDAC (Canada)—use online content and community engagement strategies to share educational resources, personal experiences, and advocacy messages, thereby broadening public understanding and reducing stigma (CHADD, 2024; Young et al., 2021). Webinars, online forums, and live Q&A sessions hosted by clinicians and ADHD advocates provide accessible information about symptoms, diagnosis pathways, and treatment options. Influential public figures like Simone Biles and Michael Phelps, alongside neurodiversity influencers on platforms such as YouTube and TikTok, have played a significant role in normalizing ADHD, helping to dismantle stigma through personal narratives. A central objective of these campaigns is to combat misinformation, particularly that ADHD often persists into adulthood and is a neurodevelopmental disorder rather than a purely behavioral issue. Advocacy initiatives collaborate with healthcare organizations to fact-check content and ensure that accurate information is disseminated online.

Schools are a critical setting for ADHD awareness raising and early intervention. Teachers are often the first to observe ADHD symptoms in students, but a lack of formal training can lead to underdiagnosis, stigma, or insufficient support (Hinshaw & Arnold, 2022). Teacher training programs aim to equip educators with skills to recognize ADHD symptoms and implement inclusive classroom practices, covering topics such as behavioral interventions, positive reinforcement, and ADHD-friendly learning accommodations (Ward et al., 2022). Extending awareness to students through peer education initiatives for example at ADHD-focused assemblies or "ADHD Simulation Days," fosters empathy and reduces stigma among classmates (Mueller et al., 2012). Early screening programs integrated into school health check-ups, as seen in countries like Finland and Canada (Njardvik et al., 2025), ensure timely identification of ADHD. Parental engagement is another vital component of school-based efforts; workshops for caregivers provide guidance on home management strategies, communication techniques, and available treatment options, creating a more supportive environment both at school and at home (Daley & Birchwood, 2010).

Healthcare outreach and community engagement efforts are essential in enhancing ADHD literacy among medical professionals and the broader public. Public health campaigns targeting general practitioners and pediatricians, to equip them with training to recognize ADHD symptoms and refer patients to specialist services. Community-outreach, frequently led by public health agencies, could include free ADHD screening events (however, as with all screening programs, it is important that referral pathways are in place for individuals with positive diagnosis). Community outreach would include distribution of educational resources and be conducted in partnership with schools and community centers to facilitate service access.

Workplace-focused campaign activities aim to improve understanding of ADHD in professional settings, promoting ADHD-friendly policies such as flexible schedules, task structuring, and environmental modifications. These efforts need to align with and promote an inclusive understanding and application of workplace legislative requirements, such as the Americans with Disabilities Act (ADA) in the United States and the Equality Act in the United Kingdom to ensure that employees with ADHD are afforded appropriate legal protections.

Comprehensive ADHD awareness campaigns have helped reduce stigma and improve societal attitudes, shifting the framing of ADHD from a behavioral problem to a neurodevelopmental condition (Lebowitz, 2016). Increasing understanding among parents, teachers, and employers has led to more supportive responses to ADHD-related challenges (Sayal et al., 2018). Regions with comprehensive awareness efforts have reported higher rates of early ADHD identification (Sayal et al., 2018), resulting in improved academic, social, and developmental trajectories for affected individuals. Importantly, public pressure generated by awareness campaigns has prompted governments to allocate additional resources toward ADHD research, healthcare services, and educational programs (Hinshaw & Scheffler, 2014). These initiatives have also contributed to wider adoption of ADHD-friendly teaching methods (Daley et al., 2014) and workplace accommodations, supporting greater inclusion and productivity for individuals with ADHD.

10.2.2 ADHD and Neurodiversity Advocacy

Collectively known as the neurodiversity movement, advocacy has been instrumental in challenging deficit-based views of ADHD, instead framing it as a natural and valuable variation in human cognition (Armstrong, 2017). By advocating for acceptance, inclusion, and systemic accommodation, this framework encourages educational, occupational, and societal structures to recognize and support individuals with ADHD (Walker et al., 2021). Neurodiversity advocates emphasize the strengths commonly associated with ADHD—including creativity, innovation, resilience, and problem-solving abilities (Sedgwick et al., 2019)—while pushing for policies that foster ADHD-friendly environments. These efforts have contributed to notable shifts in public attitudes, educational approaches, and workplace practices.

Originally rooted in the autism community, the neurodiversity movement has expanded to encompass a range of cognitive differences, including ADHD, dyslexia, and dyspraxia (Singer, 1998). Central to this perspective is the belief that ADHD represents a difference rather than a disorder, necessitating supportive accommodations instead of attempts at "fixing" individuals. Neurodiversity advocates argue that ADHD-related traits can be advantageous in the right environments. For example, distractibility may manifest as heightened pattern recognition or rapid idea generation, while impulsivity may foster risk-taking and decisiveness (Armstrong, 2017). However, advocates also highlight that societal barriers—such as rigid school or workplace structures—can create or exacerbate many of the difficulties faced by neurodivergent individuals. Organizations such as the ADHD Foundation (UK), The Neurodiversity Hub, an international initiative that supports universities and employers in creating inclusive opportunities for neurodiverse individuals, and the Neurodiversity Project have been at the forefront of promoting ADHD inclusion within this framework (Neurodiversity Hub, 2025). Their activities include raising awareness of ADHD as part of neurodivergent identity, lobbying for inclusive education policies, and supporting neurodiverse hiring practices.

Shifting perspectives on ADHD increasingly highlight the distinct strengths associated with the condition (Bailey et al., 2022). While ADHD has traditionally been pathologized within medical and educational systems, neurodiversity advocates emphasize the potential for rapid idea generation, innovative problem-solving, risk-taking, and adaptability (Sedgwick et al., 2019). For example, distractibility is reframed as heightened creativity and the ability to identify novel patterns, while impulsivity can foster decisive action in uncertain situations (The Center for ADHD, 2023). Empirical studies have shown that individuals with ADHD are disproportionately represented in entrepreneurship, the arts, and other innovation-driven sectors (White & Shah, 2011). Global corporate initiatives at companies such as Microsoft, SAP (Systems, Applications, and Products in Data Processing), and EY (Ernst & Young) have leveraged these strengths by incorporating neurodiversity hiring programs, recognizing ADHD as a valuable asset to organizational creativity and productivity (Austin & Pisano, 2017).

Growing awareness of neurodiversity has also influenced workplace policies aimed at supporting employees with ADHD. Key changes include the introduction of flexible work arrangements—such as remote work options and adaptable deadlines—to better accommodate ADHD-related challenges. Employers have also implemented structured task management tools, including Trello (a visual organizer that helps reduce overwhelm and prioritize tasks) and the Pomodoro Technique (a time-management method involving focused intervals and breaks), and introduced environmental modifications, such as quiet zones and noise-canceling equipment, to reduce distractions (Choosing Therapy, 2025; Health.com, 2024; NeuroLaunch, 2024). Additionally, mentorship and ADHD coaching programs have become increasingly common, helping employees navigate professional environments more effectively (Crook & McDowall, 2024). Both the United Kingdom and Australia have taken leadership roles in promoting neurodiverse hiring practices, with employers actively seeking to recruit and retain individuals with ADHD and related conditions. Emerging certification programs further support businesses in developing neurodiversity-friendly workplaces (Cristofaro et al., 2024).

The influence of neurodiversity advocacy has extended into education, encouraging a shift toward more inclusive and supportive learning environments for students with ADHD. Schools are increasingly adopting Universal Design for Learning (UDL), a framework that promotes flexibility in teaching methods and assessment practices to accommodate varied learning styles (Meyer et al., 2014). Strengths-based educational approaches, such as project-based learning and hands-on activities, are also gaining traction as effective methods for engaging students with ADHD (Ärlestig, 2008). Flexible assessment methods—including oral presentations, creative projects, and the use of assistive technologies—further contribute to equitable learning environments (Lynch et al., 2024). Several countries have integrated neurodiversity-focused policies into their national education systems. Finland and Denmark, for example, have introduced ADHD-inclusive school models with individualized learning plans (Egelund & Dyssegaard, 2021; Toom & Husu, 2016) while the United States ensures educational accommodations through 504 Plans (Gonzalez, 2020) and the Individuals with Disabilities Education Act (IDEA) (Dragoo, 2024).

While progress has been made, there is a need for ongoing advocacy to ensure that ADHD is fully recognized as part of the broader neurodiversity paradigm. Current priorities include clearer legal recognition of ADHD as a protected disability in certain jurisdictions and ensuring more consistent access to accommodations in both education and employment settings. Increasing ADHD representation in media and policy discourse is vital to moving beyond deficit-oriented narratives and promoting public understanding of ADHD-related strengths. Advocacy efforts also emphasize the expansion of neurodiverse hiring initiatives beyond sectors like technology and the creative industries. Finally, further research is needed to explore ADHD within a neurodiversity framework, focusing on resilience, creativity, and adaptive strategies alongside traditional clinical challenges.

10.3 Future Directions in ADHD Policy and Advocacy

As ADHD increasingly garners recognition as a condition with considerable public health impacts, the need to strengthen policy frameworks becomes ever more pressing. Persistent gaps in current systems—including diagnostic delays, unequal access to care, and inadequate legal protections—underscore the necessity for comprehensive reforms. A combination of early screening, integrated healthcare models, expanded research investment, and workplace protections will be essential to advance ADHD care and equity (Faraone et al., 2021).

Policy reforms must address the structural barriers that hinder timely diagnosis and treatment while promoting inclusion in educational and professional settings. Universal ADHD screening programs embedded within school systems for early detection and improved long-term outcomes are critical. Without timely intervention, undiagnosed ADHD can result in academic underachievement, social difficulties, and heightened risk for comorbid mental health conditions. Structured screening tools administered by teachers and school psychologists can enhance diagnostic accuracy and facilitate timely referrals for clinical evaluation. These efforts should be supported by multi-tiered intervention models that incorporate behavioral strategies, individualized education plans (IEPs), and parent engagement programs. Exemplary models exist, e.g., in Finland and Denmark where they have integrated ADHD screening into routine school health services, leading to earlier diagnoses and improved academic and psychosocial outcomes for students with ADHD (Brinkman et al., 2020).

Integrating ADHD management into primary care systems is another critical step, as over-reliance on specialist services contributes to significant delays in ADHD diagnosis and treatment, particularly in regions with shortages of child psychiatrists and neurologists. By equipping primary care providers with appropriate training and screening tools—such as the Vanderbilt ADHD Diagnostic Rating Scale (Bard et al., 2013) and the Conners Comprehensive Behavior Rating Scale (Conners et al., 1998)—health systems can decentralize ADHD care and promote more timely intervention (Kasmire et al., 2016). Establishing standardized national guidelines for ADHD management in primary care will further enhance diagnostic consistency and treatment quality (Faraone et al., 2021). In countries like Canada and Australia, primary care integration has reduced wait times and improved access to ADHD services, particularly in rural and underserved regions. The development of telehealth models also holds promise for expanding ADHD care beyond urban centers.

Expanding government funding for ADHD research is essential to address current gaps in innovation and evidence-based policy development. ADHD continues to be significantly underfunded relative to other neurodevelopmental and mental health conditions, limiting progress in treatment and support systems (Faraone et al., 2021). Priority areas for research include the neurobiological underpinnings of ADHD, the development of non-stimulant therapeutic interventions, and the longitudinal study of ADHD and appropriate intervention across the lifespan. Research that explores ADHD in later life, as well as its economic and societal impacts, will be particularly valuable for informing cost-effective policy solutions. Governments should prioritize the allocation of dedicated ADHD funding within national health budgets and partner with research institutions to expand ADHD-specific research and intervention grant opportunities. Increased international collaboration will also be key to advancing global ADHD policy and treatment innovations. The U.S. National Institute of Mental Health (NIMH), for instance, has increased its investment in ADHD research, supporting breakthroughs in non-stimulant medication and behavioral interventions (Brinkman et al., 2020).

Finally, expanding legal protections and workplace accommodations for ADHD is essential. Adults with ADHD frequently encounter workplace discrimination and limited access to necessary accommodations, contributing to career instability and financial inequity (Austin & Pisano, 2017). Recognizing ADHD as a protected disability under national employment laws would grant individuals the right to workplace accommodations. Financial incentives for employers—such as tax benefits for inclusive hiring practices—can further encourage the adoption of neurodiversity-friendly policies (Monteleone, 2016). Mandatory accommodations might include flexible work schedules, structured task management systems, access to assistive technologies, and ADHD-focused employee support programs. While the Americans with Disabilities Act (ADA) in the United States provides some level of protection, implementation and enforcement remain inconsistent. Similarly, although the United Kingdom and Australia have expanded disability rights frameworks, ADHD recognition within these laws is often restricted to severe cases. National workplace inclusion programs modeled after existing initiatives for autism (Krzeminska & Hawse, 2020) and dyslexia (FAIRFAX, 2023) could help normalize ADHD-friendly practices across a wider range of sectors.

10.4 Reducing Healthcare Disparities in ADHD Diagnosis and Treatment

Healthcare disparities continue to shape ADHD diagnosis and treatment outcomes globally. Racial, gender, and socioeconomic inequities result in delayed or missed diagnoses, reduced access to evidence-based care, and higher rates of untreated ADHD in marginalized populations. Diagnosis and treatment disproportionately favor wealthier, urban populations, leaving low-income, rural, and minority communities underserved (Brady et al., 2021). Addressing these disparities requires comprehensive policy reforms that promote equitable access to diagnosis and treatment, subsidized medications, and the expansion of telehealth services for underserved regions.

Racial, gender, and socioeconomic disparities significantly affect ADHD care access. Black, Hispanic, and Indigenous children are consistently underdiagnosed relative to White children, even though they exhibit ADHD symptoms at similar rates (Morgan et al., 2016). Misdiagnosis is common, with minority children more likely to be labeled with behavioral disorders such as Oppositional Defiant Disorder (ODD), which reduces their access to ADHD-specific interventions (Coker et al., 2016). Implicit bias within healthcare systems, compounded by barriers like lack of insurance, further limits access to appropriate treatment and medication. Gender disparities add another layer of complexity: girls with ADHD are often underdiagnosed because they typically present with inattentiveness and internalizing behaviors such as anxiety or emotional dysregulation, which may be less disruptive and therefore less likely to trigger referral (Hinshaw & Arnold, 2022). Many women are only diagnosed in adulthood, often after years of unrecognized symptoms.

Social disadvantage and socioeconomic status also plays a crucial role, with children from low-income families facing structural obstacles including reduced availability of mental health specialists, financial barriers to assessments and treatments, and under-resourced schools that often lack the capacity to provide accommodations such as IEPs.

Policy reforms to reduce these disparities should include the implementation of mandatory ADHD screening programs in public schools, ensuring early detection across all socioeconomic and racial groups. Healthcare providers should undergo implicit bias training to mitigate diagnostic inequities, particularly among racial minorities and females. Strengthening school-based mental health services in underfunded districts can further improve access to affordable ADHD assessments and interventions. For example, the U.S. Medicaid expansion has improved ADHD diagnosis rates and treatment access for children from low-income families, though disparities across racial and gender lines persist (Brady et al., 2021).

Financial barriers remain a significant obstacle to ADHD treatment, with monthly medication costs posing a major challenge for those without insurance coverage (Faraone et al., 2021). Non-stimulant medications like atomoxetine (Strattera) and guanfacine are often even more expensive and less accessible in low-income settings. In low- and middle-income countries (LMICs), access to ADHD medication is often severely limited, forcing families to seek costly imports (Chan et al., 2023). Expanding government-funded or subsidized medication programs is essential to improving affordability. The UK's National Health Service (NHS) provides ADHD medications at reduced costs, offering a model for improved access. Brazil and Argentina have also introduced national ADHD medication programs to reduce financial barriers for low-income families (Chan et al., 2023). Policy recommendations include expanding insurance coverage to fully subsidize ADHD medications, implementing government procurement programs to lower drug costs, and increasing funding for behavioral therapy to complement pharmacological treatment.

Geographic barriers also significantly affect ADHD care, particularly in rural and remote regions, where ADHD specialists are scarce. Families in these areas often face long travel distances, high costs, and prolonged wait times for diagnosis and treatment (Haimi & Lerner, 2021). Telehealth has emerged as a scalable, cost-effective solution to help bridge these gaps. Virtual ADHD assessments and remote therapy sessions allow individuals in underserved areas to access care without the logistical burdens of travel (Kenter et al., 2023). Telehealth platforms also offer digital tools for medication management and adherence monitoring, which can improve treatment outcomes while reducing patient costs. Governments should prioritize investment in telepsychiatry programs targeting rural and low-income populations. Additionally, reimbursement policies must be updated to ensure parity between in-person and telehealth ADHD consultations under both public and private insurance plans. Emerging technologies, such as AI-assisted diagnostic tools, could further empower primary care providers to deliver ADHD care remotely (Duda et al., 2016), however, need to be cognizant of and a ate ours of patient confidentiality and data integrity. Notable progress has been made in this area; for example, Australia's National Telehealth Initiative has expanded ADHD services to rural communities, improving access and reducing wait times. Similarly, the United States implemented telehealth-friendly legislation during the COVID-19 pandemic, enabling remote ADHD evaluations across multiple states (Saldarriaga et al., 2020).

10.5 Improving Educational and Workplace Support for Individuals with ADHD

Ensuring robust support systems in educational and occupational settings is essential for individuals with ADHD to thrive. However, many schools and workplaces remain ill-equipped to provide appropriate accommodations, reinforcing systemic barriers to academic success. Inflexible learning and working environments, coupled with limited awareness and inadequate legal frameworks, continue to hinder the full participation of people with ADHD in both academic and professional contexts (Brady et al., 2021). Addressing these challenges requires targeted policy recommendations and best practices that prioritize ADHD-inclusive education and employment systems.

Mandatory ADHD-specific teacher training would assist in equipping students edified educators with the knowledge and skills needed to support students effectively. Despite teachers playing a pivotal role in early identification and management of ADHD, many lack formal training on managing ADHD symptoms in the classroom (Preckel et al., 2006). This gap can lead to the misinterpretation of ADHD-related behaviors as laziness, defiance, or a lack of discipline. As a result, punitive measures such as detention or suspension are frequently overused, while evidence-based accommodations remain under-implemented (Brinkman et al., 2020). Embedding ADHD-specific training within teacher certification and professional development pathways would help to address this issue. Such training should focus on recognizing ADHD symptoms early, implementing classroom accommodations, and adopting ADHD-friendly teaching strategies—such as structured routines, additional time on assignments, movement breaks, and reducing environmental distractions. Finland and Sweden have integrated ADHD-focused modules into national teacher training curricula (Taanila et al., 2014), while the UKs Department of Education has mandated special needs training, including ADHD awareness, as part of its inclusive education strategy (Britain & Britain, 2015).

In the employment sphere, individuals with ADHD can face challenges, including rigid work environments, unrealistic productivity expectations, and stigma surrounding disclosure (Austin & Pisano, 2017). Many employers remain unaware of ADHD's impact on executive functioning, contributing to workplace cultures that fail to support neurodivergent employees adequately. To foster more inclusive workplaces, governments should enact legislation that mandates reasonable accommodations for employees with ADHD, ensuring compliance with national disability laws. Recommended accommodations include flexible work schedules, task management technologies, access to quiet workspaces, and ADHD coaching or mentorship programs (Sedgwick et al., 2019).

Leading organizations such as Microsoft, SAP, and Goldman Sachs have launched formal neurodiversity hiring programs recognizing the strengths of neurodivergent talent. Microsoft spearheads efforts through its *Neurodiversity Career Connector*, part of its broader Neurodiversity Hiring Program, which offers tailored recruitment and support pathways for neurodivergent candidates (Microsoft, 2025).

SAP's *Autism at Work* initiative, operational since 2013, has expanded to include ADHD and emphasizes inclusion through adaptations in hiring and workplace culture (Austin & Pisano, 2017). Goldman Sachs, in collaboration with Specialisterne, offers a paid internship program with mentorship and support tailored for neurodivergent individuals, including those with ADHD (Forbes, 2022). Despite these promising initiatives, broader workplace integration remains uneven. Although the Americans with Disabilities Act (ADA) legally protects employees with ADHD in the United States, enforcement and employer compliance are highly variable, resulting in inconsistent access to necessary accommodations (Blanck, 2023). To promote inclusive and ADHD-aware workplace cultures, coordinated strategies are needed to embed neurodiversity and accommodations into mainstream corporate diversity and inclusion frameworks—expanding beyond pilot programs to scalable, systemic change (Brady et al., 2021).

For individuals with severe ADHD-related impairments, financial assistance and access to disability benefits is essential. However, ADHD is often excluded from disability benefit classifications unless accompanied by comorbid conditions such as anxiety or depression. Even when ADHD is recognized, claimants frequently face a high evidentiary burden, requiring extensive documentation to prove eligibility. Policy reforms should broaden the legal recognition of ADHD as a qualifying disability, particularly when the condition substantially impairs daily functioning. Streamlining application processes for financial aid programs could alleviate barriers for individuals seeking support. Financial assistance should also extend beyond basic income supports. Recommended initiatives include grants for ADHD coaching and therapy, subsidies for assistive technologies in workplaces, and scholarships for students with ADHD to offset education-related costs (Prelock, 2021). Several countries have introduced progressive policies in this domain. For instance, Canada's disability tax credits acknowledge ADHD-related executive function challenges (Government of Canada, 2022). The UK's Personal Independence Payment (PIP) program includes ADHD under its disability benefits for severe impairments (UK Government, 2023), while the U.S. Social Security Administration (SSA) provides limited ADHD-related disability benefits, often requiring legal advocacy to navigate eligibility hurdles (Social Security Administration, 2022).

Summary

This chapter has examined the global and national policy landscape surrounding ADHD, highlighting key initiatives aimed at strengthening ADHD advocacy and care systems. Despite ADHD being formally recognized in diagnostic systems like the ICD-11 and DSM-5, it remains underrepresented in many public health frameworks. This limited prioritization has led to fragmented policies, diagnostic delays, and significant inequities in care across both high-income and low- and middle-income countries (LMICs). ADHD recognition varies widely, with particular challenges in LMICs stemming from resource limitations, cultural stigma, and a lack of trained specialists.

ADHD advocacy organizations have played a crucial role in driving awareness, shaping public policy, and fostering support networks. Digital media campaigns, school-based programs, and healthcare outreach initiatives have contributed to reducing stigma, promoting early diagnosis, and enhancing ADHD literacy among educators, healthcare providers, and the general public. The neurodiversity movement has further shifted societal perceptions of ADHD, emphasizing strengths such as creativity, adaptability, and innovation, while advocating for more inclusive policies in education and employment sectors.

To advance ADHD care globally, policy recommendations include integrating ADHD management into primary care, implementing universal screening in schools, expanding funding for ADHD research, and strengthening legal protections for ADHD in the workplace. Additional strategies are needed to reduce disparities in ADHD care, particularly among racial minorities, women, and low-income populations. Improving access to telehealth services, subsidizing ADHD medications, mandating ADHD-specific teacher training, and supporting neurodiverse hiring programs are essential next steps in creating ADHD-friendly environments. Overall, the chapter highlights that comprehensive reforms across health, education, and employment sectors are vital to reducing barriers and promoting the well-being of individuals with ADHD worldwide.

References

American Psychiatric Association. (2013). *Diagnostic and statistical manual of mental disorders* (5th ed.). American Psychiatric Publishing.

Ärlestig, H. (2008). Structural prerequisites for principals' and teachers' communication about teaching and learning issues. *Improving Schools, 11*(3), 189–203. https://doi.org/10.1177/1365480208097000

Armstrong, T. (2017). Neurodiversity: The future of special education? *Educational Leadership, 74*(7), 10–16.

Austin, R. D., & Pisano, G. P. (2017). Neurodiversity as a competitive advantage. *Harvard Business Review, 95*(3), 96–103.

Bard, D. E., Wolraich, M. L., Neas, B., Doffing, M., & Beck, L. (2013). The psychometric properties of the Vanderbilt attention-deficit hyperactivity disorder diagnostic parent rating scale in a community population. *Journal of Developmental and Behavioral Pediatrics, 34*(2), 72–82. https://doi.org/10.1097/DBP.0b013e31827a3a22

Blanck, P. (2023). On the importance of the Americans with disabilities act at 30. *Journal of Disability Policy Studies, 34*(3), 176–198.

Brady, A. M., et al. (2021). ADHD service use and barriers to care. *Journal of Attention Disorders, 25*(10), 1365–1375.

Brinkman, W. B., Epstein, J. N., & Banaschewski, T. (2020). ADHD care in the context of the COVID-19 pandemic. *Journal of Developmental & Behavioral Pediatrics, 41*(5), 377–379.

Britain, G., & Britain, G. (2015). *Special educational needs and disability code of practice: 0 to 25 years: Statutory guidance for organisations who work with and support children and Young people with special educational needs and disabilities*. Department for Education.

CHADD. (2024, October). *ADHD Awareness 2024: Awareness is key! Attention Magazine.* Retrieved from https://chadd.org/attention-article/adhd-awareness-2024-awareness-is-key/

Chan, A. Y. L., Ma, T. T., Lau, W. C. Y., Ip, P., Coghill, D., Gao, L., Jani, Y. H., Hsia, Y., Wei, L., Taxis, K., Simonoff, E., Taylor, D., Lum, T. Y., Man, K. K. C., & Wong, I. C. K. (2023). Attention-deficit/hyperactivity disorder medication consumption in 64 countries and regions from 2015 to 2019: A longitudinal study. *EClinicalMedicine, 58*, 101780. https://doi.org/10.1016/j.eclinm.2022.101780

Choosing Therapy. (2025). "*The Pomodoro Technique & ADHD: Improving Focus and Reducing Overwhelm.*" This piece highlights how organizing work into focused intervals with built-in breaks supports individuals with ADHD in managing attention, time blindness, and productivity.

Coker, T. R., et al. (2016). Racial and ethnic disparities in ADHD diagnosis and treatment. *Pediatrics, 138*(3), e20160407.

Conners, C. K., Sitarenios, G., Parker, J. D., & Epstein, J. N. (1998). The revised Conners' parent rating scale (CPRS-R): Factor structure, reliability, and criterion validity. *Journal of Abnormal Child Psychology, 26*(4), 257–268. https://doi.org/10.1023/a:1022602400621

Cortese, S., Adamo, N., Del Giovane, C., Mohr-Jensen, C., Hayes, A. J., Carucci, S., Atkinson, L. Z., Tessari, L., Banaschewski, T., Coghill, D., Hollis, C., Simonoff, E., Zuddas, A., Barbui, C., Purgato, M., Steinhausen, H. C., Shokraneh, F., Xia, J., & Cipriani, A. (2018). Comparative efficacy and tolerability of medications for attention-deficit hyperactivity disorder in children, adolescents, and adults: A systematic review and network meta-analysis. *Lancet Psychiatry, 5*(9), 727–738. https://doi.org/10.1016/s2215-0366(18)30269-4

Cristofaro, M., Giardino, P. L., Camilli, R., & Hristov, I. (2024). Unlocking the sustainability of medium enterprises: A framework for reducing cognitive biases in sustainable performance management. *Journal of Management & Organization, 30*(3), 490–520. https://doi.org/10.1017/jmo.2023.55

Crook, T., & McDowall, A. (2024). Paradoxical career strengths and successes of ADHD adults: An evolving narrative. *Journal of Work-Applied Management, 16*(1), 112–126.

Daley, D., & Birchwood, J. (2010). ADHD and academic performance: Why does ADHD impact on academic performance and what can be done to support ADHD children in the classroom? *Child: Care, Health and Development, 36*(4), 455–464. https://doi.org/10.1111/j.1365-2214.2009.01046.x

Daley, D., van der Oord, S., Ferrin, M., Danckaerts, M., Doepfner, M., Cortese, S., & Sonuga-Barke, E. J. S. (2014). Behavioral interventions in attention-deficit/hyperactivity disorder: A meta-analysis of randomized controlled trials across multiple outcome domains. *Journal of the American Academy of Child & Adolescent Psychiatry, 53*(8), 835–847.e835. https://doi.org/10.1016/j.jaac.2014.05.013

Danielson, M. L., Bitsko, R. H., Ghandour, R. M., Holbrook, J. R., Kogan, M. D., & Blumberg, S. J. (2018). Prevalence of parent-reported ADHD diagnosis and associated treatment among U.S. children and adolescents, 2016. *Journal of Clinical Child and Adolescent Psychology, 47*(2), 199–212. https://doi.org/10.1080/15374416.2017.1417860

Dragoo, K. E. (2024). *The Individuals with Disabilities Education Act (IDEA), Part C: Early Intervention for Infants and Toddlers with Disabilities.* CRS Report R43631, Version 13. Updated. *Congressional Research Service.*

Duda, M., Ma, R., Haber, N., & Wall, D. P. (2016). Use of machine learning for behavioral distinction of autism and ADHD. *Translational Psychiatry, 6*(2), e732. https://doi.org/10.1038/tp.2015.221

Egelund, N., & Dyssegaard, C. B. (2021). Special needs education and the inclusion process in Denmark: Conceptual and practical challenges at national and local levels. In *Dialogues between northern and Eastern Europe on the development of inclusion* (pp. 52–65). Routledge.

Fairfax, A. (2023). Dyslexia-Friendly Practice. *The British Dyslexia Association-Teaching Dyslexic Students: Theory and Practice*, 219.

Faraone, S. V., Banaschewski, T., Coghill, D., Zheng, Y., Biederman, J., Bellgrove, M. A., Newcorn, J. H., Gignac, M., Al Saud, N. M., Manor, I., Rohde, L. A., Yang, L., Cortese, S.,

Almagor, D., Stein, M. A., Albatti, T. H., Aljoudi, H. F., Alqahtani, M. M. J., Asherson, P., & Wang, Y. (2021). The world federation of ADHD international consensus statement: 208 evidence-based conclusions about the disorder. *Neuroscience & Biobehavioral Reviews, 128*, 789–818. https://doi.org/10.1016/j.neubiorev.2021.01.022

Forbes. (2022, April 13). Goldman Sachs is investing in neurodiverse talent with Specialisterne partnership. *Forbes*. Retrieved from https://www.forbes.com/sites/jenniferpalmer/2022/04/13/goldman-sachs-investing-in-neurodiverse-talent/

French, B., Sayal, K., & Daley, D. (2019). Barriers and facilitators to understanding of ADHD in primary care: A mixed-method systematic review. *European Child & Adolescent Psychiatry, 28*(8), 1037–1064. https://doi.org/10.1007/s00787-018-1256-3

Froehlich, T. E., Lanphear, B. P., Epstein, J. N., Barbaresi, W. J., Katusic, S. K., & Kahn, R. S. (2007). Prevalence, recognition, and treatment of attention-deficit/hyperactivity disorder in a national sample of US children. *Archives of Pediatrics & Adolescent Medicine, 161*(9), 857–864. https://doi.org/10.1001/archpedi.161.9.857

Ginsberg, Y., Quintero, J., Anand, E., Casillas, M., & Upadhyaya, H. P. (2014). Underdiagnosis of attention-deficit/hyperactivity disorder in adult patients: A review of the literature. *Prim Care Companion CNS Disord, 16*(3). https://doi.org/10.4088/PCC.13r01600

Gonzalez, I. (2020). *Section 504 of the rehabilitation act of 1973: A policy analysis*. California State University.

Government of Canada. (2022). *Disability tax credit (DTC)*. Retrieved from https://www.canada.ca/en/revenue-agency/services/tax/individuals/segments/tax-credits-deductions-persons-disabilities/disability-tax-credit.html

Health, N. I. f., & Excellence, C. (2018). *Attention deficit hyperactivity disorder: Diagnosis and management*. National Institute for Health and Care Excellence.

Health.com. (2024). *For People with ADHD, Headphones Can Make It Easier to Work or Study—Here's Why*. This article discusses how noise-canceling headphones and quieter work environments significantly improve concentration for people with ADHD by minimizing distracting stimuli.

Haimi, M., & Lerner, A. (2021). The impact of ADHD on children and families. *Frontiers in Psychiatry*, 12, 1–8.

Hinshaw, S. P., & Scheffler, R. M. (2014). *The ADHD explosion: Myths, medication, money, and today's push for performance*. Oxford University Press.

Hinshaw, S. P., & Arnold, L. E. (2022). Attention-deficit hyperactivity disorder, multimodal treatment, and longitudinal outcome: Evidence, paradox, and challenge. *Wiley Interdisciplinary Reviews: Cognitive Science, 13*(3), e1583. https://doi.org/10.1002/wcs.1583

Jensen, P. S. (2009). Book review: Barkley, R. A., murphy, K. R., & Fischer, M. (2008). ADHD in adults: What the science says. New York: Guilford. *Journal of Attention Disorders, 13*(1), 97–98. https://doi.org/10.1177/1087054709333321

Kasmire, K. E., Rogers, S. C., & Sturm, J. J. (2016). Trampoline Park and home trampoline injuries. *Pediatrics, 138*(3), e20161236. https://doi.org/10.1542/peds.2016-1236

Kenter, R. M. F., Gjestad, R., Lundervold, A. J., & Nordgreen, T. (2023). A self-guided internet-delivered intervention for adults with ADHD: Results from a randomized controlled trial. *Internet Interventions, 32*, 100614. https://doi.org/10.1016/j.invent.2023.100614

Krzeminska, A., & Hawse, S. (2020). Mainstreaming neurodiversity for an inclusive and sustainable future workforce: Autism-spectrum employees. In *Industry and higher education: Case studies for sustainable futures* (pp. 229–261). Springer.

Lebowitz, M. S. (2016). Stigmatization of ADHD: A developmental review. *Journal of Attention Disorders, 20*(3), 199–205. https://doi.org/10.1177/1087054712475211

Lynch, P., Singal, N., & Francis, G. A. (2024). Educational technology for learners with disabilities in primary school settings in low- and middle-income countries: A systematic literature review. *Educational Review, 76*(2), 405–431. https://doi.org/10.1080/00131911.2022.2035685

McKenna, K., Wanni Arachchige Dona, S., Gold, L., Silk, T. J., & Le, H. N. D. (2025). Effectiveness and cost-effectiveness of interventions to increase knowledge and awareness of attention deficit hyperactivity disorder: A systematic review. *European Child & Adolescent Psychiatry, 34*(6), 1769–1794. https://doi.org/10.1007/s00787-025-02646-4

National Institute for Health and Care Excellence. (2018). Attention deficit hyperactivity disorder: Diagnosis and management (NG87). NICE.

Meyer, A., et al. (2014). ADHD and functional impairment: A review. *Clinical Psychology Review, 34*(8), 653–667.

Microsoft. (2025). Neurodiversity hiring program. *Microsoft Careers*. Retrieved August 23, 2025, from https://careers.microsoft.com/us/en/neurodiversity

Monteleone, R. (2016). Employment for all: United States disability policy. *Tizard Learning Disability Review, 21*(3), 154–161.

Morgan, P. L., et al. (2016). Racial and ethnic disparities in ADHD diagnosis. *Pediatrics, 138*(3), e20160407.

Mueller, A. K., Fuermaier, A. B., Koerts, J., & Tucha, L. (2012). Stigma in attention deficit hyperactivity disorder. *Atten Defic Hyperact Disord, 4*(3), 101–114. https://doi.org/10.1007/s12402-012-0085-3

Neurodiversity Hub. (2025). *About us*. Retrieved August 23, 2025, from https://www.neurodiversityhub.o

NeuroLaunch. (2024). "*Transform Task Management for ADHD with Trello*." This article explains how Trello's visual format—boards, lists, and cards—helps individuals with ADHD organize tasks, break them into manageable steps, and reduce overwhelm.

NICE. (2018). *Attention deficit hyperactivity disorder: Diagnosis and management (NICE guideline NG87)*. Retrieved from https://www.nice.org.uk/guidance/ng87

Njardvik, U., Wergeland, G. J., Riise, E. N., Hannesdottir, D. K., & Öst, L. G. (2025). Psychiatric comorbidity in children and adolescents with ADHD: A systematic review and meta-analysis. *Clinical Psychology Review, 118*, 102571. https://doi.org/10.1016/j.cpr.2025.102571

Polanczyk, G., Rohde, L. A., Szobot, C., Schmitz, M., Montiel-Nava, C., & Bauermeister, J. J. (2008). ADHD treatment in Latin America and the CARIBBEAN. *Journal of the American Academy of Child & Adolescent Psychiatry, 47*(6), 721–722. https://doi.org/10.1097/CHI.0b013e31816c0008

Preckel, F., Holling, H., & Vock, M. (2006). Academic underachievement: Relationship with cognitive motivation, achievement motivation, and conscientiousness. *Psychology in the Schools, 43*(3), 401–411. https://doi.org/10.1002/pits.20154

Prelock, P. (2021). Learning disability. In *Encyclopedia of autism spectrum disorders* (pp. 2661–2668). Springer.

Saldarriaga, W., Payán-Gómez, C., González-Teshima, L. Y., Rosa, L., Tassone, F., & Hagerman, R. J. (2020). Double genetic hit: Fragile X syndrome and partial deletion of protein patched homolog 1 antisense as cause of severe autism Spectrum disorder. *Journal of Developmental & Behavioral Pediatrics, 41*(9) https://journals.lww.com/jrnldbp/fulltext/2020/12000/double_genetic_hit__fragile_x_syndrome_and_partial.7.aspx

Sayal, K., Prasad, V., Daley, D., Ford, T., & Coghill, D. (2018). ADHD in children and young people: Prevalence, care pathways, and service provision. *The Lancet Psychiatry, 5*(2), 175–186. https://doi.org/10.1016/S2215-0366(17)30167-0

Sedgwick, J. A., Merwood, A., & Asherson, P. (2019). The positive aspects of attention deficit hyperactivity disorder: A qualitative investigation of successful adults with ADHD. *ADHD Attention Deficit and Hyperactivity Disorders, 11*(3), 241–253. https://doi.org/10.1007/s12402-018-0277-6

Shaw, M., Hodgkins, P., Caci, H., Young, S., Kahle, J., Woods, A. G., & Arnold, L. E. (2012). A systematic review and analysis of long-term outcomes in attention deficit hyperactivity disorder: Effects of treatment and non-treatment. *BMC Medicine, 10*(1), 99. https://doi.org/10.1186/1741-7015-10-99

Singer, J. (1998). Odd people in: The birth of community amongst people on the autistic spectrum. *Disability & Society, 13*(4), 535–554.

Sikirica, V., Flood, E., Dietrich, C. N., Quintero, J., Harpin, V., Hodgkins, P., Skrodzki, K., Beusterien, K., & Erder, M. H. (2015). Unmet needs associated with attention-deficit/hyperactivity disorder in eight European countries as reported by caregivers and adolescents: Results from qualitative research. *Patient, 8*(3), 269–281. https://doi.org/10.1007/s40271-014-0083-y

Social Security Administration. (2022). *Disability evaluation under Social Security (Blue Book): Childhood and adult ADHD. Washington, DC.* Retrieved from https://www.ssa.gov/disability/professionals/bluebook/112-00-MentalDisorders-Childhood.htm.

Sonuga-Barke, E. J., Brandeis, D., Cortese, S., Daley, D., Ferrin, M., Holtmann, M., Stevenson, J., Danckaerts, M., van der Oord, S., Döpfner, M., Dittmann, R. W., Simonoff, E., Zuddas, A., Banaschewski, T., Buitelaar, J., Coghill, D., Hollis, C., Konofal, E., Lecendreux, M., & Sergeant, J. (2013). Nonpharmacological interventions for ADHD: Systematic review and meta-analyses of randomized controlled trials of dietary and psychological treatments. *The American Journal of Psychiatry, 170*(3), 275–289. https://doi.org/10.1176/appi.ajp.2012.12070991

Taanila, A., Ebeling, H., Tiihala, M., Kaakinen, M., Moilanen, I., Hurtig, T., & Yliherva, A. (2014). Association between childhood specific learning difficulties and school performance in adolescents with and without ADHD symptoms: A 16-year follow-up. *Journal of Attention Disorders, 18*(1), 61–72. https://doi.org/10.1177/1087054712446813

The Center for ADHD. (2023, November 21). *The creativity of ADHD*. Retrieved from https://www.thecenterforadhd.com/the-creativity-of-adhd/

Toom, A., & Husu, J. (2016). Finnish teachers as 'makers of the many' balancing between broad pedagogical freedom and responsibility. In *Miracle of education: The principles and practices of teaching and learning in Finnish schools (second revised edition)* (pp. 41–55). SensePublishers Rotterdam.

UK Government. (2023). *Personal Independence Payment (PIP)*. Retrieved from https://www.gov.uk/pip/what-youll-get

Visser, S. N., Danielson, M. L., Wolraich, M. L., Fox, M. H., Grosse, S. D., Valle, L. A., Holbrook, J. R., Claussen, A. H., & Peacock, G. (2016). Vital signs: National and state-specific patterns of attention deficit/hyperactivity disorder treatment among insured children aged 2-5 years - United States, 2008-2014. *MMWR. Morbidity and Mortality Weekly Report, 65*(17), 443–450. https://doi.org/10.15585/mmwr.mm6517e1

Walker, C. S., Walker, B. H., Brown, D. C., Buttross, S., & Sarver, D. E. (2021). Defining the role of exposure to adverse childhood experiences (ACEs) in ADHD: Examination in a national sample of US children. *Child Abuse & Neglect, 112*, 104884. https://doi.org/10.1016/j.chiabu.2020.104884.

Ward, R. J., Bristow, S. J., Kovshoff, H., Cortese, S., & Kreppner, J. (2022). The effects of ADHD teacher training programs on teachers and pupils: A systematic review and meta-analysis. *Journal of Attention Disorders, 26*(2), 225–244. https://doi.org/10.1177/1087054720972801

World Health Organization. (2021). *Comprehensive mental health action plan 2013–2030.* World Health Organization.

Wolraich, M. L., Hagan, J. F., Jr., Allan, C., Chan, E., Davison, D., Earls, M., Evans, S. W., Flinn, S. K., Froehlich, T., Frost, J., Holbrook, J. R., Lehmann, C. U., Lessin, H. R., Okechukwu, K., Pierce, K. L., Winner, J. D., & Zurhellen, W. (2019). Clinical practice guideline for the diagnosis, evaluation, and treatment of attention-deficit/hyperactivity disorder in children and adolescents. *Pediatrics, 144*(4). https://doi.org/10.1542/peds.2019-2528

Young, S., Asherson, P., Lloyd, T., Absoud, M., Arif, M., Colley, W. A., Cortese, S., Cubbin, S., Doyle, N., Morua, S. D., Ferreira-Lay, P., Gudjonsson, G., Ivens, V., Jarvis, C., Lewis, A., Mason, P., Newlove-Delgado, T., Pitts, M., Read, H., & Skirrow, C. (2021). Failure of healthcare provision for attention-deficit/hyperactivity disorder in the United Kingdom: A consensus statement. *Frontiers in Psychiatry, 12*, 649399. https://doi.org/10.3389/fpsyt.2021.649399

Chapter 11
Impact of ADHD on Sexuality

Abstract Attention-deficit/hyperactivity disorder (ADHD) influences a wide array of life domains, including sexuality and intimate relationships. While existing literature has extensively documented ADHD's impact on academic achievement, occupational functioning, and social interactions, its effects on sexual health, behaviors, and relational dynamics have received comparatively limited scholarly attention.

Core ADHD traits—such as impulsivity, inattention, and emotional dysregulation—can shape patterns of sexual behavior, influence intimacy, and affect relationship satisfaction across the lifespan. These characteristics may contribute to both challenges and risks within sexual and romantic contexts, as well as opportunities for heightened emotional intensity and spontaneity in intimate relationships.

This chapter critically explores the intersection between ADHD and sexuality, focusing on the psychological, behavioral, and relational dimensions of sexual experiences among individuals with ADHD.

11.1 Impulsivity and Risk-Taking in Sexual Behavior

Adolescents and young adults with ADHD are more likely to engage in sexual activity earlier than their neurotypical counterparts, a pattern linked to heightened impulsivity and novelty-seeking behaviors. The challenges in weighing long-term consequences, coupled with emotional impulsivity, contribute to premature sexual engagement. Studies indicate that adolescents with ADHD are approximately twice as likely to engage in sexual activity before the age of 16 years, a trend that is particularly evident among females, who face increased risks of early sexual initiation and unplanned pregnancies (Barkley et al., 2019).

The impulsivity associated with ADHD often extends into patterns of romantic and sexual relationships, with individuals frequently reporting a greater number of lifetime sexual partners than their neurotypical peers (Retz et al., 2021).

G. Ayano et al., *ADHD Across the Lifespan*, SpringerBriefs in Modern Perspectives on Disability Research,
https://doi.org/10.1007/978-981-95-8712-4_11

Sensation-seeking and difficulties maintaining long-term romantic attachments may drive this trend. For men with ADHD, casual sexual encounters and short-term relationships are more prevalent, whereas women with ADHD often experience relational instability. In both groups, low self-esteem and heightened rejection sensitivity may contribute to seeking emotional validation through sexual experiences (Barkley et al., 2019).

A key concern in ADHD-related sexual behaviors is the inconsistent use of contraceptives. Inattention, forgetfulness, and impulsivity can result in lower adherence to safe-sex practices, thereby increasing the risk of sexually transmitted infections (STIs) and unintended pregnancies (Flory et al., 2006). Research suggests that young adults with ADHD are approximately 1.5 times more likely to engage in unprotected sex compared to their neurotypical peers. For women with ADHD, inconsistent contraceptive use—including missed doses of oral contraceptives—is common, driven by executive functioning challenges and difficulties with routine adherence. This underscores the need for ADHD-specific interventions that promote structured contraceptive strategies, such as the use of digital reminders and long-acting reversible contraceptives (Retz et al., 2021).

The cumulative impact of early sexual initiation, multiple sexual partners, and inconsistent contraceptive use among individuals with ADHD presents additional public health risks. Elevated rates of STIs and unintended pregnancies highlight the need for tailored sexual health education that is sensitive to the cognitive and behavioral challenges associated with ADHD. Effective interventions should incorporate visual aids, reminder tools, and digital platforms to reinforce safe sex practices (Greijdanus et al., 2020). Additionally, discussions addressing impulsivity, emotional regulation, and risk-taking behaviors should be integrated into ADHD treatment plans. Healthcare providers play a crucial role in initiating conversations about sexual health, particularly for adolescents and young adults. Importantly, early childhood education programs can play a preventive role by embedding self-regulation, decision-making, and social-emotional learning skills into the curriculum from a young age. Such foundational skills—taught through age-appropriate classroom activities, play-based learning, and positive behavioral reinforcement—help children with ADHD develop coping strategies before they enter adolescence, a critical period when sexual health-related risk behaviors may emerge (Domitrovich et al., 2017; Denham et al., 2014). Public health programs should also emphasize the development of structured contraceptive adherence programs and behavioral strategies designed to support individuals with ADHD in managing their sexual health.

11.2 Hypersexuality and ADHD

For some individuals with ADHD, heightened sexual drive—commonly referred to as hypersexuality—can be a significant challenge, often linked to dopaminergic dysregulation. The same neurobiological mechanisms underlying ADHD-related impulsivity, reward-seeking, and difficulties with delayed gratification may also contribute to increased sexual arousal and risk-taking behaviors (Retz et al., 2021). While not universally experienced among all individuals with ADHD, hypersexuality can manifest as compulsive sexual behaviors, pornography addiction, or impulsive decision-making within intimate relationships, often resulting in emotional distress, relational instability, and increased engagement in risky sexual encounters (Barkley et al., 2019). Hypersexuality in ADHD appears to stem from a combination of neurochemical imbalances, poor impulse control, and emotional dysregulation, with sex frequently serving as a maladaptive coping strategy for managing stress, anxiety, and low self-esteem (Flory et al., 2006).

ADHD is closely associated with dysregulation of dopamine pathways, which play a critical role in reward processing, motivation, and pleasure-seeking behaviors. In the context of sexuality, dopamine dysfunction may amplify cravings for stimulation, leading to heightened sexual desire and risk-prone behaviors (Flory et al., 2006). Individuals with ADHD may experience increased sensitivity to reward stimuli, making them more prone to engage in pleasure-seeking behaviors, including sex. Difficulty delaying gratification can result in impulsive sexual decision-making, including unplanned encounters and neglect of safer-sex practices. Sensation-seeking tendencies common among individuals with ADHD can also foster a preference for novel or high-risk sexual experiences, further increasing vulnerability to negative relational and health outcomes.

Deficits in impulse control, a core characteristic of ADHD, are central to understanding compulsive sexual behavior within this population. While not all individuals with ADHD develop compulsive sexual tendencies, a significant proportion report difficulties regulating sexual behaviors. These include problematic pornography use that interferes with daily functioning and contributes to emotional distress; risky sexual behaviors such as infidelity or unplanned sexual encounters driven by impulsive decision-making; and a heightened likelihood of engaging in unprotected sex, multiple partnerships, or encounters with unfamiliar partners with limited consideration of the associated risks (Barkley et al., 2019). Co-occurring mental health conditions—including anxiety, depression, or substance use disorders—may further exacerbate the risk of compulsive sexual behavior (Retz et al., 2021). Interventions targeting ADHD symptoms, such as stimulant medication or cognitive-behavioral therapy (CBT), have been shown to improve self-regulation and reduce problematic sexual behaviors (Flory et al., 2006).

Emotional dysregulation, another defining feature of ADHD, often manifests as mood instability, difficulty managing frustration, and heightened stress sensitivity. In this context, sex may serve as a coping mechanism for individuals with ADHD to alleviate negative affect, regulate mood, or bolster self-esteem (Barkley et al., 2019). Sexual behaviors may function as a form of emotional escape, with individuals engaging in hypersexuality during periods of distress, anxiety, or low mood. Additionally, rejection sensitivity and social challenges may fuel validation-seeking behaviors, with some individuals relying on sexual encounters to compensate for feelings of inadequacy or relational insecurity (Flory et al., 2006). Difficulties establishing emotional intimacy may also lead to prioritization of physical over emotional connection, contributing to instability in romantic and sexual relationships.

Effective management of hypersexuality in individuals with ADHD requires a multi-pronged approach that addresses both neurobiological and behavioral factors. Pharmacological treatments, including stimulant (e.g., methylphenidate, amphetamines) and non-stimulant medications (e.g., atomoxetine), may enhance impulse control and executive functioning, reducing compulsive tendencies, including hypersexual behavior (Retz et al., 2021). Cognitive-behavioral therapy (CBT) is particularly effective in helping individuals with ADHD develop self-awareness, regulate emotional responses, and adopt healthier coping mechanisms. Techniques such as impulse-control training and mindfulness can reduce engagement in risky sexual behaviors. Sexual health education tailored to ADHD should include psychoeducation on safe sex practices, boundary setting, and strategies for building emotionally supportive relationships. Couples counseling may also be beneficial for addressing relational challenges rooted in emotional dysregulation. Additionally, non-clinical strategies—such as adopting structured daily routines, engaging in alternative stress-relieving activities (e.g., exercise, creative outlets), and avoiding high-risk situations (e.g., limiting exposure to triggering stimuli)—can further support individuals in managing hypersexuality (Kafka, 2010).

11.3 ADHD and Sexual Dysfunction

While some individuals with ADHD experience heightened sexual desire and impulsivity, others report various forms of sexual dysfunction, including difficulties with arousal, focus, emotional connection, and overall sexual satisfaction. ADHD-related symptoms—such as inattentiveness, mind-wandering, emotional detachment, and impulsivity—can negatively affect sexual intimacy, leading to frustration within romantic relationships and impairing sexual well-being (Barkley et al., 2019). Furthermore, pharmacological treatments for ADHD, including both stimulant and non-stimulant medications, may have side effects such as reduced libido, delayed orgasm, or erectile dysfunction (Retz et al., 2021). These overlapping challenges underscore the complex interplay between ADHD symptomatology, treatment, and sexual functioning.

One of the most frequently reported difficulties among individuals with ADHD is sustaining attention and arousal during sexual activity (Chen et al., 2018). Inattentiveness and distractibility can extend into intimate moments, disrupting sexual engagement and satisfaction. Mind-wandering during sex may reduce a person's ability to remain fully present with their partner, impacting physical and emotional connection. Executive functioning deficits may further contribute to difficulties initiating intimacy or maintaining sexual focus. Individuals with ADHD often describe disruptions in arousal mid-activity, or find themselves distracted by intrusive, unrelated thoughts. These attentional lapses can result in challenges with orgasm or diminished enjoyment of sexual experiences (Flory et al., 2006). For couples, these issues can lead to relational strain, miscommunication, or feelings of rejection, highlighting the need for open conversations about ADHD's influence on intimacy and sexual dynamics.

Emotional dysregulation, a hallmark feature of ADHD, may also impair the capacity for deep emotional connection during sexual encounters. Some individuals with ADHD experience emotional detachment during intimacy, characterized by a preoccupation with external distractions and difficulty interpreting non-verbal cues from their partner (Retz et al., 2021). For others, ADHD may contribute to the formation of short-term, intense relationships that quickly fade due to inconsistent emotional engagement. Additionally, rejection sensitivity dysphoria (RSD)—commonly associated with ADHD—can heighten anxiety about sexual performance or partner satisfaction, sometimes leading to avoidance of intimacy altogether (Barkley et al., 2019). Addressing RSD and related interpersonal challenges requires a life-course approach that integrates early screening, individualized coping strategies, and sustained access to both pharmacological (e.g., stimulants, non-stimulants) and non-pharmacological interventions (e.g., cognitive-behavioral therapy, social skills training). Advances in medical research are refining treatment protocols to improve not only symptom control but also quality of life outcomes across developmental stages. Importantly, untreated ADHD and associated conditions like RSD can contribute to significant economic costs over the lifespan, driven by reduced relationship stability, lower productivity, and increased healthcare utilization, whereas timely and sustained treatment can yield substantial cost savings and long-term psychosocial benefits (Daley & Birchwood, 2010; Faraone et al., 2021). Strategies to enhance emotional connection in individuals with ADHD include mindfulness techniques to stay present during intimacy, regular emotional check-ins with partners, and the integration of affectionate, non-sexual physical touch to foster intimacy beyond sexual interactions.

Challenges related to attention, emotional regulation, and impulsivity may contribute to lower sexual satisfaction among individuals with ADHD and their partners. These difficulties may manifest as inconsistent sexual desire, relational misunderstandings, or conflict over intimacy frequency and quality. Partners of individuals with ADHD may misinterpret inattentiveness during intimacy as disinterest or rejection, which can erode relational trust and emotional security. Likewise, impulsivity and emotional fluctuations can create instability in relationships, reinforcing a cycle of frustration and miscommunication (Flory et al., 2006). Over time, these dynamics may negatively affect relationship satisfaction and long-term stability, underscoring the importance of mutual understanding and proactive relational strategies.

While pharmacological treatments for ADHD are effective in improving core symptoms such as impulsivity, attention deficits, and emotional dysregulation, they may also contribute to sexual dysfunction in some individuals. Stimulant medications, including methylphenidate and amphetamines, may improve focus and impulse control, leading to enhanced emotional engagement during sexual activity. However, they are also associated with decreased libido in certain individuals (Retz et al., 2021). Non-stimulant medications, such as atomoxetine or guanfacine, may stabilize mood and reduce hyperactivity and can have side effects such as erectile dysfunction, delayed orgasm, or reduced sexual interest (Bieś et al., 2025). While some individuals report that ADHD medication improves their capacity for emotional and relational connection, others experience diminished sexual desire or satisfaction as a side effect. Strategies to mitigate medication-related sexual dysfunction include adjusting medication dosages or timing, exploring alternative pharmacological options, and behavioral interventions such as CBT or sex therapy.

11.4 Emotional Dysregulation and Intimacy

Emotional dysregulation is a core characteristic of ADHD that can significantly impact intimacy and emotional connectedness within romantic and sexual relationships. Heightened emotional reactivity, mood instability, and impulsive emotional responses often create relational environments that feel unpredictable and overwhelming for both individuals with ADHD and their partners (Barkley et al., 2019). People with ADHD can experience emotions more intensely than neurotypical individuals, which may lead to difficulty modulating affection, frustration, and perceived rejection. This intensity can manifest in relational patterns characterized by cycles of heightened passion followed by emotional withdrawal, contributing to tension and instability within intimate partnerships (Eakin et al., 2004).

Individuals with ADHD may fluctuate between intense expressions of affection and periods of frustration or disengagement. These shifts may occur rapidly and without clear external triggers, making the emotional climate of relationships feel volatile. Partners often report difficulty predicting or managing these emotional shifts, leading to relational stress and miscommunication (Flory et al., 2006). To mitigate these patterns, emotional self-awareness practices—such as identifying common emotional triggers—and the use of structured relationship check-ins may help regulate emotional highs and lows.

Inattentiveness and distractibility can make it challenging for individuals with ADHD to sustain emotional engagement in relationships. Moments of perceived inattentiveness, missed emotional cues, or lapses in follow-through on romantic commitments can leave partners feeling disconnected or unimportant (Retz et al., 2021). Active listening strategies and the deliberate scheduling of distraction-free quality time can foster deeper emotional presence and help reduce miscommunication. By intentionally creating spaces for emotional connection, individuals with ADHD may enhance intimacy and strengthen relational bonds.

Some individuals with ADHD may rely heavily on their partners for emotional regulation, creating dynamics that may become co-dependent over time (Eakin et al., 2004). While seeking reassurance and emotional grounding is common in close relationships, over-reliance can place strain on partners, who may feel responsible for managing the other's mood (Barkley et al., 2019). Building emotional self-sufficiency through independent coping strategies—such as journaling, mindfulness, or exercise—and engaging in therapy to develop emotional regulation skills can help alleviate this imbalance and promote relational resilience (Mitchell et al., 2017).

Rejection Sensitivity Dysphoria (RSD) is a phenomenon frequently reported in individuals with ADHD, characterized by heightened sensitivity to perceived criticism or rejection. Although targeted interventions to address RSD exist, formal training for educators and school staff remains largely unavailable or inaccessible within current work environments. Effective strategies should incorporate dedicated classroom relief time for teachers to participate in ADHD-specific training, structured diagnostic support for parent–teacher dyads, and integration of RSD-related content into professional development (PD) days. Such measures would enhance early identification, improve communication between families and schools, and ensure that interventions are informed, timely, and responsive to the unique emotional challenges faced by students with ADHD. Moreover, embedding social-emotional learning (SEL) curricula in early childhood education can foster self-regulation, emotion awareness, and resilience—foundational skills that buffer challenges like RSD and enhance long-term functioning. Meta-analytic evidence confirms SEL strengthens emotional competencies and academic outcomes (Durlak et al., 2011), and recent controlled interventions (e.g., Fun FRIENDS program) demonstrate efficacy in preschool settings (Hosokawa et al., 2024).

Even minor relational disagreements may elicit intense emotional reactions, defensive behaviors, or emotional withdrawal in individuals with RSD (Flory et al., 2006). Beyond school and workplace accommodations, personal strategies can help mitigate these responses, such as practicing a brief pause before reacting to perceived rejection, seeking clarification during emotionally charged interactions, and engaging in therapeutic interventions to build resilience and enhance conflict resolution skills (Galloway & Newman, 2017).

Emotional impulsivity is another ADHD-related trait that can impact intimacy. Individuals may respond to emotional triggers with spontaneous, sometimes regrettable, words or actions, potentially damaging trust and stability within relationships (Retz et al., 2021). Over time, partners may feel compelled to avoid sensitive topics or adopt a hypervigilant stance to prevent emotional escalation. Developing de-escalation techniques, such as pausing before responding and employing calm communication methods, may help individuals with ADHD reduce emotional impulsivity and foster healthier relational dynamics.

A multifaceted approach is essential to addressing emotional instability within ADHD-affected relationships. Cognitive Behavioral Therapy (CBT) and couples therapy can equip individuals and their partners with practical tools to improve emotional regulation and relational communication. Mindfulness practices and meditation may also enhance emotional awareness and impulse control, while

ADHD medications can help stabilize mood and reduce emotional reactivity in some cases (Mitchell et al., 2017). Encouraging individuals with ADHD to adopt independent coping strategies—such as stress-reducing activities or personal development pursuits—can further promote emotional balance and self-regulation.

Summary

This chapter has explored the intersection between ADHD and sexuality, highlighting how core ADHD symptoms—such as impulsivity, inattention, and emotional dysregulation—shape sexual behaviors, intimacy, and relationship satisfaction across the lifespan. Individuals with ADHD are more likely to engage in early sexual activity, experience heightened impulsivity in sexual decision-making, and face elevated risks of sexually transmitted infections and unintended pregnancies due to inconsistent contraceptive use. These behaviors are linked to challenges with self-regulation, sensation-seeking, and executive dysfunction.

For some, ADHD is associated with hypersexuality, including compulsive sexual behaviors, pornography addiction, and risk-taking in intimate relationships. This pattern is often driven by dopaminergic dysregulation and emotional instability. Others may experience sexual dysfunction, such as difficulties sustaining arousal, focus, or emotional engagement during sexual activity. ADHD medications can also contribute to sexual side effects, including reduced libido and orgasmic challenges.

Emotional dysregulation has a significant impact on intimacy and relational dynamics, contributing to cycles of passion, conflict, and emotional withdrawal. Rejection Sensitivity Dysphoria (RSD), impulsivity in emotional expression, and difficulties with sustained emotional closeness often strain ADHD-affected relationships.

The chapter emphasizes the importance of tailored interventions—such as ADHD-specific sexual health education, cognitive-behavioral therapy, mindfulness, and medication management—to address these challenges. By fostering awareness and providing structured support, individuals with ADHD and their partners can improve sexual health, relationship stability, and emotional intimacy.

References

Barkley, R. A., & Fischer, M. (2019). Hyperactive child syndrome and estimated life expectancy at young adult follow-up: The role of ADHD persistence and other potential predictors *Journal of Attention Disorders, 23*(9), 907–923. https://doi.org/10.1177/1087054718816164

Bieś, R., Szewczyk, Z., Warchala, A., Martyniak, E., & Krzystanek, M. (2025). The impact of methylphenidate on sexual functions: A systematic review of benefits and risks. *Pharmaceuticals (Basel), 18*(5). https://doi.org/10.3390/ph18050718

Chen, M. H., Hsu, J. W., Huang, K. L., Bai, Y. M., Ko, N. Y., Su, T. P., Li, C. T., Lin, W. C., Tsai, S. J., Pan, T. L., Chang, W. H., & Chen, T. J. (2018). Sexually transmitted infection among adolescents and young adults with attention-deficit/hyperactivity disorder: A Nationwide longitudinal study. *Journal of the American Academy of Child and Adolescent Psychiatry, 57*(1), 48–53. https://doi.org/10.1016/j.jaac.2017.09.438

Daley, D., & Birchwood, J. (2010). ADHD and academic performance: Why does ADHD impact on academic performance and what can be done to support ADHD children in the classroom? *Child: Care, Health and Development, 36*(4), 455–464. https://doi.org/10.1111/j.1365-2214.2009.01046.x

Denham, S. A., Bassett, H. H., & Zinsser, K. (2014). Early childhood teachers as socializers of young children's emotional competence. *Early Childhood Education Journal, 42*(2), 137–143. https://doi.org/10.1007/s10643-013-0584-2

Domitrovich, C. E., Durlak, J. A., Staley, K. C., & Weissberg, R. P. (2017). Social-emotional competence: An essential factor for promoting positive adjustment and reducing risk in school children. *Child Development, 88*(2), 408–416. https://doi.org/10.1111/cdev.12739

Durlak, J. A., Weissberg, R. P., Dymnicki, A. B., Taylor, R. D., & Schellinger, K. B. (2011). The impact of enhancing students' social and emotional learning: A meta-analysis of school-based universal interventions. *Child Development, 82*(1), 405–432. https://doi.org/10.1111/j.1467-8624.2010.01564.x

Eakin, L., Minde, K., Hechtman, L., Ochs, E., Krane, E., Bouffard, R., Greenfield, B., & Looper, K. (2004). The marital and family functioning of adults with ADHD and their spouses. *Journal of Attention Disorders, 8*(1), 1–10. https://doi.org/10.1177/108705470400800101

Faraone, S. V., Banaschewski, T., Coghill, D., Zheng, Y., Biederman, J., Bellgrove, M. A., Newcorn, J. H., Gignac, M., Al Saud, N. M., Manor, I., Rohde, L. A., Yang, L., Cortese, S., Almagor, D., Stein, M. A., Albatti, T. H., Aljoudi, H. F., Alqahtani, M. M. J., Asherson, P., & Wang, Y. (2021). The world federation of ADHD international consensus statement: 208 evidence-based conclusions about the disorder. *Neuroscience & Biobehavioral Reviews, 128*, 789–818. https://doi.org/10.1016/j.neubiorev.2021.01.022

Flory, K., Molina, B. S. G., Pelham, W. E., Jr., Gnagy, E., & Smith, B. (2006). Childhood attention-deficit/hyperactivity disorder predicts risky sexual behavior in young adulthood. *Journal of Clinical Child and Adolescent Psychology, 35*(4), 571–577. https://doi.org/10.1207/s15374424jccp3504_8

Galloway, H., & Newman, E. (2017). Is there a difference between child self-ratings and parent proxy-ratings of the quality of life of children with a diagnosis of attention-deficit hyperactivity disorder (ADHD)? A systematic review of the literature. *ADHD Attention Deficit and Hyperactivity Disorders, 9*(1), 11–29. https://doi.org/10.1007/s12402-016-0210-9

Greijdanus, H., de Matos Fernandes, C. A., Turner-Zwinkels, F., Honari, A., Roos, C. A., Rosenbusch, H., & Postmes, T. (2020). The psychology of online activism and social movements: Relations between online and offline collective action. *Current Opinion in Psychology, 35*, 49–54.

Hosokawa, R., Matsumoto, Y., Nishida, C., Funato, K., & Mitani, A. (2024). Enhancing social-emotional skills in early childhood: Intervention study on the effectiveness of social and emotional learning. *BMC Psychology, 12*(1), 761. https://doi.org/10.1186/s40359-024-02280-w

Kafka, M. P. (2010). Hypersexual disorder: A proposed diagnosis for DSM-V. *Archives of Sexual Behavior, 39*(2), 377–400. https://doi.org/10.1007/s10508-009-9574-7

Mitchell, J. T., McIntyre, E. M., English, J. S., Dennis, M. F., Beckham, J. C., & Kollins, S. H. (2017). A pilot trial of mindfulness meditation training for ADHD in adulthood: Impact on Core symptoms, executive functioning, and emotion Dysregulation. *Journal of Attention Disorders, 21*(13), 1105–1120. https://doi.org/10.1177/1087054713513328

Retz, W., Ginsberg, Y., Turner, D., Barra, S., Retz-Junginger, P., Larsson, H., & Asherson, P. (2021). Attention-deficit/hyperactivity disorder (ADHD), antisociality and delinquent behavior over the lifespan. *Neuroscience & Biobehavioral Reviews, 120*, 236–248. https://doi.org/10.1016/j.neubiorev.2020.11.025

Chapter 12
Public Perceptions and Diagnostic/Health Perspectives of ADHD

Abstract This chapter critically examines the evolving public perceptions and diagnostic frameworks surrounding Attention-Deficit/Hyperactivity Disorder (ADHD). Despite widespread scientific agreement on ADHD as a legitimate neurodevelopmental condition, public understanding of the disorder remains fragmented, often influenced by cultural narratives, societal stigma, and divergent health system practices.

The chapter explores how ADHD is perceived across different societies, how stigma and misconceptions influence diagnosis and treatment-seeking behaviors, and how historical and contemporary debates shape public and clinical discourses on ADHD. In parallel, the chapter reviews the evolution of ADHD diagnostic criteria, considering both the medicalization of attention and behavioral difficulties and the influence of healthcare system structures on diagnosis rates and treatment access.

Finally, attention is given to disparities in how ADHD is diagnosed and managed across diverse socio-cultural and healthcare contexts, highlighting the ongoing tensions between clinical perspectives and public attitudes.

12.1 Common Misconceptions About ADHD

Despite an extensive body of research confirming ADHD as a neurodevelopmental condition underpinned by genetic and neurobiological mechanisms, public understanding of ADHD remains clouded by persistent myths. These misconceptions contribute to widespread stigma, delayed diagnoses, and disparities in access to appropriate treatment (Barkley, 2021). Misunderstandings are particularly pronounced among adults, females, and minority populations, whose symptoms are frequently misattributed to personality traits or environmental factors (Nussbaum, 2011). This section critically examines several of the most prevalent myths about ADHD and presents the scientific evidence that refutes them.

A common and harmful misconception is that ADHD reflects laziness or a lack of personal motivation. This myth dismisses the well-established neurobiological

G. Ayano et al., *ADHD Across the Lifespan*, SpringerBriefs in Modern Perspectives on Disability Research,
https://doi.org/10.1007/978-981-95-8712-4_12

underpinnings of ADHD, including structural and functional differences in brain regions associated with executive function, impulse control, and reward processing (Faraone et al., 2021). In reality, ADHD-related procrastination, forgetfulness, and inconsistent task completion arise from deficits in executive functioning—particularly difficulties with initiation, planning, and sustaining effort (Barkley, 2021). Rather than reflecting apathy, individuals with ADHD frequently exert disproportionate cognitive and emotional effort to achieve everyday tasks, often resulting in mental fatigue and frustration.

Although public discourse often emphasizes "over-diagnosis," the preponderance of evidence points to underdiagnosis in key subgroups—especially girls/women and adults. Contributing factors include less disruptive inattentive/internalizing presentations that draw fewer referrals; misattribution of symptoms to anxiety, depression, or personality; masking/compensation until environmental demands increase (e.g., secondary school, university, parenthood, menopause); overshadowing by comorbidities; referral tools historically normed on hyperactive male samples (Quinn & Madhoo, 2014); and, in adults, the requirement to document childhood onset, which further delays recognition (Morgan et al., 2016). While ADHD diagnosis rates have increased globally, these trends largely reflect improved awareness and recognition rather than excessive pathologizing of normative behaviors. Indeed, untreated ADHD is associated with substantial risks, including academic failure, employment instability, and comorbid mental health conditions (Faraone et al., 2021).

A longstanding belief is that ADHD is a disorder confined to childhood, with symptoms dissipating over time. However, longitudinal studies consistently demonstrate that ADHD frequently persists into adulthood, albeit with shifting symptomatology. Hyperactivity may decline, while difficulties with attention, executive functioning, and emotional regulation often endure (Biederman et al., 2012). The persistence of ADHD beyond childhood is increasingly recognized, although many adults remain undiagnosed or misdiagnosed with conditions such as anxiety or depression (Kooij et al., 2019). This misconception contributes to delayed interventions, leaving adults with ADHD vulnerable to relationship difficulties, underemployment, and chronic stress.

Another enduring myth attributes ADHD to poor parenting, lack of discipline, or excessive screen exposure. While environmental factors can influence the severity of ADHD symptoms, the disorder is highly inheritable, with twin studies estimating a heritability rate of approximately 80% (Thapar et al., 2013). Neuroimaging research further supports ADHD's biological basis, identifying structural abnormalities in neural circuits associated with attention regulation and impulse control (Cortese et al., 2018). Parenting style and screen time may exacerbate symptoms but do not constitute causal factors. Importantly, this misconception places undue blame on caregivers, diverting attention from the need for appropriate clinical intervention and support (Faraone et al., 2021).

Persistent misconceptions about ADHD perpetuate stigma and can hinder access to effective care. Although public awareness has improved in recent years (Mueller et al., 2012) misinformation continues to delay diagnoses and deter individuals from seeking support, especially in marginalized populations. Efforts to improve public understanding should prioritize evidence-based education, challenge deficit-focused narratives, and promote ADHD recognition across the lifespan and diverse demographic groups.

12.2 Stigma and Its Impact on Diagnosis and Treatment

Although ADHD is increasingly recognized within medical and scientific circles as a legitimate neurodevelopmental disorder, social stigma remains a significant barrier to timely diagnosis, effective treatment, and broader societal acceptance. Many individuals with ADHD experience internalized stigma or anticipate discrimination, which can deter them from seeking formal assessment or disclosing their diagnosis (Hamed et al., 2015). This section examines how stigma intersects with gender, culture, and adulthood, shaping the diagnostic and treatment trajectories of individuals with ADHD.

Fear of being labeled as lazy, disorganized, or incompetent contributes to significant delays in ADHD diagnosis, particularly among adults, women, and racial minorities. Anticipated stigma prevents individuals from pursuing assessments or disclosing their condition in academic, professional, and social contexts (Quinn & Madhoo, 2014). Misconceptions about ADHD as a character flaw—rather than a neurological condition—further fuel these concerns. In professional settings, fears of being perceived as unreliable or unproductive often lead to non-disclosure, which in turn hinders access to workplace accommodations. Similarly, parents may delay seeking evaluations for their children out of fear that a diagnosis will result in negative labeling or reduced expectations. Interventions to combat this stigma could include targeted social marketing health campaigns, workplace education, and advocacy to normalize ADHD as a valid medical condition requiring appropriate support and intervention (Lebowitz, 2013).

ADHD in females is frequently underdiagnosed or misdiagnosed due to differences in symptom presentation and social expectations. Girls and women are more likely to exhibit inattentive symptoms—such as disorganization and internalized restlessness—rather than hyperactivity, which tends to prompt clinical attention more readily in boys (Quinn & Madhoo, 2014). In addition, females are more likely to engage in social masking—overcompensating through perfectionism or social mimicry—which can obscure ADHD symptoms and lead to alternative diagnoses such as anxiety or mood disorders (Young et al., 2020). Clinicians and educators may fail to recognize the gendered expression of ADHD, contributing to diagnostic disparities and delayed interventions.

Systemic inequities in healthcare access and implicit biases contribute to ADHD underdiagnosis among racial and ethnic minority groups. Black, Hispanic, and Indigenous children are less likely to be diagnosed with ADHD and more likely to be labeled with disruptive behavioral disorders, such as oppositional defiant disorder (ODD) or conduct disorder (CD) (Morgan et al., 2016). Unconscious bias operates through subtle mechanisms—teachers and clinicians may apply higher symptom thresholds, frame identical behaviors as "defiance" rather than inattention, or favor disciplinary routes over mental-health referrals—leading to systematic under-identification at equivalent symptom burden (Coker et al., 2016; Paidipati et al., 2017). Bias can also shape how parent/teacher rating scales are completed and interpreted, amplifying misclassification and diagnostic overshadowing (Paidipati et al., 2017). Language barriers, cultural stigma surrounding mental health, and a historical mistrust of healthcare institutions exacerbate these disparities (Hamed et al., 2015). Addressing these challenges necessitates a focus on cultural competence in healthcare settings, improved outreach to underserved communities, and bias-awareness training for professionals involved in school-based referrals and clinical evaluations. Practical mitigations include universal school and primary-care screening, bilingual assessors and interpreters, and routine equity audits that track referral, diagnosis, and treatment rates by race/ethnicity to identify and close gaps (Coker et al., 2016; Zhao et al., 2023).

Adults with ADHD continue to encounter skepticism regarding the legitimacy of their diagnosis. Despite the growing recognition of ADHD as a lifelong condition, the prevailing belief that ADHD "should be outgrown" persists, contributing to diagnostic gaps and inadequate treatment access for adults (Kooij et al., 2019). In employment settings, concerns about stigma lead some adults to conceal their ADHD diagnosis, avoiding requests for accommodations such as flexible deadlines or structured workflows. This dynamic contributes to underperformance, workplace stress, and challenges in self-advocacy. Shifting public perceptions of adult ADHD requires both a revision of diagnostic frameworks to better reflect adult symptomatology and greater employer engagement with neurodiversity initiatives.

Reducing ADHD-related stigma is critical to improving diagnosis rates, treatment access, and quality of life for affected individuals. Future efforts should focus on raising public awareness through culturally sensitive education campaigns, training healthcare providers to recognize ADHD presentations across gender, age, and cultural contexts, and encouraging employers to adopt ADHD-inclusive policies and promote neurodiversity in the workplace. By dismantling stigma and addressing systemic biases, healthcare systems and societies can ensure more equitable access to ADHD diagnosis, treatment, and accommodations.

12.3 Cross-Cultural Views on ADHD

ADHD is recognized globally as a neurodevelopmental disorder; however, its conceptualization, diagnosis, and management vary widely across cultural contexts. While Western healthcare systems largely frame ADHD through a biomedical lens, many non-Western societies interpret ADHD behaviors within cultural, educational, or moral frameworks. These differences contribute to variations in diagnosis rates, treatment preferences, and public acceptance worldwide (Hamed et al., 2015). This section provides a comparative analysis of ADHD across Western, Asian, Middle

Eastern, and European regions, emphasizing how cultural beliefs and healthcare infrastructures influence ADHD recognition and treatment.

In countries such as the United States, the United Kingdom, Canada, and Australia, ADHD is well-established within medical and educational systems as a neurodevelopmental disorder. These countries adopt a predominantly biomedical approach to ADHD, supported by structured diagnostic and treatment frameworks (Faraone et al., 2021). Key features include the widespread use of DSM or ICD diagnostic criteria, high public awareness and routine school-based screening, and legal protections under disability rights legislation that support educational and occupational accommodations. Widespread use of stimulant medications, including methylphenidate and amphetamines, is often combined with behavioral interventions (Hinshaw & Scheffler, 2014). While this approach has fostered early identification and support systems, concerns persist regarding potential overdiagnosis and an over-reliance on pharmacotherapy. Nonetheless, underdiagnosis remains a challenge, particularly for females, adults, and minority populations (Quinn & Madhoo, 2014).

In contrast, many Asian and Middle Eastern countries approach ADHD from a more behavioral or moralistic standpoint, often perceiving symptoms such as inattentiveness and hyperactivity as reflections of poor discipline or familial dysfunction (Hamed et al., 2015). Cultural influences in these regions include a preference for discipline-based strategies, prioritizing strict parenting or educational regimens over medical intervention, and a cultural emphasis on academic achievement that can stigmatize behaviors perceived as disruptive or underperforming. Additionally, mental health stigma contributes to reluctance in seeking psychiatric evaluations or disclosing neurodevelopmental conditions. Limited access to ADHD-trained clinicians and culturally appropriate mental health services further exacerbates diagnostic and treatment challenges. While urban areas in countries such as China, Japan, and South Korea have begun integrating Western diagnostic and treatment models (ref), ADHD remains underdiagnosed in rural settings, where social stigma and parental expectations present significant barriers.

Across Europe, ADHD medication use has risen over the past 15–20 years, but levels and growth vary markedly by country and age group, with Nordic countries (e.g., Sweden, Denmark, Iceland) showing sustained increases—including in adults—while parts of Southern and Central Europe remain more conservative in both diagnosis and prescribing; overall European use is still moderate relative to the United States, reflecting practice differences rather than prevalence alone (Bachmann et al., 2017; Karlstad et al., 2016). Guidelines are not uniform: most European guidance endorses stimulants as first-line pharmacotherapy when impairment persists, but differs on the timing and priority of psychosocial interventions—NICE (UK) places medication earlier for school-age children than some continental guidance, whereas German, Dutch, and Spanish guidelines more strongly emphasize parent-training/psychoeducation first—though all stress multimodal care across the lifespan (NICE, 2018; Banaschewski et al., 2018; Döpfner et al., 2018; NVvP, 2015; Ministerio de Sanidad, 2017). For adults, an updated European consensus likewise supports stimulants as first-line within individualized pathways that integrate psychoeducation and psychological therapies, helping to explain both rising adult prescribing in the North and persistent intra-European variation (Kooij et al., 2019).

Global prescription trends further illustrate disparities in ADHD management. The United States continues to lead in stimulant prescriptions, driven by both high diagnostic rates and broader cultural acceptance of pharmacological treatments, whereas Europe and many other regions lag significantly behind (Bachmann et al., 2017; Dutta et al., 2022; Gu et al., 2022). European countries demonstrate moderate prescribing patterns, often contingent on national guidelines and clinician discretion, while many Asian and Middle Eastern countries exhibit limited stimulant use due to regulatory restrictions, lower public acceptance, and fewer trained specialists (Hamed et al., 2015). These disparities reflect broader sociocultural and systemic factors, including healthcare accessibility, mental health literacy, and cultural narratives about behavioral and cognitive functioning.

To address international disparities, efforts should focus on expanding culturally sensitive ADHD education initiatives to reduce stigma, increasing the availability of ADHD-trained professionals in under-resourced regions, and encouraging global collaboration to align diagnostic standards and improve treatment access. By enhancing cross-cultural awareness and addressing systemic barriers, ADHD care can become more equitable and responsive to the diverse needs of global populations.

12.4 Evolution of ADHD Diagnostic Criteria

The conceptualization and diagnostic framework for ADHD have evolved markedly over recent decades. Early diagnostic systems largely prioritized hyperactivity, overlooking key features such as inattention and executive dysfunction. Subsequent updates to the DSM and ICD frameworks have broadened recognition of ADHD, emphasizing its persistence across the lifespan and its heterogeneity in symptom presentation (Faraone et al., 2021). This section traces the historical development of ADHD diagnostic criteria, focusing on key changes that have influenced clinical practice and public understanding.

The introduction of ADHD into formal diagnostic systems began with the DSM-III (1980) and ICD-9 (1979), where the disorder was termed "Hyperkinetic Reaction of Childhood" (American Psychiatric Association, 1980). These early classifications defined ADHD primarily by observable hyperactive and impulsive behaviors, positioning ADHD as a childhood-specific condition and reinforcing misconceptions that symptoms resolve with age. They lacked criteria for inattentiveness, leading to underdiagnosis of children—particularly females—who presented with non-hyperactive symptoms (Barkley, 2015). As a result, early models disproportionately identified hyperactive males while neglecting those with predominantly inattentive or internalizing symptom profiles (Quinn & Madhoo, 2014).

A decade later in DSM-IV (1994) and ICD-10 (1992) introduced major revisions by acknowledging symptom heterogeneity and establishing ADHD subtypes (American Psychiatric Association, 1994). These subtypes included Predominantly Inattentive Type, Predominantly Hyperactive-Impulsive Type, and Combined Type. These updates improved the recognition of ADHD in females and individuals exhibiting inattentiveness, disorganization, or executive functioning deficits without marked hyperactivity. However, the frameworks still primarily focused on childhood diagnosis, with adult ADHD continuing to receive limited attention in clinical settings (Asherson et al., 2016). Although the broadened diagnostic framework helped diversify the clinical understanding of ADHD, it maintained a child-centered diagnostic threshold.

The DSM-5 (2013) and ICD-11 (2022) shifted ADHD diagnostics toward a lifespan perspective, recognizing its persistence into adulthood (American Psychiatric Association, 2013). Key changes included acknowledgment that ADHD frequently endures into adolescence and adulthood, affecting occupational, relational, and daily functioning domains. These frameworks adopted lower symptom thresholds for adults (e.g., five symptoms required instead of six) to account for age-related symptom manifestation changes (Faraone et al., 2021). They also offered greater consideration of gender-specific ADHD presentations, improving detection in women and girls, who often exhibit internalizing symptoms such as anxiety, emotional dysregulation, and social withdrawal (Quinn & Madhoo, 2014). These changes have contributed to more accurate diagnosis and treatment of adults and females with ADHD, supporting a move toward equitable clinical recognition. These revisions likely produced a modest increase in adult case identification—especially among individuals who previously fell just short of DSM-IV thresholds—yet reviews suggest that recent growth in adult diagnoses is driven at least as much by heightened awareness, screening, and service access as by the criteria change itself (Faraone et al., 2021; Kooij et al., 2019).

Modern clinical models now extend beyond traditional DSM/ICD criteria to encompass additional domains. Executive dysfunction—deficits in working memory, time management, task initiation, and organizational skills—is recognized as a core ADHD impairment, affecting academic and occupational success (Brown, 2013). Emotional dysregulation, while not yet formalized within diagnostic manuals, is increasingly acknowledged as a clinically significant feature of ADHD, encompassing emotional impulsivity and mood lability (Barkley, 2015).

Advances in neuroimaging have revealed structural and functional alterations in ADHD-related brain networks, particularly in the prefrontal cortex and dopaminergic pathways, reinforcing its classification as a neurodevelopmental disorder (Faraone et al., 2021). These contemporary understandings align clinical assessment more closely with real-world ADHD presentations, offering a more holistic approach to diagnosis and intervention.

12.5 Challenges in ADHD Diagnosis

The diagnosis of Attention-Deficit/Hyperactivity Disorder (ADHD) presents significant clinical complexities. Despite advances in the understanding of ADHD as a neurodevelopmental condition, the absence of a definitive biomarker, compounded by diagnostic biases and symptom overlap with other psychiatric disorders, continues to affect the accuracy and timeliness of diagnosis (Faraone et al., 2021). ADHD remains a clinically diagnosed condition, reliant on behavioral assessment tools, patient history, and symptom checklists aligned with DSM-5 or ICD-11 criteria (Asherson et al., 2016).

Clinical interviews and behavioral rating scales, such as the Conners' Rating Scale (Conners et al., 1998) and the ADHD Rating Scale (Amador-Campos et al., 2016), are subject to self-reporting inaccuracies and observer bias, particularly in adult populations (Barkley, 2015). Symptom subjectivity further complicates diagnosis, as individuals may mask symptoms or lack insight into executive dysfunction. Cultural and gender-based disparities in symptom interpretation contribute to a systemic under-recognition of inattentive-type ADHD, especially among women and culturally diverse populations (Quinn & Madhoo, 2014). Emerging solutions include growing interest in the development of neuroimaging markers and genetic testing protocols aimed at providing greater diagnostic objectivity, as well as enhanced clinician training focusing on diverse ADHD symptom presentations to mitigate diagnostic disparities (Hinshaw & Scheffler, 2014).

Historically regarded as a childhood-limited condition, ADHD in adulthood remains underdiagnosed and under-treated (Kooij et al., 2019). Masking behaviors, such as over-structuring and overcompensation, often obscure symptom recognition. Adults frequently present with secondary symptoms, including anxiety or depression, that clinicians may prioritize diagnostically, leaving ADHD undetected (Asherson et al., 2016). Limited professional knowledge of adult-specific ADHD symptomatology, such as emotional dysregulation and chronic disorganization, contributes to diagnostic oversight (Faraone et al., 2021). The absence of timely diagnosis in adults is associated with poorer occupational and relational outcomes, financial instability, and heightened psychosocial stress. Recommendations to address this challenge include expanding ADHD screening protocols within adult mental health and primary care settings and providing broader public and professional education to dismantle the misconception that ADHD is exclusively a childhood disorder (Fayyad et al., 2017).

ADHD symptomatology shares substantial commonalities with other psychiatric and neurodevelopmental disorders, complicating differential diagnosis. For example, anxiety disorders share symptoms of inattention and restlessness, but anxiety is situation-dependent while ADHD is trait-based (Lahey & Willcutt, 2010). Depression includes symptoms of low motivation and poor focus, but ADHD is characterized by hyperactivity, whereas depression often involves psychomotor retardation. Autism Spectrum Disorder (ASD) shares executive dysfunction and social challenges, but ASD often includes sensory sensitivities and rigid routines.

Bipolar disorder involves impulsivity and mood instability, yet bipolar mood episodes are episodic, while ADHD mood shifts are brief and reactive (Yerys et al., 2019). The co-occurrence of ADHD with mood and anxiety disorders can obscure its detection, and clinicians may erroneously attribute executive dysfunction to anxiety or mood disorders, particularly in adult populations. Proposed interventions include comprehensive psychological evaluations that incorporate developmental history and functional impairment assessments (APA, 2013). Additionally, training in differential diagnosis and comorbidity awareness is critical to improving diagnostic precision.

12.6 Healthcare System Barriers to ADHD Diagnosis and Treatment

Despite growing recognition of ADHD as a lifelong neurodevelopmental disorder, significant healthcare system limitations continue to delay diagnosis and restrict access to treatment, particularly among adults, low-income individuals, and populations residing in underserved regions. These systemic barriers—ranging from lengthy waiting periods and financial constraints to shortages of trained specialists and insufficient adult ADHD services—pose considerable challenges for individuals seeking appropriate evaluation and care.

In many public healthcare systems, ADHD diagnostic services are overburdened, resulting in prolonged delays for assessments and subsequent interventions. For example, within the UKs National Health Service (NHS), individuals may wait between 6 months and 2 years for an ADHD assessment, with some experiencing even longer delays (Gibb et al., 2018). Similarly, public healthcare systems in Canada and Australia face extended wait times, prompting many to seek costly private assessments. In the United States, while wait times vary by region, they are often exacerbated by a shortage of ADHD specialists and heightened demand for services. These delays can have serious consequences, including the deterioration of academic and occupational functioning, an elevated risk of misdiagnosis, and a disproportionate impact on individuals from lower socioeconomic backgrounds who are less likely to afford private alternatives. To address this challenge, healthcare systems could expand ADHD screening protocols within primary care, empowering general practitioners to conduct initial assessments and triage more complex cases to specialists. In addition, integrating digital assessments and telehealth services may help alleviate in-person bottlenecks, while increased investment in public ADHD clinics could help meet rising demand.

Beyond delays in access, financial barriers also represent a major obstacle to equitable ADHD care. Diagnostic assessments, medications, and ongoing behavioral therapies often impose substantial out-of-pocket costs on families, particularly in systems where ADHD care is not fully covered by insurance or public health funding (Gibb et al., 2018). These financial burdens contribute to lower diagnosis rates among low-income populations and exacerbate healthcare disparities. Untreated ADHD may also result in higher long-term costs due to associated mental health conditions, workplace instability, and interactions with the criminal justice system. To reduce cost-related barriers, governments could expand publicly funded ADHD services, subsidize treatment costs, and integrate ADHD evaluations into routine primary care, eliminating the need for expensive specialist referrals.

Many healthcare systems lack a sufficient number of professionals trained specifically in ADHD diagnosis and management, further limiting service accessibility. While pediatric ADHD services are relatively more common, adult ADHD specialists remain scarce, especially in non-metropolitan areas. As a result, general practitioners, who often lack ADHD-specific training, are tasked with managing patients who may require specialized care. This shortage disproportionately affects rural and under-resourced communities and contributes to longer wait times and diminished quality of care. Addressing this issue requires training more general practitioners and primary care physicians to conduct ADHD assessments and initiate treatment plans. In addition, embedding ADHD-focused training within medical and psychiatric education and expanding telemedicine platforms could facilitate specialist access in underserved regions.

A further barrier is the persistent focus on pediatric ADHD, which leaves many adults underdiagnosed and without adequate support. While pediatric ADHD clinics are widespread, adult-focused services are comparatively rare, complicating the transition from child to adult care. Adults with ADHD are frequently referred to general mental health services where specific ADHD expertise may be lacking (Asherson et al., 2010). Inadequate insurance coverage for adult ADHD treatment and limited availability of workplace accommodations further hinder effective care. This gap in adult services contributes to elevated rates of undiagnosed ADHD in adulthood, reduced educational and career outcomes, and increased risk of comorbid mental health conditions. A more comprehensive response would involve establishing dedicated adult ADHD clinics, expanding insurance coverage for adult evaluations and treatment, and implementing workplace ADHD support programs.

Summary

This Chapter examined how public perceptions, diagnostic criteria, and systemic healthcare barriers shape the understanding and management of ADHD globally. The chapter began by identifying persistent misconceptions about ADHD, including beliefs that it is caused by laziness, poor parenting, or is overdiagnosed, which continue to fuel stigma and hinder accurate diagnosis—especially among females, adults, and minority populations. Stigma was shown to exacerbate diagnostic and treatment disparities, reinforcing gender and cultural biases that delay timely care and contribute to the underrecognition of ADHD symptoms in girls and racial minorities, often due to symptom masking and social expectations. Additionally, the chapter highlighted the lack of awareness and stigma surrounding adult ADHD as factors that impede diagnosis and workplace accommodations, further marginalizing affected individuals. Cross-cultural differences in the conceptualization and management of ADHD were also addressed, noting that Western countries typically adopt a medicalized model with structured support systems, while many Asian and Middle Eastern cultures interpret ADHD behaviors within behavioral or moralistic frameworks, leading to underdiagnosis and limited treatment access. European approaches were characterized as more heterogeneous, with some nations favoring behavioral interventions over pharmacological treatments.

The chapter also traced the historical evolution of ADHD diagnostic criteria, from early hyperactivity-focused models to modern frameworks, such as the DSM-5 and ICD-11, which acknowledge ADHD as a lifelong condition with heterogeneous presentations. Despite these advancements, diagnostic challenges remain—particularly the absence of objective tests, underdiagnosis in adults, and frequent symptom overlap with conditions such as anxiety, depression, autism, and bipolar disorder, complicating differential diagnosis. The chapter concluded by exploring systemic healthcare barriers, including long wait times for ADHD assessments, high costs of diagnosis and treatment, shortages of trained specialists, and inadequate adult ADHD services. To address these issues, recommendations included expanding publicly funded ADHD services, integrating ADHD screening into primary care, enhancing clinician training, and establishing dedicated adult ADHD clinics. These measures aim to improve equitable access to timely diagnosis, treatment, and long-term support for individuals with ADHD across diverse populations.

References

Amador-Campos, J. A., Nuño, L., & Gómez-Benito, J. (2016). The Conner's adult ADHD rating scales-long self-report and observer forms: Validation of the Catalan version. *Journal of Psychopathology and Behavioral Assessment, 38*(2), 209–215. https://doi.org/10.1007/s10862-015-9518-6

American Psychiatric Association. (1980). *Diagnostic and statistical manual of mental disorders (3rd ed.)*. Washington, DC: APA.

American Psychiatric Association. (1994). *Diagnostic and statistical manual of mental disorders (4th ed.)*. Washington, DC: APA.

APA. (2013). Diagnostic and statistical manual of mental disorders. *American Psychiatric Association, 21*(21), 591–643.

Asherson, P., Adamou, M., Bolea, B., Muller, U., Morua, S. D., Pitts, M., Thome, J., & Young, S. (2010). Is ADHD a valid diagnosis in adults? Yes. *Bmj, 340*, c549. https://doi.org/10.1136/bmj.c549

Asherson, P., Buitelaar, J., Faraone, S. V., & Rohde, L. A. (2016). Adult attention-deficit hyperactivity disorder: Key conceptual issues. *World Psychiatry, 15*(3), 245–248. https://doi.org/10.1002/wps.20344

Bachmann, C. J., Philipsen, A., & Hoffmann, F. (2017). ADHD in Germany: Trends in diagnosis and pharmacotherapy. *Deutsches Ärzteblatt International, 114*(9), 141–148. https://doi.org/10.3238/arztebl.2017.0141. https://www.aerzteblatt.de/int/article.asp?id=186559

Banaschewski, T., et al. (2018). European ADHD Guidelines Group recommendations. *European Child and Adolescent Psychiatry, 27*, 1467–1480. https://doi.org/10.1007/s00787-018-1129-4

Barkley, R. A. (2015). *Attention-deficit hyperactivity disorder: A handbook for diagnosis and treatment (4th ed.)*. New York: Guilford Press.

Barkley, R. A. (2021). *Taking charge of adult ADHD (2nd ed.)*. New York: Guilford Press.

Biederman, J., Petty, C. R., Evans, M., Small, J., & Faraone, S. V. (2012). How persistent is ADHD? A controlled 10-year follow-up study of boys with ADHD. *Psychiatry Research, 198*(3), 508–512. https://doi.org/10.1016/j.psychres.2012.01.010

Brown, T. E. (2013). *A new understanding of ADHD in children and adults: Executive function impairments*. New York: Routledge.

Coker, T. R., Elliott, M. N., Toomey, S. L., Schwebel, D. C., Cuccaro, P., Tortolero Emery, S., Davies, S. L., Visser, S. N., & Schuster, M. A. (2016). Racial and Ethnic Disparities in ADHD Diagnosis and Treatment. Pediatrics, 138(3). https://doi.org/10.1542/peds.2016-0407

Cortese, S., Adamo, N., Del Giovane, C., Mohr-Jensen, C., Hayes, A. J., Carucci, S., Atkinson, L. Z., Tessari, L., Banaschewski, T., Coghill, D., Hollis, C., Simonoff, E., Zuddas, A., Barbui, C., & Cipriani, A. (2018). Comparative efficacy and tolerability of medications for attention-deficit hyperactivity disorder in children, adolescents, and adults: A systematic review and network meta-analysis. *The Lancet Psychiatry, 5*(9), 727–738. https://doi.org/10.1016/S2215-0366(18)30269-4

Conners, C. K., Sitarenios, G., Parker, J. D. A., & Epstein, J. N. (1998). The revised Conners' parent rating scale (CPRS-R): Factor structure, reliability, and criterion validity. *Journal of Abnormal Child Psychology, 26*(4), 257–268. https://doi.org/10.1023/A:1022602400621

Döpfner, M., et al. (2018). Guidelines for ADHD in children and adolescents. *European Child and Adolescent Psychiatry, 27*, 1059–1088. https://doi.org/10.1007/s00787-018-1104-0

Dutta, C. N., Christov-Moore, L., Ombao, H., & Douglas, P. K. (2022). Neuroprotection in late life attention-deficit/hyperactivity disorder: A review of pharmacotherapy and phenotype across the lifespan. *Frontiers in Human Neuroscience, 16*, 938501. https://doi.org/10.3389/fnhum.2022.938501

Faraone, S. V., Banaschewski, T., Coghill, D., Zheng, Y., Biederman, J., Bellgrove, M. A., Newcorn, J. H., Gignac, M., Al Saud, N. M., Manor, I., Rohde, L. A., Cortese, S., Almagor, D., Stein, M. A., Albatti, T. H., Aljoudi, H. F., Alqahtani, M. M. J., Asherson, P., Atwoli, L., & Wang, Y. (2021). The World Federation of ADHD International Consensus Statement: 208 evidence-based conclusions about the disorder. *Neuroscience & Biobehavioral Reviews, 128*, 789–818. https://doi.org/10.1016/j.neubiorev.2021.01.022

Fayyad, J., Sampson, N. A., Hwang, I., Adamowski, T., Aguilar-Gaxiola, S., Al-Hamzawi, A., Andrade, L. H. S. G., Borges, G., de Girolamo, G., Florescu, S., Gureje, O., Haro, J. M., Hu, C., Karam, E. G., Lee, S., Navarro-Mateu, F., O'Neill, S., Pennell, B.-E., Piazza, M., & on behalf of the, W. H. O. W. M. H. S. C. (2017). The descriptive epidemiology of DSM-IV adult ADHD in the World Health Organization world mental health surveys. *ADHD Attention Deficit and Hyperactivity Disorders, 9*(1), 47–65. https://doi.org/10.1007/s12402-016-0208-3

Gibb, A. C. N., Crosby, M. A., McDiarmid, C., Urban, D., Lam, J. Y. K., Wales, P. W., Brockel, M., Raval, M., Offringa, M., Skarsgard, E. D., Wester, T., Wong, K., de Beer, D., Nelson, G., & Brindle, M. E. (2018). Creation of an enhanced recovery after surgery (ERAS) guideline for neonatal intestinal surgery patients: A knowledge synthesis and consensus generation approach and protocol study. *BMJ Open, 8*(12), e023651. https://doi.org/10.1136/bmjopen-2018-023651

Gu, L., Yang, L., Wang, L., Guo, Y., Wei, B., & Li, H. (2022). Understanding the spatial diffusion dynamics of the COVID-19 pandemic in the city system in China. *Social Science & Medicine, 302*, 114988. https://doi.org/10.1016/j.socscimed.2022.114988

Hamed, A. M., Kauer, A. J., & Stevens, H. E. (2015). Why the diagnosis of attention deficit hyperactivity disorder matters. *Frontiers in Psychiatry, 6*, 168. https://doi.org/10.3389/fpsyt.2015.00168

Hinshaw, S. P., & Scheffler, R. M. (2014). *The ADHD explosion: Myths, medication, money, and today's push for performance*. Oxford: Oxford University Press.
Karlstad, Ø., Zoëga, H., Furu, K., Bahmanyar, S., Martikainen, J. E., Kieler, H., & Pottegård, A. (2016). Use of drugs for ADHD among adults-a multinational study among 15.8 million adults in the Nordic countries. *European Journal of Clinical Pharmacology, 72*(12), 1507–1514. https://doi.org/10.1007/s00228-016-2125-y
Kooij, J. J. S., Bijlenga, D., Salerno, L., Jaeschke, R., Bitter, I., Balázs, J., Thome, J., Dom, G., Kasper, S., Nunes Filipe, C., Stes, S., Mohr, P., Leppämäki, S., Casas, M., Bobes, J., McCarthy, J. M., Richarte, V., Kjems Philipsen, A., Pehlivanidis, A., & Asherson, P. (2019). Updated European consensus statement on diagnosis and treatment of adult ADHD. *European Psychiatry, 56*(1), 14–34. https://doi.org/10.1016/j.eurpsy.2018.11.001
Lahey, B. B., & Willcutt, E. G. (2010). Predictive validity of a continuous alternative to nominal subtypes of attention-deficit/hyperactivity disorder for DSM–V. *Journal of Clinical Child & Adolescent Psychology, 39*(6), 761–775. https://doi.org/10.1080/15374416.2010.517173
Lebowitz, M. S. (2013). Stigmatization of ADHD: A developmental review. *Journal of Attention Disorders, 20*(3), 199–205. https://doi.org/10.1177/1087054712475211
Mueller, A. K., Fuermaier, A. B. M., Koerts, J., & Tucha, L. (2012). Stigma in attention deficit hyperactivity disorder. *ADHD Attention Deficit and Hyperactivity Disorders, 4*(3), 101–114. https://doi.org/10.1007/s12402-012-0085-3
National Institute for Health and Care Excellence (NICE). (2018). Attention deficit hyperactivity disorder: Diagnosis and management (NG87). London: NICE.
Nussbaum, N. L. (2011). ADHD and female specific concerns: A review of the literature and clinical implications. *Journal of Attention Disorders, 16*(2), 87–100. https://doi.org/10.1177/1087054711416909
NVvP (Dutch Psychiatric Association). (2015). Multidisciplinary guideline ADHD. Utrecht: NVvP.
Ministerio de Sanidad. (2017). Guía de práctica clínica sobre el trastorno por déficit de atención con hiperactividad (TDAH). Madrid: Ministry of Health, Spain.
Morgan, P. L., Staff, J., Hillemeier, M. M., Farkas, G., & Maczuga, S. (2016). Racial and ethnic disparities in ADHD diagnosis from kindergarten to eighth grade. *Pediatrics, 138*(3), e20160407. https://doi.org/10.1542/peds.2016-0407
Paidipati, C. P., Brawner, B., Eiraldi, R., & Deatrick, J. A. (2017). Parent and family processes related to ADHD Management in Ethnically Diverse Youth. *Journal of the American Psychiatric Nurses Association, 23*(2), 90–112. https://doi.org/10.1177/1078390316687023
Quinn, P. O., & Madhoo, M. (2014). A review of attention-deficit/hyperactivity disorder in women and girls: Uncovering this hidden diagnosis. *The Primary Care Companion for CNS Disorders, 16*(3), PCC.13r01596. https://doi.org/10.4088/PCC.13r01596
Thapar, A., Cooper, M., Eyre, O., & Langley, K. (2013). Practitioner review: What have we learnt about the causes of ADHD? *Journal of Child Psychology and Psychiatry, 54*(1), 3–16. https://doi.org/10.1111/j.1469-7610.2012.02611.x
Yerys, B. E., et al. (2019). Executive functioning in ADHD and related conditions. *Neuropsychology Review, 29*(2), 123–140. https://doi.org/10.1007/s11065-019-09403-3
Young, S., Adamo, N., Ásgeirsdóttir, B. B., Branney, P., Beckett, M., Colley, W., Cubbin, S., Deeley, Q., Farrag, E., Gudjonsson, G., Hill, P., Hollingdale, J., Kilic, O., Lloyd, T., Mason, P., Paliokosta, E., Perecherla, S., Sedgwick, J., Skirrow, C., & Woodhouse, E. (2020). Females with ADHD: An expert consensus statement taking a lifespan approach providing guidance for the identification and treatment of attention-deficit/ hyperactivity disorder in girls and women. *BMC Psychiatry, 20*(1), 404. https://doi.org/10.1186/s12888-020-02707-9
Zhao, X., Hayes, T., Timmons, A. C., Wu, W., & Frazier, S. L. (2023). Unpacking inequities in ADHD diagnosis: Examining individual-level race/ethnicity and state-level online information-seeking patterns. *Administration and Policy in Mental Health, 50*(4), 576–590. https://doi.org/10.1007/s10488-023-01259-w

Chapter 13
Future Directions in ADHD Research and Public Health

Abstract This chapter explores the future directions for ADHD research and public health, highlighting both persistent gaps and emerging priorities. Despite decades of scientific progress, key areas remain under-researched, particularly concerning ADHD in adults, females, older populations, and individuals from non-Western contexts. These gaps hinder the development of equitable interventions and contribute to disparities in diagnosis and treatment outcomes globally.

The chapter outlines pressing research needs, including investigations into the neurobiological underpinnings of ADHD across the lifespan, culturally sensitive diagnostic frameworks, and gender-specific symptomatology. In addition, it examines novel scientific developments, such as advances in neuroimaging, genetics, digital health technologies, and transdiagnostic approaches that promise to refine both diagnosis and treatment.

Finally, the chapter proposes public health strategies to reduce healthcare disparities and improve long-term outcomes for individuals with ADHD. These include scaling up early intervention programs, increasing global access to evidence-based treatments, promoting neurodiversity awareness, and fostering cross-sector collaboration between health care, education, and employment sectors. By addressing these areas, future ADHD research and public health policy can ensure more inclusive, effective, and globally responsive care systems.

13.1 Unanswered Questions and Emerging Research Areas in ADHD

Despite significant advances in understanding ADHD, numerous research gaps remain, particularly concerning its progression across the lifespan and its broader impact on cognitive, mental health, and social outcomes. Much of the existing literature focuses on short-term interventions in childhood and adolescence, leaving unanswered questions about ADHD's long-term trajectory and its interaction with aging processes (Faraone et al., 2021). Addressing these gaps through robust

G. Ayano et al., *ADHD Across the Lifespan*, SpringerBriefs in Modern Perspectives on Disability Research,
https://doi.org/10.1007/978-981-95-8712-4_13

longitudinal studies is crucial for informing public health strategies and tailoring interventions across the lifespan.

1. *The Need for Long-Term ADHD Studies*

   ADHD symptoms persist into adulthood in approximately 50–60% of cases (Biederman et al., 2012), yet research on ADHD's presentation and impact during midlife and older adulthood remains scarce. Questions remain about how ADHD manifests during the 40s, 50s, and beyond, whether it contributes to heightened risk of cognitive decline or neurodegenerative disorders such as Alzheimer's disease, and how early-life interventions influence long-term occupational and social functioning. Furthermore, the evolution of ADHD symptoms with age—whether attentional deficits and impulsivity diminish or transform—remains poorly understood. Some preliminary evidence also suggests potential overlap between ADHD and mild cognitive impairment (MCI) due to shared executive dysfunction profiles (Caye et al., 2016). An important question is about the long-term safety and health outcomes of stimulant and non-stimulant medications across the lifespan are also underexplored. To address these gaps, future research should prioritize longitudinal cohort studies, including neuroimaging, to track brain structure and function changes over time. Comparative studies examining career trajectories, financial stability, and social integration would further clarify ADHD's lifelong impact.
2. *ADHD and Aging: Cognitive Decline, Executive Functioning, and Mental Health*

   ADHD's interaction with the aging process is an emerging research area. While traditionally categorized as a neurodevelopmental disorder, ADHD may exacerbate age-related cognitive decline through persistent deficits in executive functioning (Caye et al., 2016). Preliminary studies suggest that ADHD might increase susceptibility to early cognitive decline, though further validation in larger cohorts is required.

   Current evidence remains inconclusive as to whether ADHD elevates the risk of neurodegenerative diseases, such as Alzheimer's, or if compensatory strategies help mitigate age-related challenges (Callahan et al., 2017; Levine et al., 2023). Additionally, ADHD in older adults is associated with higher rates of comorbid mental health conditions, including anxiety, depression, and substance use disorders (Faraone et al., 2021). Understanding ADHD's interaction with late-life psychosocial factors—such as social isolation, emotional regulation challenges, and late-onset depression—will be essential for developing targeted interventions. Research focusing on the lived experience, carers, and service providers would assist with this. A systems perspective (Luke & Stamatakis, 2012) drawing in systems science methodologies would support the prioritization of action and provide context for government policy. A research focus inequality is essential as undiagnosed ADHD in older adults can adversely affect quality of life, employment stability, financial security, and relationships. More research is needed to design support services that address these challenges effectively. This might include the use of qualitative methodologies to explore patient journey pathways, treatment activation.

3. *The Long-Term Impact of Early ADHD Interventions*
   While early ADHD diagnosis and treatment improve short-term outcomes, research into the long-term benefits of these interventions remains limited. Most studies focus on symptom reduction during childhood or adolescence, leaving it unclear whether early treatment influences life trajectories into adulthood (Moffitt et al., 2015). Key questions include whether early intervention enhances career success, financial independence, and relationship stability. Untreated ADHD is consistently linked to lower educational attainment, higher unemployment, and income disparities (Biederman et al., 2012). Longitudinal studies could determine whether early interventions mitigate these risks. ADHD's association with higher divorce rates, relational conflict, and parenting difficulties (Faraone et al., 2021) also highlights the need to assess whether early therapeutic strategies—including behavioral therapies and medications—enhance long-term relationship quality and family dynamics. Moreover, given the frequent comorbidity between ADHD and conditions such as depression, anxiety, and substance use disorders, research should examine whether early ADHD treatment reduces the risk of secondary mental health issues later in life. Future studies should include retrospective cohort comparisons of individuals treated in childhood versus those diagnosed in adulthood and examine the lasting neurodevelopmental effects of ADHD treatment on brain maturation.

13.2 ADHD in Understudied Populations

Despite increasing recognition of ADHD as a lifelong and globally prevalent disorder, certain populations remain significantly underrepresented in ADHD research. Historically, studies have predominantly focused on male children in Western contexts, leaving substantial knowledge gaps regarding ADHD's manifestation and management in females, non-Western cultures, and individuals at the intersection of multiple marginalized identities. Addressing these gaps is crucial to advancing equitable, culturally informed ADHD care and policy.

1. *ADHD in Females: The Role of Hormones and Gender Differences*
   ADHD has long been conceptualized as a predominantly male disorder, with diagnostic rates favoring boys by a ratio of approximately 2:1 or 3:1 (Quinn & Madhoo, 2014). However, emerging research highlights that ADHD is substantially under-diagnosed in females due to gender-specific symptom presentations and hormonal fluctuations that may exacerbate symptoms (Hinshaw et al., 2022). Hormonal changes during puberty, menstruation, pregnancy, and menopause can influence dopamine regulation and executive functioning, yet little research has explored their impact on ADHD symptom severity or treatment efficacy. Inattentive symptoms, more common in females, are often less disruptive in educational settings and may be misattributed to personality traits or mood disorders, leading to misdiagnoses such as anxiety, depression, or borderline

personality disorder (Quinn & Madhoo, 2014). This diagnostic gap can result in delays in appropriate ADHD treatment and support.

Future research should prioritize developing gender-sensitive diagnostic criteria and screening tools that account for hormonal influences. Longitudinal studies examining ADHD symptom trajectories in relation to hormonal transitions, as well as clinical trials exploring treatment adaptations during key hormonal phases, are critically needed.

2. *ADHD in Non-Western Cultures: Global Disparities in Research and Treatment*

   ADHD research has historically centered on North America and Europe, resulting in limited understanding of ADHD in non-Western contexts. Reported prevalence rates are generally lower in these regions, often reflecting underdiagnosis due to stigma, limited healthcare infrastructure, and differing cultural conceptualizations of ADHD (Hamed et al., 2015).

   In many Asian and Middle Eastern cultures, ADHD symptoms are frequently interpreted through behavioral or moralistic lenses rather than as indicators of a neurodevelopmental disorder. Discipline-based strategies often take precedence over medical interventions, and mental health stigma further reduces help-seeking behaviors (Hamed et al., 2015).

   Disparities in healthcare access and the shortage of ADHD-trained clinicians exacerbate these challenges, particularly in low- and middle-income countries. Future research should prioritize cross-cultural studies comparing ADHD prevalence, diagnostic criteria, treatment approaches, and healthcare access across global regions (Faraone et al., 2021; Sayal et al., 2010). Qualitative research exploring cultural beliefs and attitudes toward ADHD will be critical to tailoring effective public health initiatives and interventions.

3. *Intersectionality in ADHD Research: Race, Gender, and Socioeconomic Status*

   ADHD research has often neglected the intersection of race, ethnicity, gender, and socioeconomic status in shaping ADHD diagnosis and treatment outcomes. Marginalized communities—including Black, Hispanic, Indigenous, and lower-income populations—face systemic barriers that contribute to underdiagnosis and under-treatment (Morgan et al., 2016). For example, ADHD symptoms in Black and Hispanic children are more likely to be interpreted as behavioral problems rather than neurodevelopmental challenges, resulting in higher rates of conduct disorder or oppositional defiant disorder diagnoses and disproportionate school disciplinary actions (Morgan et al., 2016).

   Socioeconomic status further compounds these disparities. Low-income families often face financial obstacles, such as the high cost of private assessments, medications, and therapies. Additionally, rural and underserved areas typically lack ADHD specialists, leading to diagnostic delays and reduced access to care. Cultural stigma and mistrust of healthcare systems may further discourage families from pursuing ADHD evaluations or treatment.

Future research should prioritize large-scale epidemiological studies to assess how race, gender, and socioeconomic status influence ADHD diagnosis and treatment. Policy-focused research is also needed to investigate strategies for reducing disparities, such as implementing culturally competent training for healthcare providers, expanding ADHD screening in schools, and increasing access to affordable ADHD services.

13.3 Advances in Neurobiology and Precision Medicine

Recent breakthroughs in genetics, neuroimaging, and pharmacology are transforming our understanding of ADHD, paving the way for more targeted and individualized treatment approaches (Faraone et al., 2021) These advances offer the potential to move beyond the current trial-and-error approach to ADHD management and toward interventions tailored to each individual's unique biological profile.

Genetic research has highlighted ADHD as one of the most heritable neuropsychiatric conditions, with twin studies estimating heritability rates of approximately 70–80% (Faraone et al., 2021). While the genetic basis of ADHD is well established, ongoing research is focusing on identifying specific gene variants that contribute to symptom variability and treatment response. Genome-wide association studies have identified multiple gene variants linked to ADHD, particularly those involved in dopamine regulation, neurotransmitter function, and brain development (Demontis et al., 2019). Although polygenic risk scores are being developed to assess individual ADHD risk, they are not yet widely used in clinical settings. Notably, genetic influences on medication response are under investigation, with variants in dopamine receptor genes such as DRD4 and DRD5 showing potential associations with differential responses to stimulant and non-stimulant medications. As this field matures, genetic testing could guide early ADHD risk assessment, inform personalized medication selection, and improve understanding of ADHD subtypes at the genetic level.

In parallel, neuroimaging research is deepening our understanding of ADHD's impact on brain structure and function, supporting differential diagnosis and potentially informing individualized treatment plans (Cortese et al., 2018). Studies using functional magnetic resonance imaging (fMRI), electroencephalography (EEG), and positron emission tomography (PET) consistently reveal structural and functional brain differences in individuals with ADHD, including smaller prefrontal cortex volume, delayed cortical maturation, and reduced connectivity in executive function networks (Hoogman et al., 2017; Lay et al., 2023; Sutcubasi et al., 2020). Functional MRI studies highlight dopamine-related reward processing and attention network differences that may underlie core ADHD symptoms such as impulsivity and distractibility. EEG research suggests that theta/beta wave ratios could serve as diagnostic markers for ADHD, though further validation is needed. Incorporating neuroimaging findings into clinical practice could enhance diagnostic accuracy, distinguish ADHD from conditions with overlapping symptoms, such as autism spectrum disorder or bipolar disorder, and guide treatment monitoring.

Precision medicine approaches aim to tailor ADHD treatment based on genetic, neurological, and metabolic profiles, offering the potential to revolutionize ADHD care (Faraone et al., 2021), although are likely to be available in wealthy countries and to wealthy individuals due to their cost. Pharmacogenetic research is exploring genetic markers such as catechol-O-methyltransferase (COMT), dopamine receptor D4 (DRD4), and the dopamine transporter gene (SLC6A3/DAT1) to predict individual responses to specific medications. Additionally, metabolic factors, including gut microbiome composition and individual metabolic rates, may influence how patients respond to medication and experience side effects. Beyond pharmacological interventions, non-pharmacological strategies such as neurofeedback, dietary modifications, and cognitive training are being investigated as complementary or alternative approaches, particularly for individuals who do not respond optimally to medication. Although ADHD is highly heritable, with twin studies estimating heritability at around 70–80% (Faraone & Larsson, 2019), behavioral interventions remain critical in mitigating symptom burden and improving daily functioning. Nutritional strategies, including elimination diets and supplementation approaches, have shown small but significant benefits in subgroups of patients (Sonuga-Barke et al., 2013). Importantly, long-term multimodal management—including both pharmacological and behavioral treatments—has been associated with improved educational attainment, employment outcomes, and reduced healthcare costs across the lifespan (Jensen et al., 2007). As this body of research grows, clinicians may increasingly integrate neuroimaging and genetic data into ADHD assessments, enabling more personalized, effective treatment plans that reduce side effects and enhance patient outcomes.

In summary, advances in genetics, neuroimaging, and precision medicine hold promise for transforming ADHD diagnosis and treatment. By integrating biological insights into clinical practice, these developments have the potential to revolutionize ADHD care, offering more precise, effective, and individualized interventions for people living with ADHD.

Continuous update of population representative monitoring and surveillance is recommended to assess ADHD prevalence and associations.

13.4 Innovations in ADHD Treatment Approaches

While stimulant medications remain the cornerstone of ADHD treatment, emerging innovations are expanding therapeutic options beyond traditional pharmacology. Novel interventions such as neurofeedback, digital therapeutics, psychedelic-assisted therapy, and integrated care models are redefining ADHD management. These strategies aim to enhance executive functioning, emotional regulation, and long-term outcomes across diverse patient populations.

Neurofeedback has gained prominence as a non-invasive intervention enabling individuals to train their brain activity in real-time, enhancing attention, impulse control, and executive functioning. This method employs EEG-based feedback to help patients self-regulate atypical neural patterns commonly associated with ADHD. Complementary techniques such as transcranial magnetic stimulation (TMS) and transcranial direct current stimulation (tDCS) are under investigation for their potential to modulate brain activity and alleviate ADHD symptoms. Early findings are promising, though these modalities are currently used as adjunctive treatments due to variability in their long-term efficacy. Future developments may include portable neurofeedback devices enabling home-based training, as well as the integration of TMS and tDCS to enhance cognitive rehabilitation for patients unresponsive to conventional medications.

Psychedelic-assisted therapy is also being explored as a potential treatment for ADHD, particularly in addressing emotional dysregulation. Compounds such as psilocybin, MDMA, and LSD are under investigation for their capacity to enhance neuroplasticity, self-awareness, and emotional stability in neurodiverse populations. Preliminary research suggests that psychedelics may foster improvements in cognitive flexibility and resilience, with psilocybin being studied for its potential to promote introspection and MDMA-assisted therapy evaluated for its anxiolytic and self-regulatory effects in ADHD populations. Despite these promising directions, much remains unknown regarding the mechanisms underlying these therapies, and current trials are in early stages. Future research may focus on developing microdosing protocols and psychedelic-assisted psychotherapy frameworks tailored to ADHD-related emotional challenges. Rigorous safety and efficacy studies are essential before clinical adoption can be considered.

Digital therapeutics, including mobile applications, virtual reality (VR), and AI-enhanced cognitive training programs, offer promising avenues for strengthening executive function and attention control in ADHD populations. Interventions such as EndeavorRx, an FDA-approved game-based application, have demonstrated efficacy in improving working memory and attentional capacity (Kollins et al., 2020). AI-driven cognitive training platforms further personalize interventions by dynamically adjusting task difficulty in response to user performance. Although these tools hold substantial potential, sustained user engagement and long-term cognitive benefits require further empirical validation. Looking ahead, the future of digital therapeutics may include VR-based simulations of real-world executive function challenges, as well as mobile platforms that provide continuous behavioral coaching and symptom tracking.

Integrated care models are increasingly recognized as essential in ADHD treatment paradigms, reflecting a shift toward multimodal approaches that address behavioral, psychological, and lifestyle factors. Comprehensive interventions incorporating diet, exercise, sleep optimization, and behavioral coaching have demonstrated efficacy as adjuncts to medication management. ADHD coaching, in particular, has shown promise in improving executive functioning and self-regulation among adults and university students. Emerging integrated care models may include multidisciplinary ADHD clinics that offer pharmacological treatment, neurofeedback, cognitive training, and behavioral therapies under one roof. Telehealth-based coaching and lifestyle-focused programs, including dietary interventions and mindfulness practices, are also being incorporated into holistic care frameworks, further supporting individuals with ADHD in achieving sustainable symptom management and improved quality of life.

13.5 ADHD in Understudied Populations

While ADHD research has expanded globally, key populations remain underrepresented in both clinical and public health studies. Much of the existing research has concentrated on male children in North America and Europe, leaving critical gaps in understanding ADHD among females, non-Western populations, and individuals from diverse racial, ethnic, and socioeconomic backgrounds. These disparities contribute to delayed diagnoses, misdiagnoses, and unequal access to treatment, reinforcing systemic inequities in health care.

ADHD in females has historically been overlooked, with diagnosis ratios favoring males at approximately 2:1 or 3:1 (Quinn & Madhoo, 2014). Contemporary evidence, however, highlights significant underdiagnosis in females, partly due to gender-specific symptom expression and the influence of hormonal fluctuations on executive functioning and emotional regulation (Hinshaw et al., 2022). Estrogen and progesterone levels, for example, impact dopamine pathways linked to ADHD symptomatology, leading to cyclical variations in symptom severity across the menstrual cycle, pregnancy, and menopause. Females often present with inattentive-type ADHD, characterized by internalizing symptoms such as anxiety, daydreaming, and low self-esteem—features less likely to prompt clinical attention. Consequently, many women receive diagnoses late in life, often after years of being misdiagnosed with mood or personality disorders. Future research must develop gender-sensitive diagnostic criteria, evaluate treatment efficacy across hormonal stages, and address the unique psychosocial challenges faced by females with ADHD.

In non-Western cultures, ADHD research remains limited, hindering understanding of its prevalence and management in regions such as Africa, Asia, Latin America, and the Middle East (Hamed et al., 2015). This gap is especially evident in adults, including midlife populations (40 years and older), where ADHD remains under-recognized and understudied despite growing evidence of its persistence into later adulthood (Ayano et al., 2023).

In these areas, ADHD is often underdiagnosed due to cultural beliefs that frame inattentiveness or hyperactivity as behavioral or disciplinary issues rather than as a neurodevelopmental condition. Stigma, limited mental health literacy, and a lack of ADHD-trained clinicians further hinder diagnosis and treatment. Additionally, disparities in healthcare infrastructure and resource constraints restrict access to pharmacological and behavioral interventions. Cross-cultural epidemiological studies and qualitative research into local perceptions of ADHD are essential to inform culturally responsive diagnostic tools and treatment strategies. Health policy analyses could also elucidate how systemic factors in low- and middle-income countries shape ADHD care.

Intersectionality further complicates ADHD research, as disparities in diagnosis and treatment are compounded by the interaction of race, gender, and socioeconomic status. Minority populations, including Black, Hispanic, and Indigenous children, are less likely to be diagnosed with ADHD compared to White children, despite exhibiting similar symptom prevalence (Morgan et al., 2016).

ADHD-related behaviors in minority youth are often misinterpreted as oppositional or delinquent, leading to punitive disciplinary measures such as suspensions or involvement with the juvenile justice system. Socioeconomic barriers, including limited access to specialists, high costs of private evaluations, and restricted insurance coverage, exacerbate inequities in diagnosis and treatment. Implicit bias among healthcare providers may also contribute to these disparities (Hinshaw et al., 2022). Addressing these challenges requires large-scale epidemiological research to document disparities, community-based studies to explore cultural stigma, and policy-driven solutions aimed at promoting equitable access to ADHD care.

13.6 ADHD in Public Health Policy

ADHD isotopes public health concern due to its profound implications for education, employment, health care, and social well-being. Despite growing recognition of ADHD as a lifelong neurodevelopmental condition, many healthcare systems and public institutions continue to underprioritize ADHD in policy and practice. This underrepresentation has led to insufficient accommodations, limited research funding, and persistent stigma. Advancing public health responses to ADHD will require coordinated strategies across workplaces, government funding initiatives, and public awareness campaigns.

Although ADHD is widely acknowledged as a neurodevelopmental disorder, legal and institutional accommodations in professional environments remain inconsistent and often inadequate. While ADHD is recognized under the Americans with Disabilities Act (ADA) in the United States, the Equality Act in the United Kingdom, and the Disability Discrimination Act in Australia, its designation as a disability frequently depends on the severity of functional impairment (Biederman et al., 2021). As a result, many individuals with ADHD struggle with executive functioning, time management, and emotional regulation in the workplace but face systemic barriers to obtaining reasonable adjustments. Moreover, fear of stigma and discrimination deters many from disclosing their diagnosis to employers (Faraone et al., 2021). Policy reforms should mandate clearer guidelines for ADHD-inclusive workplace accommodations, expand legal protections to recognize the broader impact of executive dysfunction, and implement employer education programs on neurodiversity. Effective workplace accommodations may include flexible schedules, access to quiet workspaces, structured task management tools, and regular performance feedback.

Despite its high prevalence, ADHD research receives disproportionately less funding than other neurodevelopmental and mental health conditions (Faraone et al., 2021). This underfunding constrains progress in developing diagnostic tools, personalizing treatments, and understanding long-term outcomes. Furthermore, many individuals face significant barriers to accessing ADHD services, including prolonged wait times, high out-of-pocket costs, and limited public healthcare coverage for pharmacological and behavioral treatments (Hinshaw & Scheffler, 2014). To address these gaps, governments should prioritize increased funding for ADHD research, including large-scale studies on biological markers, comorbidities, and treatment efficacy. Policies should also expand government-subsidized ADHD services, enhance school-based screening programs for early identification, and invest in training healthcare professionals to better recognize and manage ADHD across the lifespan. These measures will reduce disparities and improve access to effective care.

Public misconceptions surrounding ADHD remain widespread, perpetuating stigma and contributing to delayed diagnoses and reduced treatment engagement. Common myths, such as equating ADHD with laziness or poor parenting, persist despite substantial scientific evidence confirming ADHD as a neurobiological condition characterized by executive dysfunction and altered dopamine regulation (Barkley, 2021). Targeted public health campaigns are critical to counteracting misinformation and fostering understanding of ADHD as a chronic, lifelong disorder. National awareness efforts should focus on improving public knowledge of ADHD symptoms, particularly in adults, and highlighting the evidence base supporting pharmacological and behavioral interventions. School-based programs can play a vital role in educating teachers, students, and parents, while workplace initiatives should promote neurodiversity-friendly practices. Digital platforms and social media campaigns can amplify these messages, sharing the lived experiences of individuals with ADHD to humanize the condition and reduce stigma.

Summary

This chapter emphasizes the critical need for advancing ADHD research and public health strategies to address persistent knowledge gaps and improve outcomes. Despite growing awareness of ADHD as a lifelong neurodevelopmental condition, questions about its trajectory into midlife and late adulthood, treatment efficacy, and social impact remain underexplored. The chapter calls for longitudinal studies to understand ADHD's progression across the lifespan, particularly regarding cognitive decline, occupational challenges, and mental health in diverse adult populations.

Recognizing disparities in diagnosis and treatment, the chapter highlights the importance of including underrepresented groups—such as females, non-Western populations, and individuals from varied racial and socioeconomic backgrounds—in ADHD research. Addressing these disparities is essential for ensuring equitable access to care and support.

The chapter also advocates for the integration of scientific innovations, including genetic research to identify ADHD biomarkers, advanced neuroimaging for precise diagnostics, and the incorporation of precision medicine into ADHD care. These approaches can move ADHD treatment beyond the current trial-and-error model toward more personalized, effective interventions.

Finally, the chapter outlines key public health policy recommendations, including expanding workplace accommodations, increasing government funding for ADHD research and services, and launching targeted public awareness campaigns to reduce stigma. Together, these strategies aim to create a future where ADHD is managed through evidence-based, personalized care supported by inclusive policies and global health initiatives.

References

Ayano, G., Tsegay, L., Gizachew, Y., Necho, M., Yohannes, K., Abraha, M., Demelash, S., Anbesaw, T., & Alati, R. (2023). Prevalence of attention deficit hyperactivity disorder in adults: Umbrella review of evidence generated across the globe. *Psychiatry Research, 328*, 115449. https://doi.org/10.1016/j.psychres.2023.115449

Barkley, R. A. (2021). Taking Charge of Adult ADHD. 2nd ed. New York: Guilford Press.

Biederman. J, DiSalvo, M., Green, A., Woodworth, K. Y., Gilfix, T., Law, C., Gabrieli, J., & Faraone, S. V. (2021). Rates of switching stimulants in consecutively referred medication-naïve adults with attentiondeficit/hyperactivity disorder. *Acta Psychiatrica Scandinavica, 144*(6), 626–634. https://doi.org/10.1111/acps.13370

Biederman, J., Petty, C. R., Evans, M., Small, J., & Faraone, S. V. (2012). How persistent is attention-deficit/hyperactivity disorder? A controlled 10-year follow-up study of boys with ADHD. *Psychiatry Research,198*(3), 508–512. https://doi.org/10.1016/j.psychres.2012.01.010

Callahan, B. L., Bierstone, D., Stuss, D. T., & Black, S. E. (2017). Adult ADHD: Risk factor for dementia or phenotypic mimic? *Frontiers in Aging Neuroscience, 9*, 260. https://doi.org/10.3389/fnagi.2017.00260

Caye, A., Swanson, J. M., Thapar, A., Sibley, M. H., Arseneault, L., Hechtman, L., Arnold, L. E., Niclasen, J., Moffitt, T. E., & Rohde, L. A. (2016). Life span studies of ADHD—Conceptual challenges and predictors of persistence and outcome. *Current Psychiatry Reports, 18*, 111. https://doi.org/10.1007/s11920-016-0750-x

Cortese, S., Adamo, N., Del Giovane, C., Mohr-Jensen, C., Hayes, A. J., Carucci, S., Atkinson, L. Z., Tessari, L., Banaschewski, T., Coghill, D., Hollis, C., Simonoff, E., Zuddas, A., Barbui, C., & Cipriani, A. (2018). Comparative efficacy and tolerability of medications for ADHD in children, adolescents, and adults: A systematic review and network meta-analysis. *The Lancet Psychiatry, 5*(9), 727–738. https://doi.org/10.1016/S2215-0366(18)30269-4

Demontis, D., Walters, R. K., Martin, J., Mattheisen, M., Als, T. D., Agerbo, E., Baldursson, G., Belliveau, R., Bybjerg-Grauholm, J., Bækvad-Hansen, M., Cerrato, F., Chambert, K., Churchhouse, C., Dumont, A., Eriksson, N., Gandal, M., Goldstein, J., Grove, J., Gudmundsson, O. O., & Neale, B. M. (2019). Discovery of the first genome-wide significant risk loci for ADHD. *Nature Genetics, 51*, 63–75. https://doi.org/10.1038/s41588-018-0269-7

Faraone, S. V., & Larsson, H. (2019). Genetics of attention deficit hyperactivity disorder. *Molecular Psychiatry, 24*(4), 562–575. https://doi.org/10.1038/s41380-018-0070-0

Faraone, S. V., Banaschewski, T., Coghill, D., Zheng, Y., Biederman, J., Bellgrove, M. A., Newcorn, J. H., Gignac, M., Al Saud, N. M., Manor, I., Rohde, L. A., Yang, L., Cortese, S., Almagor, D., Stein, M. A., Albatti, T. H., Aljoudi, H. F., Alqahtani, M. M. J., Asherson, P., … Wang, Y. (2021). The world federation of ADHD international consensus statement: 208 evidence-based conclusions about the disorder. *Neuroscience & Biobehavioral Reviews, 128*, 789–818. https://doi.org/10.1016/j.neubiorev.2021.01.022

Hamed, A. M., Kauer, A. J., Stevens, H. E. (2015). Why the diagnosis of attention deficit hyperactivity disorder matters. *Frontiers in Psychiatry, 6*, 168. https://doi.org/10.3389/fpsyt.2015.00168

Hinshaw, S. P., Nguyen, P. T., O'Grady, S. M., & Rosenthal, E. A. (2022). Annual research review: Attention-deficit/hyperactivity disorder in girls and women. *Journal of Child Psychology and Psychiatry, 63*(4), 484–496. https://doi.org/10.1111/jcpp.13480

Hinshaw, S. P., & Scheffler, R. M. (2014). *The ADHD Explosion: Myths, Medication, Money, and Today's Push for Performance*. Oxford: Oxford University Press.

Hoogman, M., Bralten, J., Hibar, D. P., Mennes, M., Zwiers, M. P., Schweren, L. S. J., van Hulzen, K. J. E., Medland, S. E., Shumskaya, E., Jahanshad, N., Zeeuw, P. D., Szekely, E., Sudre, G., Wolfers, T., Onnink, A. M. H., Dammers, J. T., Mostert, J. C., Vives-Gilabert, Y., Kohls, G., … Franke, B. (2017). Subcortical brain volume differences in participants with attention deficit hyperactivity disorder in children and adults: A cross-sectional mega-analysis. *The Lancet Psychiatry, 4*(4), 310–319. https://doi.org/10.1016/S2215-0366(17)30049-4

Jensen, P. S., Arnold, L. E., Swanson, J. M., Vitiello, B., Abikoff, H. B., Greenhill, L. L., Hechtman, L., Hinshaw, S. P., Pelham, W. E., Wells, K. C., Conners, C. K., Elliott, G. R., Epstein, J. N., Hoza, B., March, J. S., Molina, B. S. G., Newcorn, J. H., Severe, J. B., Wigal, T., … Hur, K. (2007). *3-year follow-up of the NIMH MTA study*. Lippincott Williams & Wilkins. https://doi.org/10.1097/CHI.0b013e3180686d48

Kollins, S. H., DeLoss, D. J., Cañadas, E., Lutz, J., Findling, R. L., Keefe, R. S. E., Epstein, J. N., Cutler, A. J., & Faraone, S. V. (2020). A novel digital intervention for ADHD improves attention in children. *The Lancet Digital Health, 2*(4), e168–e178. https://doi.org/10.1016/S2589-7500(20)30034-X

Lay, B. P. P., Koya, E., Hope, B. T., Esber, G. R., & Iordanova, M. D. (2023). The recruitment of a neuronal ensemble in the central nucleus of the amygdala during the first extinction episode has persistent effects on extinction expression. *Biological Psychiatry, 93*(4), 300–308. https://doi.org/10.1016/j.biopsych.2022.07.021

Levine, S. Z., Rotstein, A., Kodesh, A., Sandin, S., Lee, B. K., Weinstein, G., Schnaider Beeri, M., & Reichenberg, A. (2023). Adult attention-deficit/hyperactivity disorder and the risk of dementia. *JAMA Network Open, 6*(10), e2338088–e2338088. https://doi.org/10.1001/jamanetworkopen.2023.38088

Luke, D. A., & Stamatakis, K. A. (2012). Systems science methods in public health: Dynamics, networks, and agents. *Annual Review of Public Health, 33*, 357–376. https://doi.org/10.1146/annurev-publhealth-031210-101222

Moffitt, T. E., Houts, R., Asherson, P., Belsky, D. W., Corcoran, D. L., Hammerle, M., Harrington, H., Hogan, S., Meier, M. H., Polanczyk, G. V., Poulton, R., Ramrakha, S., Sugden, K., Williams, B., Rohde, L. A., & Caspi, A. (2015). Is adult ADHD a childhood-onset neurodevelopmental disorder? *American Journal of Psychiatry, 172*(10), 967–977. https://doi.org/10.1176/appi.ajp.2015.14101266

Morgan, P. L., Staff, J., Hillemeier, M. M., Farkas, G., & Maczuga, S. (2016). Racial and ethnic disparities in ADHD diagnosis from kindergarten to eighth grade. Pediatrics, 138(3), e20160407. https://doi.org/10.1542/peds.2016-0407

Sayal, K., Owen, V., White, K., Merrell, C., Tymms, P., & Taylor, E. (2010). Impact of early school-based screening and intervention programs for ADHD on children's outcomes and access to services: Follow-up of a school-based trial at age 10 years. *Archives of Pediatrics & Adolescent Medicine, 164*(5), 462–469. https://doi.org/10.1001/archpediatrics.2010.40

Sonuga-Barke, E. J., Brandeis, D., Cortese, S., Daley, D., Ferrin, M., Holtmann, M., Stevenson, J., Danckaerts, M., van der Oord, S., Döpfner, M., Dittmann, R. W., Simonoff, E., Zuddas, A., Banaschewski, T., Buitelaar, J., Coghill, D., Hollis, C., Konofal, E., Lecendreux, M., … Sergeant, J. (2013). Nonpharmacological interventions for ADHD: Systematic review and meta-analyses of randomized controlled trials of dietary and psychological treatments. *The American Journal of Psychiatry, 170*(3), 275–289. https://doi.org/10.1176/appi.ajp.2012.12070991

Sutcubasi, B., Metin, B., Kurban, M. K., Metin, Z. E., Beser, B., & Sonuga-Barke, E. (2020). Resting-state network dysconnectivity in ADHD: A system-neuroscience-based meta-analysis. *The World Journal of Biological Psychiatry, 21*(9), 662–672. https://doi.org/10.1080/15622975.2020.1775889

Quinn, P. O., & Madhoo, M. (2014). A review of attention-deficit/hyperactivity disorder in women and girls: Uncovering this hidden diagnosis. *Primary Care Companion CNS Disorders, 16*(3), PCC.13r01596. https://doi.org/10.4088/PCC.13r01596

MIX
Papier aus verantwortungsvollen Quellen
Paper from responsible sources
FSC® C105338

If you have any concerns about our products,
you can contact us on
ProductSafety@springernature.com

In case Publisher is established outside the EU,
the EU authorized representative is:
Springer Nature Customer Service Center GmbH
Europaplatz 3, 69115 Heidelberg, Germany

Printed by Libri Plureos GmbH
in Hamburg, Germany